HOSPITAL AND WELFARE LIBRARY SERVICES

HOSPITAL AND WELFARE LIBRARY SERVICES
An International Bibliography

Compiled and edited by

EILEEN E CUMMING ALA

Based on Work Begun by Mona E Going FLA for the International Federation of Library Associations, Sub-Section of Libraries in Hospitals

The Library Association/London

Published 1977 by The Library Association
7 Ridgmount Street, London WC1E 7AE

ISBN 0 85365 139 6

British Library Cataloguing in Publication Data:

Cumming, Eileen Elizabeth
   Hospital and welfare library services: an
international bibliography.
   1. Hospital libraries.   2. Libraries and
the handicapped.
   I. Title   II. Library Association
016.0276'6   Z675.H7

ISBN 0-85365-139-6

Set in 10 on 11pt Monotype Garamond 156 and
made and printed in Great Britain by
The Garden City Press Limited
Letchworth, Hertfordshire SG6 1JS

As chairman of the Libraries in Hospitals Sub-Section of the International Federation of Library Associations it gives me pleasure and satisfaction to write a foreword to the most ambitious and extended enterprise of the Sub-Section.

With pleasure because, being a hospital librarian myself, I am aware of the value of being able to consult a complete survey of thoughts and experiences in hospital librarianship in other parts of the world. For librarians in countries where services for patients in hospitals and for the elderly and handicapped in institutions and in the community are not yet recognised as an essential part of their work, this bibliography might be of some help to get services started. For others, it can open up new vistas and be a stimulus to discover new ways of working.

My satisfaction stems from the fact that the sub-section's correspondents, nearly all fieldworkers who realised the importance of this enterprise and the ultimate gain to themselves, have co-operated to bring the building materials together, rough building materials, which had to be checked and put into order.

Elsewhere you will read about the history of this bibliography's compilation. With gratitude and respect I mention here the names of the pioneer, Mona Going, who started the work in earnest, and of Eileen Cumming, who with her feeling for accuracy and perfection, and with admirable perseverance, spent so much time on its achievement.

May *Hospital and Welfare Library Services: an International Bibliography* find its way in the world to raise the standard of library services and, in consequence, to brighten and enlarge the lives of patients, the handicapped and the elderly, of every nationality.

Petra B Leeuwenburgh

Président de la sous-section des Bibliothèques dans les hôpitaux de la Fédération Internationale des Associations de Bibliothècaires, j'ai le plaisir et la satisfaction de vous présentér le projet le plus ambitieux et le plus vaste de la sous-section.

Etant bibliothécaire d'hôpital moi-même, mon plaisir provient de ma capacité personnelle d'apprécier l'utilité de pouvoir consulter à volonté un répertoire complet des réflexions et expériences faites en bibliothéconomie d'hôpital dans d'autres parties du monde.

Dans les pays où les services pour malades hospitalisés, pour personnes âgées et pour personnes handicapées en institut ou dans la communauté, ne sont pas reconnus, cet ouvrage peut être un outil de départ utile. Pour les autres, cette bibliographie peut ouvrir de nouveaux horizons et stimuler le désir de découvrir d'autres méthodes de travail.

Ma satisfaction provient de la coopération donnée par les correspondants de la sous-section, presque tous eux-mêmes bibliothécaires d'hôpital, qui ont réalisé l'importance et l'utilité de ce travail et ont donc apporté les matériaux de base qui ont ensuite dû être vérifiés et répertoriés.

L'histoire de cette compilation vous sera décrite plus loin mais je voudrais mentionner ici avec gratitude et respect les noms de Mona Going qui a eu le courage de commencer ce travail, et de Eileen Cumming qui l'a mené à bonne fin grâce à sa capacité d'exactitude, son désir de perfection et son admirable persévérance.

Puisse *Hospital and Welfare Library Services – an International Bibliography* améliorer les normes de ces services bibliothécaires spécifiques et aider à donner de la joie aux malades, handicapés et personnes âgées de toutes les nationalités.

Petra B. Leeuwenburgh

VORWORT

Als Vorsitzende der Untersektion 'Bibliotheken in Krankenhäusern' des Internationalen Verbandes der Bibliothekar-Vereine darf ich mit Freude und Befriedigung das Vorwort zu diesem vielversprechenden und ausführlichen Unternehmen der Untersektion schreiben.

Mit Freude, weil ich als Krankenhausbibliothekarin die Möglichkeit besonders zu schätzen weiß, eine vollständige Zusammenfassung aller Überlegungen und Erfahrungen im Krankenhaus-Bibliothekswesen in anderen Teilen der Welt zu Rate ziehen zu können. Für Bibliothekare in Ländern, in denen die Dienste für Krankenhauspatienten und alte und behinderte Menschen in Heimen noch nicht als wesentlicher Teil ihrer Arbeit erkannt werden, möge diese Bibliographie Anstoß sein, die Arbeit zu beginnen. Für andere kann sie neue Aussichten eröffnen und ein Anreiz sein, neue Wege für die Arbeit zu entdecken.

Meine Befriedigung stützt sich auf die Tatsache, daß die Korrespondenten der Untersektion – fast alle Praktiker, die die Bedeutung dieses Unternehmens und den letzlichen Gewinn für sich selbst erkannten – mitgewirkt haben, das Material zusammenzutragen – Rohmaterial, das geprüft und geordnet werden mußte.

An anderer Stelle können Sie über die Geschichte der Zusammenstellung dieser Bibliographie nachlesen. Mit Dankbarkeit und Hochachtung erwähne ich hier die Namen der Pionierin, Mona Going, die das Werk begann und von Eileen Cumming, die mit ihrem Gefühl für Genauigkeit und Perfektion und mit bewundernswerter Beharrlichkeit so viel Zeit für seine Fertigstellung aufwandte.

Möge *Hospital and Welfare Library Services – an International Bibliography* ihren Weg in die Welt finden, um den Standard der Bibliotheksdienste zu heben und als Folge davon, das Leben von Patienten, behinderten und alten Menschen jeder Nationalität zu erhellen und zu bereichern.

Petra B. Leeuwenburgh

CONTENTS

Foreword   v

Introduction   1

Abbreviations   15

Bibliography 1863–1972   17

Author Index   153

Geographical Index   166

Subject Index   169

CONTENU

Préface   v

Introduction   1

Abréviations   15

Bibliographie 1863–1972   17

Index par auteur   153

Index par région géographique   166

Index par sujet traité   170

INHALTSVERZEICHNIS

Vorwort   v

Einführung   1

Abkürzungen   15

Bibliographie 1863–1972   17

Verfasser-Register   153

Geographisches Register   166

Schlagwort-Register   171

Historical background

The suggestion that an international bibliography on hospital libraries should be compiled was first made at a meeting of the Sub-Committee of Hospital Libraries during the IFLA Council in London in 1948. It was proposed that each country should be responsible for preparing the section relating to its own literature and that a general editor should be designated. The bibliography was further discussed at the meetings in 1949 and 1950, when some duplicated lists were circulated, but no published work resulted.

The subject was raised again in Sofia in 1963 when it was decided to bring it forward to the 1966 meeting in The Hague. The present work stems directly from that meeting. There, Miss Mona Going who was already collecting material on her own behalf, was asked to undertake the compilation of the bibliography for the Sub-Section. The International Correspondents were asked to help Miss Going by submitting the relevant items from their own countries. The present editor's involvement began in 1968 when Miss Going asked her for assistance in scanning the literature.

A work of this nature based on international co-operation has many problems and the bibliography grew rather haphazardly. At Copenhagen in 1969 a recommendation from Miss Going that the present editor collect references from 1968 onwards to form a second publication was approved. However, in 1971, when the total number of entries had reached approximately 850, Miss Going decided to hand over the work completely for checking and completion. At this point it was decided to exclude references to medical and nursing libraries and to concentrate on services to patients. The completed bibliography has a total of 2164 entries.

Purpose

The aim in compiling this bibliography was to provide as comprehensive a list as possible of books and articles relating to library services to the sick and handicapped throughout the world. It is hoped that it will prove a useful source of reference, that it will pinpoint areas where nothing or little has been written, or is being done, and will thereby stimulate interest in the practice of hospital librarianship.

Scope

The entries refer to the different aspects of library service to patients in all types of hospitals, to the housebound, the elderly, the physically handicapped (blind, deaf, etc.) and to the mentally disordered (i.e. mentally ill and mentally handicapped) whether in hospital or in the community. Lists of 'easy readers' and books for backward children have been included as it was thought that these would be useful for those interested in book selection for the mentally handicapped.

Articles on library provision to meet the professional reading needs of hospital staff have been included only where a substantial part of the article relates also to services to patients.

Hospital and Welfare Library Services

Period covered

The earliest reference, dated 1863, is to the catalogue of the patients' library in Murray Royal Psychiatric Hospital, Perthshire; the latest entries are dated 1972.

Sources

The international correspondents of the Sub-Section have sent material relating to their own countries for inclusion. In addition, the major indexing and abstracting journals listed below have been consulted:

Hospital Abstracts
Hospital Literature Index
Library Literature
Library Science Abstracts
Library and Information Science Abstracts

Arrangement

A chronological arrangement has been chosen as it was thought that this would show the historical and comparative development of hospital libraries in the different countries through the literature, and would be useful to research workers, teachers and students.

Entries are arranged by year of publication and within each year the order is alphabetical by author, or by title in the case of anonymous items. Each entry has been assigned a running number for ease of reference from the indexes.

Alphabetisation

An important point in the alphabetisation is that letters in the Scandinavian language which are additional to the English language have been arranged in Anglicised form. This means, for example, that Åhlin does not appear after Ziegler but after Ackerknecht and before Ahlnäs and Höök appears between Holmström and Hoover. I apologise to my Scandinavian friends and colleagues for the inconvenience this will cause in their use of the index, but as the additional letters are filed in a different order in each language this seemed to be the safest solution.

Entries

As far as possible the following bibliographical details have been given:

1. for each periodical article – author, title of article, title of periodical (*in italic*), volume number, part number (in parenthesis), date of issue, year and pages.

2. for each book – author, title of book (*in italic*), edition, place of publication, publisher, date, and either the total number of pages or the relevant pages.

In both instances the title of non-English language material has been translated into English, and is given in square brackets immediately after the title of the article or the book. In a few entries, where the the original title was not available from the source, the title is given in English only and reference made to the original language.

There is no annotation but where an abstract has been published in, for example, *Hospital Abstracts* or *Library Science Abstracts*, this is cited at the end of the entry.

Analytical entries for collected works and conference papers have been included with reference from the main entry to the contents.

Indexes

There are three indexes – author, geographical and subject.

Author index
In the author index names of personal and corporate authors, joint authors and translators are listed in one alphabetical order. (For note on alphabetisation see above, p. 2). Under each name the numbers of the relevant entries are entered in sequence.

Geographical index
In an international bibliography such as this it was felt important to include a geographical index. Entry is made under the country whose practice or philosophy is being described and not by the nationality of the author. The fact that a country is not represented does not necessarily mean that there is no hospital library service but only that no references have been traced.

Subject index
The use of broad general headings has been unavoidable but, where appropriate, items are entered under more than one heading; thus an article on book selection for the blind is entered under BOOK SELECTION and BLIND AND PARTI-ALLY SIGHTED; an article on bibliotherapy in a children's hospital is entered under CHILDREN and BIBLIOTHERAPY.

Critical comment

In a work of this nature produced by co-operative effort there must inevitably be unevenness in coverage and inaccuracies are bound to occur. The major part of the editing has been done outwith working hours over a long period of time and this has created problems. Unfortunately the editor has not been able to see personally a large amount of the material included, and this also accounts for the fact that no entries have been annotated nor the literature evaluated. Some attempt has been made to overcome this lack of annotation by referring to a published abstract where possible.

In the subject index many items have had to be indexed from the abstract or by relying on the terms used in the indexes to the literature. Some of the older material has not been indexed as it was felt safer to exclude it rather than index it inaccurately.

Most of the terms used are very broad, in particular, HOSPITAL LIBRARIES,

SERVICES TO PATIENTS IN GENERAL. This heading covers the type of general article on the establishment and development of a hospital library service, descriptive articles on services to patients and handicapped readers, and articles describing the service in one hospital. Unfortunately, this means a large sequence of numbers are under one heading. The only way in which they can be subdivided for consultation is chronologically – the lower numbers relate to the early material the higher numbers to more recent items.

This work undoubtedly has shortcomings; nevertheless as the first major guide to the literature it should have an important role. It is intended to publish supplements. Critical comment which will make these supplements more useful will be welcomed as will further references both retrospective and current.

Acknowledgements

This bibliography could not have been produced without a great deal of co-operative effort and many people have contributed to it. It is impossible to mention them all individually but I should like at least to thank the following.

The International Correspondents of the Sub-Section who have sent contributions to Miss Going and to myself; in particular, the Comtesse I. G. Du Monceau de Bergendal of Belgium, and Fraulein Hannelore Schmidt of the German Federal Republic, who not only sent entries but also translated this introduction and the terms used in the subject index;

Frank Hogg of the College of Librarianship, Wales, for making it possible for me to consult long runs of *Library Literature* at home, without which the bibliography would be much shorter;

My colleagues at the Scottish Health Service Centre for their help and support, especially Miss Antonia Bunch who provided some of the early British references including the first item.

Most of all I am grateful to Miss Mona Going, who laid the foundation, who has maintained her interest and given me advice, and to Miss M. Joy Lewis, past Chairman, Miss Petra Leeuwenburgh, present Chairman, and Mrs. Jean Clarke, Secretary of the Sub-Section, for their contributions and for their patient understanding and constant encouragement and support through the completion stages of this work.

Finally, I should like to record my thanks to Mrs. Maureen Ferguson who, in preparing the typescript, coped so admirably with my manuscript in a variety of unfamiliar languages.

Eileen E. Cumming
Edinburgh
June 1975

Passé historique

L'idée de la nécessité de compiler une bibliographie des bibliothèques d'hôpitaux a été exprimée pour la première fois à une réunion de la sous-commission des bibliothèques d'hôpitaux lors du Conseil de l'IFLA tenu à Londres en 1948. On a proposé que chaque pays soit responsable de la préparation d'un chapitre relatif à sa propre littérature mais qu'un rédacteur en chef soit désigné. Cette même bibliographie a encore été discutée dans les années 1949 et 1950, lorsque certaines listes ont circulé en plusieurs exemplaires, mais aucune publication n'en a résulté.

Le projet a été discuté de nouveau à Sofia en 1963 lorsque l'on a décidé de mettre la question à l'ordre du jour de la réunion de 1966 à La Haye. Le travail actuel en est le résultat direct. A La Haye, l'on a demandé à Mademoiselle Mona Going, qui avait déjà réuni des données à titre personnel, de se charger de la compilation de la bibliographie pour la sous-section. Il avait été demandé aux correspondants internationaux d'aider Mademoiselle Going en lui soumettant les données relatives à leur pays respectif. Le rédacteur actuel a commencé à s'attacher à la tâche en 1968, lorsque Mademoiselle Going lui a demandé son aide pour la vérification des articles.

Un travail de cette espèce basée sur une coopération internationale rencontre de nombreux problèmes et la bibliographie a grandi un peu au hasard. Une recommandation de Mlle Going par laquelle il était demandé au rédacteur actuel de collationner les références depuis 1968 pour une seconde publication, a été approuvée à Copenhagen en 1969. Mais, en 1971, lorsque le nombre d'articles avait déjà totalisé environ 850 entrées, Mlle Going a décidé de lui repasser tout-à-fait la main pour la vérification et l'achèvement du travail.

C'est à ce moment-là que l'on a décidé d'exclure toutes références aux bibliothèques médicales ou à celles destinées au personnel infirmier, et de concentrer les efforts sur les services destinés aux malades. La bibliographie complète comprend un total de 2.164 articles.

But

Le but de cette compilation était de fournir le liste la plus complète possible des livres et articles traitant des services bibliothécaires destinés aux malades et handicapés à travers le monde. Il est à espérer qu'il pourra être une source utile de références, qu'il mettra en évidence les zones sur lesquelles rien ou peu n'a été écrit, et par ce fait même stimulera l'intérêt dans la pratique de la bibliothéconomie d'hôpital.

Portée

Les entrées ont trait aux différents aspects des services de bibliothèques destinés aux malades dans toutes les catégories d'hôpitaux, aux personnes âgées, aux handicapés physiques (aveugles, sourds, etc.) et aux handicapés mentaux hospitalisés ou non. Des listes de livres faciles à lire et de livres destinés aux enfants retardés ont été incluses car il a été estimé que ces listes pourraient être utiles aux personnes intéressées par la sélection de livres pour les handicapés mentaux.

Hospital and Welfare Library Services

Les articles sur des livres destinés à satisfaire les besoins professionnels du personnel des hôpitaux n'ont été inclus que lorsqu'une partie importante de l'article traitait du service aux malades.

Période couverte

La première entrée en date de 1863, a trait au catalogue de la bibliothèque destinée aux malades du Murray Royal Psychiatric Hospital du Perthshire; les dernières entrées datent de 1972.

Sources

Les correspondants internationaux de la sous-section ont envoyé les articles intéressant leur propre pays. En plus de cela, l'on a consulté les principaux journaux faisant de l'indexation et des résumés:

Hospital Abstracts
Hospital Literature Index
Library Literature
Library Science Abstracts
Library and Information Science Abstracts

Disposition

Une disposition chronologique a été choisie car il a été estimé que ceci montrerait, à travers la littérature, le développement historique et comparatif des bibliothèques d'hôpitaux des différents pays et serait utile aux chercheurs, professeurs et étudiants.

Les entrées ont été rangées par année de publication et à l'intérieur de chaque année, l'on a suivi l'ordre alphabétique par auteur, ou par titre dans le cas des articles anonymes. Chaque entrée a été chiffrée pour faciliter les références à l'index.

Alphabetisation

Il faut remarquer un point important de l'alphabetisation: les lettres des langues scandinaves qui n'existaient pas dans la langue anglaise, ont été mises sous une forme anglicisée.

Cela veut dire par exemple que Åhlin n'apparait pas après Ziegler mais après Ackernecht et avant Ahlnäs, et que Höök apparait entre Holmström et Hoover.

Je m'excuse auprès de mes amis et collègues scandinaves des inconvénients que ceci peut leur causer dans l'emploi de l'index, mais comme les lettres supplémentaires sont classées dans un ordre différent dans chaque langue, ceci semblait la solution la plus satisfaisante.

Entrées

Les détails bibliographiques suivants ont été donnés autant que possible:

6

1. Pour chaque article de périodique: l'auteur, le titre de l'article, le titre du périodique (en italique), le numéro du tome, le numéro du paragraphe (entre parenthèses), la date de parution, l'année et les pages.

2. Pour chaque livre: l'auteur, le titre du livre (en italique), l'édition, le pays de publication, l'éditeur, la date et soit le nombre total de pages soit les pages intéressant les bibliothèques d'hôpitaux.

Dans les deux cas, le titre en langue non-anglaise a été traduit en anglais mais est inscrit entre crochets juste après le titre de l'article ou du livre. Dans quelques cas, le titre d'origine n'ayant pas été donné, le titre est donné uniquement en anglais avec une référence à la lanque d'origine.

Il n'y a pas d'annotations mais si un résumé a été publié comme par exemple dans *Hospital Abstracts* ou *Library Science Abstracts*, ce sera cité à la fin de chaque entrée.

Les entrées analytiques pour les oeuvres complètes et les documents de conférences ont été incluses avec référence à l'entrée principale du sujet.

Indexation

Il y a trois indexations: par auteur, par région géographique et par sujet.

Index par auteur

Dans l'index par auteur, les noms des auteurs, des auteurs collectifs, des auteurs associés et des traducteurs sont inscrits dans le même ordre alphabétique. (Pour les explications sur l'alphabétisation, voir plus haut p. 6). Sous chaque nom d'auteur les numéros des entrées relatives sont y inscrits dans l'ordre.

Index par région géographique

Dans une bibliographie internationale comme celle-ci, l'on a considéré qu'il était important d'inclure un index par région géographique. L'entrée est faite sous le nom du pays dont les pratiques ou la philosophie sont en train d'être décrites et non d'après la nationalité d l'auteur.

Le fait qu'un pays ne soit pas représenté dans la liste ne veut pas dire nécessairement qu'il n'y existe pas de services de bibliothèques d'hôpitaux, mais uniquement que l'on n'a pas trouvé de références à ceux-ci.

Index par sujet

L'emploi de titres généraux était inévitable mais, si nécessaire, certaines rubriques sont cataloguées sous plus d'un titre par exemple un article sur la sélection de livres pour les aveugles est entré sous SÉLECTION DES LIVRES et AVEUGLES ET AMBLYOPES; un article sur la bibliothérapie dans un hôpital pour enfants est entré sous ENFANTS et BIBLIOTHÉRAPIE.

Commentaire critique

Il est inévitable que des inégalités d'étendue d'information et des inexactitudes se glissent dans un travail de cette nature produit par un effort coopératif.

La plus grande partie de la compilation a été faite en dehors des heures de travail et étalée sur une longue période de temps, ce qui a créé inévitablement certains problèmes. Le rédacteur n'a malheureusement pas eu l'occasion de voir lui-même une grande partie du matériel répertorié, ce qui explique le fait que les entrées n'ont pu être annotées ni la littérature évaluée. Des efforts ont été faits pour parer à ce manque d'information en se référant à un résumé publié chaque fois que c'était possible.

Dans l'index par sujet, certains articles ont dû être répertoriés en se basant sur des résumés ou en se référant aux termes employés dans l'index de la littérature. Certains articles très anciens n'ont pas été indexes, car il a été estimé préférable de les exclure plutôt que de les indexer d'une façon inexacte.

La plupart des termes sont employés au sens large, surtout en Bibliothèques d'Hôpitaux – Services aux malades en général. Ce titre couvre les articles de type général sur l'établissement et le développement d'un service de bibliothèque d'hôpital, les articles décrivant les services aux lecteurs malades et handicapés, et les articles décrivant le service organisé dans un hôpital particulier. Ceci veut malheureusement dire qu'un grand nombre d'articles paraissent sous un seul titre, la seule façon dont on puisse les subdiviser pour s'y référer est par ordre chronologique, les chiffres les plus bas étant attribués aux articles les plus anciens, les chiffres les plus élevés à des articles plus récents.

Ce travail présente inévitablement des lacunes, mais par le simple fait d'être le premier guide complet de ce genre de littérature, il est appelé à jouer un rôle important.

Des suppléments sont envisagés. Des commentaires critiques rendant ces suppléments plus utiles de même que des références supplémentaires rétrospectives ou courantes seront les bienvenus.

Remerciements

Cette bibliographie n'aurait pas pu être écrite sans un grand effort coopératif auquel ont participé de nombreuses personnes. Il est impossible de les mentionner toutes individuellement mais je voudrais au moins remercier les suivants:

Les correspondants internationaux de la sous-section qui ont envoyé des contributions à Mademoiselle Going ou à moi-même, en particulier la Ctesse I. G. Du Monceau de Bergendal, de Belgique, et Mlle Hannelore Schmidt, de la République Fédérale Allemande, qui ont non seulement envoyé des documents mais aussi traduit cette introduction et les termes employés dans l'index.

Monsieur Frank Hogg du College of Librarianship, Wales, qui m'a permis de consulter à domicile de longs extraits de la *Library Literature*, sans l'aide duquel cette bibliographie aurait été moins étendue.

Mes collègues du Scottish Health Service Centre et plus spécialement Mlle Antonia Bunch qui a fourni certaines des plus anciennes références britanniques et en particulier la première.

Mais je voudrais surtout exprimer ma reconnaissance à Mlle Mona Going qui a jeté les bases de ce travail, a continué à s'y intéresser et m'a prodigué ses conseils, à l'anciennce présidente Mlle M. J. Lewis, à la présidente actuelle Mlle Petra Leeuwenburgh et à la secrétaire de sous-section Mme Jean Clarke. Leur contribution, leur compréhension patiente et leurs encouragements constants m'ont soutenue pendant toutes les étapes d'achèvement de ce travail.

Je voudrais finalement remercier aussi Mme Maureen Ferguson qui, en préparant la typographie, a su si admirablement se débrouiller dans une variété de langues qui ne lui étaient pas familières.

Eileen E. Cumming
Edinbourg
Juin 1975

Entstehungsgeschichte

Die Anregung, eine internationale Bibliographie über Krankenhausbibliotheken zusammenzustellen, wurde das erste Mal auf dem Treffen des Sub-Komitees 'Krankenhausbibliotheken' während des IFLA-Kongresses 1948 in London gegeben. Vorgeschlagen wurde, daß jedes Land für das Zusammentragen seiner eigenen einschlägigen Literatur verantwortlich sein und ein Herausgeber ernannt werden sollte. Die Bibliographie wurde sodann auf den Sitzungen 1949 und 1950 diskutiert, wo einige vervielfältigte Listen zirkulierten, aber keine Veröffentlichung erfolgte. Das Thema wurde 1963 in Solfia erneut aufgegriffen – und man entschied, die Arbeit bis zum Treffen 1966 in Den Haag voranzutreiben. Das vorliegende Werk stützt sich unmittelbar auf die in Den Haag erzielten Ergebnisse. Dort wurde Miss Mona Going – sie hatte bereits auf eigene Initiative hin Material gesammelt – gebeten, die Zusammenstellung der Bibliographie für die Sub-Section zu übernehmen. Die internationalen Korrespondenten wurden daraufhin aufgefordert, Miss Going zu helfen und die entsprechenden Veröffentlichungen ihrer Länder vorzulegen. 1968 begann Miss Going mit der Prüfung der eingegangenen Beiträge.

Ein Werk dieser Art, das auf internationaler Zusammenarbeit basiert, wirft viele Probleme auf – und so wuchs die Bibliographie ziemlich langsam. Eine Empfehlung von Miss Going, Beiträge von 1968 aufwärts für eine zweite Veröffentlichung zu sammeln, wurde 1969 in Kopenhagen gebilligt. 1971 jedoch, als die Zahl der Eingänge annähernd 850 erreicht hatte, entschied Miss Going, das Werk komplett herauszugeben. Auch entschloss man sich nun, Beiträge über medizinische und Krankenpflege-Fachbibliotheken auszuschliessen und sich auf Patientenbibliotheken zu beschränken. Die Bibliographie umfasst 2164 Beiträge.

Zweck

Diese Bibliographie bezweckt die Bereitstellung einer möglichst unfassenden Liste von Büchern und Zeitschriftenartikeln über Bibliotheksdienste für Kranke und Behinderte aus aller Welt. Man hofft, daß es sich als brauchbares Nachschlagewerk erweisen wird, daß es auf Arbeitsbereiche aufmerksam macht, über die bisher nichts oder nur wenig geschrieben wurde oder getan wird, und es will deshalb das Interesse für die praktische Arbeit in Krankenhausbibliotheken wecken.

Bereich

Die Beiträge beziehen sich auf verschiedene Aspekte des Bibliotheksdienstes für Patienten in allen Arten von Krankenhäusern, für hausgebundene, alte, körperlich behinderte (Blinde, Taube, etc.) und geistig behinderte Menschen sowohl im Krankenhaus als auch in der Gemeinde. Bücherlisten für 'einfache Leser' und zurückgebliebene Kinder wurden mit einbezogen in der Annahme, daß sie für jene nützlich sein dürften, die sich für die Buchauswahl für geistig Behinderte interessieren.

Beiträge über die Bereitstellung von Fachliteratur für das Krankenhauspersonal wurden nur berücksichtigt, wenn sich der wesentliche Teil des Artikels auf die Bibliotheksdienste für Patienten bezog.

Zeitraum

Der erste Beitrag von 1863 ist der Katalog der Patientenbibliothek des Murray Royal Psychiatric Hospital in Perthshire, die letzten Beiträge stammen aus dem Jahre 1972.

Quellen

Die internationalen Korrespondenten der Sub-Section haben Material aus ihren Ländern eingesandt. Zusätzlich wurden die folgenden Zeitschriften und Nachschlagewerke ausgewertet:

Hospital Abstracts
Hospital Literature Index
Library Literature
Library Science Abstracts
Library and Information Science Abstracts

Anordnung

Gewählt wurde eine chronologische Anordnung, da man annahm, daß diese die historische und vergleichende Entwicklung der Krankenhausbibliotheken in den verschiedenen Ländern an Hand der Literatur am besten aufzeigt und für Forscher, Lehrer und Studenten nützlich wäre.

Die Beiträge wurden nach dem Jahr der Veröffentlichung und innerhalb jeden Jahres alphabetisch nach dem Verfasser oder bei anonymen Schriften nach dem Titel geordnet. Jeder Beitrag hat eine laufende Nummer, um das Nachschlagen im Register zu erleichtern.

Alphabetisierung

Bei der Alphabetisierung erscheinen Buchstaben der skandinavischen Sprachen, die im Englischen hinzugefügt werden, in anglisierter Form. Das bedeutet, daß zum Beispiel Åhlin nicht nach Ziegler erscheint, sondern nach Ackerknecht und vor Ahlnäs, Höök kommt zwischen Holström und Hoover. Ich bitte meine skandinavischen Freunde und Kollegen wegen der Schwierigkeiten, die dadurch für sie bei der Benutzung des Registers auftreten, um Entschuldigung; aber da die zusätzlichen Zeichen in jeder Sprache in verschiedenen Ordnungssystemen erscheinen, schien dies die sicherste Lösung.

Beiträge

Soweit wie möglich wurden folgende bibliographische Details angegeben:

1. für jeden Zeitschriften-Artikel – Verfasser, Titel des Artikels, Name der Zeitschrift (in Kursivschrift), Nummer des Jahrgangs, Nummer des Heftes (in Klammer), Erscheinungsdatum, Erscheinungsjahr und Seitenzahl.

2. für jedes Buch – Verfasser, Titel (in Kursivschrift), Auflage, Verlagsort, Verlag,

Erscheinungsjahr und entweder die vollständige Seitenzahl oder die zutreffenden Seiten.

In allen Fällen wurden die 'nicht-englischen' Titel ins Englische übersetzt und in eckiger Klammer unmittelbar nach dem Originaltitel angegeben. Bei einigen Beiträgen, wo der Originaltitel nicht ermittelt werden konnte, wurde der Titel nur in Englisch aufgeführt und Hinweise auf die Originalsprache gemacht.

Anmerkungen fehlen; nur wenn Auszüge veröffentlicht wurden, wird dies am Ende des Beitrages erwähnt, zum Beispiel *Hospital Abstracts* oder *Library Science Abstracts*.

Bei Beiträgen in Sammelwerken und Konferenz-Papieren begnügte man sich mit einem Hinweis auf das Hauptwerk.

Register

Es gibt drei Arten von Register: Verfasser-, geographisches- und Schlagwort-Register.

Verfasser-Register
Im Verfasser-Register sind die Namen der Autoren und Körperschaften, der Mitverfasser und Übersetzer in einer alphabetischen Ordnung aufgeführt (Anmerkungen über die Alphabetisierung siehe Seite 11). Unter jedem Namen sind die Nummern der zutreffenden Beiträge nacheinander verzeichnet.

Geographisches-Register
In einer internationalen Bibliographie wie dieser ist es wichtig, ein geographisches-Register vorzufinden. Der Beitrag steht unter dem Land, dessen Praxis oder Anschauung beschrieben wird und nicht unter der Nationalität des Autors. Die Tatsache, daß ein Land nicht aufgeführt ist, bedeutet nicht unbedingt, daß es dort keinen Krankenhausbibliotheksdienst gibt, sondern nur, daß keine schriftlichen Unterlagen ermittelt werden konnten.

Schlagwort-Register
Der Gebrauch von allgemein gültigen Schlagwörtern war unvermeidbar, doch wo es angemessen schien, wurden, Beiträge unter mehr als einem Schlagwort eingetragen, so zum Beispiel ein Artikel über die Buchauswahl für Blinde unter BUCHAUSWAHL und BLINDE UND SEHBEHINDERTE; ein Artikel über Bibliotherapie in einem Kinderkrankenhaus unter KINDER und BIBLIO-THERAPIE.

Kritische Bemerkungen

Bein einem Werk dieser Art, das in kooperativer Zusammenarbeit entstanden ist, müssen zwangsläufig Unebenheiten und Ungenauigkeiten in Kauf genommen werden. Der größte Teil des Redigierens wurde außerhalb der Dienststunden über einen längeren Zeitraum hinweg geleistet – und das verursachte einige Probleme. Unglücklicherweise konnte der Herausgeber einen großen Teil des aufgeführten Materials nicht persönlich einsehen und dies ist auch der Grund, warum weder Beiträge annotiert noch genaue Literaturhinweise gemacht werden konnten. Soweit möglich wurde versucht, diese Annotations-Lücken durch Hinweise auf veröffentlichte Besprechungen zu schließen.

Für das Schlagwort-Register wurden viele Begriffe Nachschlagewerken entnommen oder die Terminologie, die in den Literaturverzeichnissen üblich ist, verwandt. Einige der älteren Beiträge wurden nicht ins Register aufgenommen, da es korrekter schien, sie auszuschließen als ungenau zu sein.

Die meisten Begriffe sind sehr breit zu verstehen, insbesondere KRANKEN-HAUSBIBLIOTHEKEN, DIENSTE FÜR PATIENTEN IN ALLGEMEINEN KRANKENHÄUSERN. Unter diesem Schlagwort findet man die Hauptartikel über Einrichtung und Entwicklung des Krankenhausbibliothekswesens, Darstellungen über Dienste für Patienten und behinderte Leser und Artikel, die die Bibliotheksarbeit in einem bestimmten Krankenhaus beschreiben. Leider stehen hier unter einem Schlagwort eine große Anzahl von Nummern. Die einzige Möglichkeit der Unterteilung ist die chronologische – die niedrigen Nummern beziehen sich auf das ältere Material, die höheren Nummern auf die jüngsten Beiträge.

Dieses Werk hat zweifellos Unzulänglichkeiten; trotzdem sollte es als erster größerer Literaturführer über Krankenhausbibliotheksarbeit eine wichtige Rolle spielen.

Es ist beabsichtigt, Nachträge zu veröffentlichen. Kritische Bemerkungen, die diese Nachträge noch brauchbarer machen könnten, sowie weitere ältere und neuere Beiträge sind willkommen.

Dank an die Mitarbeiter

Diese Bibliographie hätte ohne kooperative Bemühungen nicht herausgebracht werden können; viele Personen haben sich daran beteiligt. Es ist unmöglich, sie alle namentlich aufzuführen; doch möchte ich wenigstens folgenden Kollegen besonders danken:

Den internationalen Korrespondenten der Sub-Section, die ihre Veröffentlichungen eingesandt haben, insbesondere Comtesse I. G. Du Monceau de Bergendal aus Belgien und Fräulein Hannelore Schmidt aus der Bundesrepublik Deutschland, die nicht nur Beiträge geschickt, sondern auch diese Einführung und die Begriffe für das Schlagwort-Register übersetzt haben;

Frank Hogg vom College of Librarianship Wales, der es mir möglich machte, die *Library Literature* für längere Zeit zuhause einzusehen, ohne die die Bibliographie wesentlich kürzer geworden wäre;

Meinen Kollegen vom Scottish Health Service Centre für ihre Hilfe und Unterstützung, besonders Miss Antonia Bunch, die einige der frühen britischen Artikel, einschließlich des ersten Beitrages lieferte.

Am meisten aber bin ich Miss Mona Going, die den Graundstein legte, ihr Interesse weiterhin bezeugte und Ratschläge gab, Miss M. Joy Lewis, der früheren

Präsidentin, Miss Petra Leeuwenburgh, der gegenwärtigen Präsidentin und Mrs. Jean Clarke, der Sekretärin der Sub-Section für ihre Unterstützung, ihr geduldiges Verständnis und ihre beständige Ermutigung und Förderung in allen Stadien dieser Arbeit zu Dank verpflichtet.

Nicht zuletzt möchte ich meinen Dank Mrs. Maureen Ferguson abstatten, die die Niederschrift vorbereitete und von meinem Manuskript so vortrefflich in den verschiedenen, ihr nicht vertrauten Sprachen abschrieb.

Eileen E. Cumming
Edinburgh
Juni 1975

AHIL Quarterly	(Association of Hospital and Institution Libraries) Quarterly
AIB Boll.	Associazione Italiana Biblioteche Bolletino d'Informazioni
ALA Bull.	American Library Association Bulletin
Am. Libr.	American Libraries
Aslib Proc.	Aslib Proceedings
Assistant Librn.	Assistant Librarian
Aust. Libr. J.	Australian Library Journal
Aust. Sch. Librn.	Australian School Librarian
Bull. Bib. Fr.	Bulletin des Bibliothèques de France
Bull. Med. Libr. Ass.	Bulletin of the Medical Library Association
Can. Libr. J.	Canadian Library Journal
Cath. Libr. Wld.	Catholic Library World
Hosp. Abstr.	Hospital Abstracts
Int. Libr. Rev.	International Library Review
Law Libr. J.	Law Library Journal
Libr. Ass. Rec.	Library Association Record
Libr. Inf. Bull.	Library and Information Bulletin (Library Association)
Libr. J.	Library Journal
Lisa	Library and Information Science Abstracts
LSA	Library Science Abstracts
PLA Bull.	(Pennsylvania Library Association) Bulletin
S. Afr. Libr.	South African Libraries
Scandinavian Publ. Libr. Q.	Scandinavian Public Library Quarterly
Spec. Libr.	Special Libraries
Tex. Libr.	Texas Libraries
Unesco Bull. Libr.	Unesco Bulletin for Libraries
Wilson Libr. Bull.	Wilson Library Bulletin

1863

1 *Catalogue of the library of Murray's Royal Institution, Perth*; compiled by M. W. J. No. 1 – Jan. 1863. Perth, printed by Robert Whittet, 1863.

1872

2 Books for hospital patients. [Royal Infirmary of Edinburgh – patients' Library.] *Lancet*, Oct. 5 1872, 503 – 504.

1895

3 TYLOR, Dorothy. Hospital libraries. (Paper read before eighteenth annual meeting of the Library Association, Cardiff, 1895.) *Library*, 7 (83) Nov. 1895, 347 – 352.

1899

4 LOOMIS, M. L. W. Plan for a hospital library. *Libr. J.*, 24 1899, 110.

1904

5 Hospital libraries in the field. *Libr. Ass. Rec.*, 6 May 15 1904, 261 – 262. Transl. from the Russian newspaper *Novoe Vremya* of April 24 1904, by Major W. H. Salmon.

1907

6 CAREY, M. E. Libraries in state institutions: the book as a tool. *Minnesota Public Library Commission Notes*, 2 1907, 67 – 70; also in *ALA Bull.*, 1 1907, conference no. 101 – 108; and in *Public Libraries*, 12 1907, 127 – 128.

1908

7 LAQUER, B. Über die Versorgung von Krankenhäusern und Heilstätten mit guten Buchern. [Using good books in hospital and sanatoria care.] *Berliner Klinische Wochenschrift*, 45 1908, 1188.

8 Reading in bed. *Lancet*, ii 1908, 1089.

9 SCHULTZE, Ernst. Über Notwendigkeit und Nutzen von Krankenhaus-Büchereien. [On the necessity and use of hospital libraries.] *Archiv f. Volkswohlfahrt*, 1 1907/08, 813 – 819.

1909

10 LEAGUE OF LIBRARY COMMISSIONS. Report of committee on commission work in state institutions. *ALA Bull.*, 3 1909, 339 – 348.

1910

11 MOORE, A. C. Work with children from institutions for the deaf and dumb. *Libr. J.*, 35 1910, 158 – 159.

1911

12   JONES, Edith Kathleen. Libraries for the patients in hospitals for the insane. *Libr. J.*, 36 1911, 637 – 639; also in *American Journal of Insanity*, 68 July 1911, 95 – 101.

13   JONES, Edith Kathleen. *The library of McLean hospital, Waverley, Massachusetts.* [Waverley, Mass.] 1911.

1912

14   JONES, Edith Kathleen. Library work among the insane: paper at 34th annual meeting ALA Ottawa, June/July 1912. *ALA Bull.*, 6 July 1912, 320 – 324; also in *New York Libraries*, 3 1912, 239 – 241.

15   JONES, Edith Kathleen. State control of state hospital libraries. *American Journal of Insanity*, April 1912, 709 – 714.

16   ROBINSON, J. A. Libraries in Iowa state institutions. *Iowa Library Commission Quarterly*, 6 1912, 252 – 256.

1913

17   CHROMSE, Irene. Zur Frage der Krankenhausbücherei. [On the question of hospital libraries.] *Zeitschrift für Krankenpflege*, Berlin, 35 1913, 175 – 186.

18   CHUTE, G. What a library can mean to an institution child. *Minnesota Public Library Commission Notes*, 4 1913, 1 – 3.

19   JONES, Edith Kathleen. *One thousand books for the hospital library selected from the shelf-list of the library of McLean Hospital, Waverley, Massachusetts*; additions and annotations, M. E. Carey, F. Waugh and J. A. Robinson. Chicago, American Library Association Publishing Board, 1913.

20   JONES, Edith Kathleen. Some problems of the institution library organizer in the state hospitals. *ALA Bull.*, 7 1913, 369 – 374.

21   State hospitals for the insane summarized reports. *New York Libraries*, 3 1913, 244 – 246.

22   TUCK, L. C. The library at the school for the deaf. *Minnesota Public Library Commission Notes*, 4 1913, 5 – 6.

1914

23   JONES, Edith Kathleen. Value of the library in the hospital for mental disease. *Maryland Psychiatric Quarterly*, 4 July 1914, 8 – 13.

1915

24   CAREY, M. E. Libraries and their management in state hospitals. *Modern Hospital*, 5 (6) Dec. 1915, 407 – 410; also in *Libr. J.*, 41 1916, 854 – 855; and in *American Library Annual*, 1916 – 1917, 61 – 62.

25   JONES, Edith Kathleen. *The hospital library* . . . St. Louis, Modern Hospital Publishing Co., 1915.

26 JONES, Edith Kathleen. On books and reading: outline of a course of lectures for nurses in hospitals. *American Journal of Insanity*, 72 (2) Oct. 1915, 297 – 303.

27 ROBINSON, J. A. Book influences for defectives and dependents: helping those who cannot help themselves. *ALA Bull.*, 7 1915, 177 – 182.

1916

28 CAREY, M. E. In the land of the counterpane: books for crippled children's library. *Nurse*, Dec. 1916, 389 – 391.

29 CAREY, M. E. Traveling libraries in hospitals. *Modern Hospital*, 6 1916, 298 – 299.

30 CLARK, P. O. A hospital circulating library; the ladies' auxiliary the proper body to have charge – some suggestions as to management. *Modern Hospital*, 7 1916, 445 – 446.

31 HOLLAND, Clive. The romance and pathos of trench and hospital libraries. [Books in demand by soldiers at the front.] *Chambers's Journal*, Dec. 1 1916, 781 – 784.

32 JONES, Edith Kathleen. Hospital libraries: their relation to patients and training schools. *National League of Nursing 22 Annual Proceedings*, 1916, 184 – 190.

33 JONES, Edith Kathleen. Importance of organized libraries in institutions. *Libr. J.*, 41 (7) July 1916, 459 – 462.

34 JONES, Edith Kathleen. What can I find to read aloud? Some books for the convalescent patient. *Nurse*, 4 (2) Feb. 1916, 79 – 88.

35 MACLEAN, Margaret. Minnesota school for feebleminded and colony for epileptics: the children's library. *Modern Hospital*, 6 1916, 368 – 369.

36 ROBINSON, G. S. Institution libraries of Iowa. *Modern Hospital*, 6 Feb. 1916, 131 – 132.

37 SCOTT, Carrie E. *compiler. Manual for institution libraries*. Chicago, American Library Association, 1916. 38 pp. (Library handbook, 10).

1917

38 AMERICAN LIBRARY ASSOCIATION. Report of the committee on libraries in hospitals, charitable and correctional institutions. *ALA Bull.*, 11 1917, 312 – 313.

39 BURGOYNE, M. H. Story of an institutional library, developed from small beginnings and conducted by patients at low cost. *Modern Hospital*, 8 1917, 251 – 253.

40 GASKELL, H. M. *The Red Cross and Order of St. John war library*. London [1917]. 8 pp.

41 JONES, Edith Kathleen. Hospital libraries: their relation to patients and training schools. *Libr. J.*, 42 (6) June 1917, 493 – 495.

42 JONES, Edith Kathleen. Hospital library economics. *Proceedings of the Alienists and Neurologists of America*, 6 1917, 171 – 176.

43   KOCH, Theodore Wesley. *Books in camp, trench and hospital* . . . London, J. M. Dent & Sons, 1917. 48 pp. Reprinted from *Libr. J.,* 42 (7) July 1917, 507 – 514; (8) Aug. 1917, 591 – 598; (10) Oct. 1917, 778 – 790.

1918

44   AMERICAN LIBRARY ASSOCIATION. Hospital librarians round table meeting. *Libr. J.,* 43 1918, 614.

45   CAREY, M. E. From camp to camp: the work of a field representative. *ALA Bull.,* 12 1918, 225 – 226.

46   CAREY, M. E. What a man reads in hospital. Paper read at ALA conference Saratoga Springs, July 2 1918. *Libr. J.,* 43 (8) Aug. 1918, 565 – 567; abstr. in *ALA Bull.,* 12 1918, 222; also abstr. in *Public Libraries,* 23 Oct. 1918, 364 – 365.

47   COCHRAN, M. R. State institution libraries in Ohio. *Libr. J.,* 43 1918, 486 – 488.

48   DOREN, E. C. The war hospital library service at Dayton, Ohio. *Bulletin of Bibliography,* 10 1918, 3 – 4.

49   JONES, Edith K[athleen]. What a base hospital librarian should know: outline of a course of training. Paper read at ALA conference Saratoga Springs, July 2 1918. *Libr. J.,* 43 (8) Aug. 1918, 568 – 572; also in *ALA Bull.,* 12 1918, 226 – 231.

50   KOCH, Theodore Wesley. *War service of the American Library Association.* Washington, ALA War Service, 1918, 34 – 37.

51   PRESTON, Nina K. Michigan school for the deaf library. *Libr. J.,* 43 (10) Oct. 1918, 749 – 750.

52   TAPPERT, K. Base hospital library, U.S. Camp Upton, N.Y. (correspondence). *Iowa Library Commission Quarterly,* 8 (7) July/Aug./Sept. 1918, 107 – 108.

53   WEBSTER, Caroline. Hospital library service: its organization. Paper read at ALA conference Saratoga Springs, July 2 1918. *ALA Papers and Proceedings,* 1918, 231 – 235; also in *Libr. J.,* 43 (8) Aug. 1918, 563 – 565.

54   WILLIAMS, Nellie. The library from the patients' point of view. *Chicago Medical Recorder,* 40 1918, 64 – 68.

55   Work in a hospital library. *Library Occurrent,* 5 1918, 83 – 86.

1919

56   AMERICAN LIBRARY ASSOCIATION. War Service. *Hospital library handbook.* [Washington] 1919. 26 pp.

57   COWLEY, Amy. Hospital library service at Fort Sheridan, Illinois. *Minnesota Department of Education Library Notes and News,* 6 (1) March 1919, 4.

58   DALE, M. Notes from a base hospital library (Camp Kearny, California). *News Notes of California Libraries,* 14 1919, 1 – 5.

59   DOUD, Margery, *compiler. Five hundred books for hospital patients, compiled at the request of Barnes Hospital, St. Louis.* St. Louis, St. Louis Public Library, 1919.

60 GREEN, Elizabeth. Can start hospital library modestly. *Hospital Management,* 3 Dec. 1919, 40.

61 GREEN, Elizabeth. A hospital library and some of its by-products. *Modern Hospital,* 12 March 1919, 161; repr. in *Public Libraries,* 24 (6) June 1919, 240 – 242.

62 Hospital librarians round table meeting. *ALA Bull.,* 13 1919, 399; also in *Libr. J.,* 44 1919, 603.

63 Hospital libraries. *Minnesota Department of Education Library Notes and News,* 6 (4) Dec. 1919, 65 – 66.

64 Hospital libraries. [American Library Association war service.] *ALA Bull.,* 13 1919, 202 – 204.

65 Hospital library service of public library of Sioux City, Iowa. *Public Libraries,* 24 1919, 418 – 419.

66 ISOM, M. F. Hospital libraries in France. *Pacific Northwest Library Association Proceedings,* 1919, 11 – 19.

67 KOCH, Theodore Wesley. *Books in the war: the romance of library war service.* Boston & New York, Houghton Mifflin, 1919, 145 – 161 American hospital libraries; 162 – 174 Books for the sick and wounded; 244 – 263 British hospital libraries.

68 MILAM, C. H. Hospital libraries. *ALA Papers and Proceedings,* Asbury Park, 1919, 202 – 203.

69 PATTEN, K. Hospital library service at Fort Snelling. *Minnesota Department of Education Library Notes and News,* 6 (1) March 1919, 2 – 3.

70 SCHWAB, S. I. *and* GREEN, Elizabeth. Therapeutic use of a hospital library. *Hospital Social Service Quarterly,* 1 Aug. 1919, 147 – 157.

71 SHELLENBERGER, Grace. Library service in a reconstruction hospital. *Iowa Library Commission Quarterly,* 8 (10) April/May/June 1919, 150 – 152.

72 SUMNER, C. W. Hospital library service, Sioux City, Iowa. *Public Libraries,* 24 (10) Dec. 1919, 418 – 419.

73 WRIGHT, R. W. Glimpses of U.S. Army Hospital Library, no. 24, Parkview, Pa. *Vermont Library Bulletin,* 15 (1) June 1919, 3 – 4.

1920

74 BANGS, J. K. My silent servants. *Bookman,* 52 Dec. 1920, 305 – 310.

75 BARKER, Mary H. The use of books in the hospital. *Modern Hospital,* 14 1920, 353 – 356.

76 CAREY, M. E. A library in Nebraska State Hospital. *Public Libraries,* 25 1920, 203.

77 ELLIOTT, J. E. The relation of the library to the hospital. *Modern Hospital,* 14 June 1920, 432 – 435.

78 HUXLEY, Florence A. A.L.A. work on Ellis Island. *Libr. J.,* 45 (8) April 15 1920, 350 – 352.

79   JONES, Caroline. A.L.A. hospital service in New York State. *Libr. J.*, 45 (11) June 1920, 491 – 493.

80   KOELHER, Elizabeth. Library in a tubercular hospital. *Special Libraries*, 11 1920, 148 – 149.

81   MILAM, C. H. Hospitals. *ALA Papers and Proceedings*, Colorado Springs, 1920, 232.

82   RANKIN, E. J. The Oteen Library. *North Carolina Library Bulletin*, 4 1920, 84 – 86.

83   Report of A.L.A. Committee on transfer of library war service activities. *Libr. J.*, 45 1920, 941.

84   SUMNER, C. W. A hospital library service. *Hospital & Social Service Quarterly*, 2 Aug. 1920, 283 – 288.

85   SUMNER, C. W. Hospital library service: a new department of public library work. *Wilson Bulletin*, 1 (20) May 1920, 480 – 482.

86   WEBSTER, Caroline. Is hospital library work worth while? *Libr. J.*, 45 (4) Feb. 15 1920, 167 – 168.

1921

87   DRAKE, Ruth B. An experiment in library work in a hospital for mental disease. *Mental Hygiene*, 5 Jan. 1921, 130 – 138.

88   HAMLIN, Donelda R. The hospital library and service bureau. *Spec. Libr.*, 12 1921, 103 – 105.

89   MILAM, C. H. What a hospital library service may accomplish. *Nation's Health*, 3 Nov. 1921, 627 – 629.

90   O'CONNOR, R. A. The Sioux City Library hospital service: some questions answered. *Libr. J.*, 46 (5) March 1 1921, 205 – 207.

91   O'CONNOR, R. A. *Two hundred books for everyday use in the hospital*. Sioux City Public Library, 1921.

92   SCHWAB, S. I. *and* GIFFORD, E. R. Book therapy in the Barnes hospital, St. Louis. *Modern Hospital*, 17 Aug. 1921, 134 – 136.

93   STRAUSS, H. Über Bibliotheken für Kranke. [Libraries for the sick.] *Zeitschrift für Krankenpflege*, 43 1921, 191.

94   SUMNER, C. W. Bringing books to hospitals. *Modern Hospital*, 16 Feb. 1921, 142 – 143.

95   SWEET, Louise. Library work in a tubercular hospital. *Libr. J.*, 46 (5) March 1 1921, 208.

96   THAYER, Mrs. Nathaniel. Library in the general hospital. *ALA Bull.*, 15 1921, 204 – 205.

97   WEBSTER, Caroline. ALA hospital service. *Libr. J.*, 46 (7) April 1 1921, 305 – 307.

1922

98   EASTMAN, L. A. Here we are. *Modern Hospital*, 18 (4) April 1922, 359 – 360.

99   JONES, Edith Kathleen. The growth of the hospital library. *Modern Hospital*, 18 May 1922, 452 – 454.

100   JONES, Edith Kathleen. The library in the mental hospital. *Modern Hospital*, 18 June 1922, 535 – 536.

101   JONES, Perrie. Reading: a doctor's prescription in the hospitals of St. Paul. *Modern Hospital*, 19 1922, 229 – 230.

102   LAVINDER, C. H. Hospital library service. *ALA Bull.*, 16 1922, 276 – 281.

103   O'CONNOR, R. A. Library work in hospitals. *Iowa Library Commission Quarterly*, 9 1922, 71 – 74; also in *Public Libraries*, 27 (1) Jan. 1922, 26 – 27.

104   STOCKETT, J. C. Hospital library at U.S. Veterans' Hospital 37, Waukesha, Wisconsin. *Wisconsin Library Bulletin*, 18 1922, 263 – 265.

105   STOCKETT, J. C. Hospital library work. *Wisconsin Library Bulletin*, 18 1922, 109 – 113.

106   SWEET, Louise. Amenities of library work in a hospital for the tuberculous. *Modern Hospital*, 19 1922, 527 – 528.

107   WEBSTER, Caroline. Hospital libraries. *Public Libraries*, 47 Aug. 1922, 662.

108   WEBSTER, Caroline. Hospital libraries prove popular. *Spec. Libr.*, 13 June 1922, 89 – 90.

1923

109   BLEDSOE, E. P. The library as a therapeutic agent. *ALA Bull.*, 17 1923, 238 – 239.

110   GREEN, Elizabeth *and* GIFFORD, E. R. Two hundred and fifty books for ward patients. *Modern Hospital*, 20 1923, 582 – 583.

111   JONES, Edith Kathleen, *editor. The hospital library, comprising articles on hospital library service, organization and book selection* ... Chicago, American Library Association, 1923. 190 pp.

112   JONES, Perrie. Arousing the library profession to meet the peculiar needs of the hospital library. *ALA Bull.*, 17 1923, 236 – 237.

113   JONES, Perrie. Books at the bedside. *Survey*, 50 1923, 544 – 545.

114   MILLER, M. P. D. The therapeutic value of well chosen books in a neuropsychiatric hospital. *Modern Hospital*, 21 1923, 384 – 386; abstr. in *ALA Bull.*, 17 1923, 235 – 236.

115   SINGLEY, Louise. Library service in a tuberculosis hospital. *Modern Hospital*, 20 April 1923, 362 – 364.

116   POMEROY, Elizabeth. The veterans' hospital library service. *Hospital Buyer*, June 1923, 51 – 54, 98.

1924

117   HOOVER, A. F. Library work in hospital. *Illinois Libraries*, 6 1924, 130 – 131.

118   RUSSELL, W. L. The library in the modern hospital. *Libr. J.*, 49 1924, 1063 – 1067.

1925

119   CAREY, M. E. Even as you and I. *Minnesota Library Notes & News*, 8 1925, 51 – 52.

120   COLLINS, H. O. What constitutes a good hospital library. *Modern Hospital*, 25 1925, 495 – 496.

121   DUBOIS, Isabel. Value of naval hospital librarians. *U.S. Naval Medical Bulletin*, 23 Nov. 1925, 403 – 406.

122   The hospital library. *Wilson Bulletin*, 2 1925, 403 – 406, 410 – 411.

123   JACKSON, J. A. Therapeutic value of books. *Modern Hospital*, 25 1925, 50 – 51.

124   JANES, L. A. Hospital library service at Fond du Lac. *Wisconsin Library Bulletin*, 21 1925, 68 – 69.

125   JONES, Edith Kathleen. Hospital library service in New England. *Boston Medical and Surgical Journal*, 192 1925, 1093 – 1094.

126   JONES, Perrie. Cost of hospital library service: a new way to aid recovery. *Trained Nurse*, 75 1925, 366 – 368.

127   JONES, Perrie. Hospital library service in Minnesota. *Minnesota Medicine*, 8 1925, 451 – 452.

128   JONES, Perrie. The mutual interest of the medical worker and the hospital librarian. *Trained Nurse*, 75 1925, 153 – 155; also in *Hospital Social Service*, 11 1925, 84 – 88.

129   MCCARDLE, S. E. What the library did for patients at Fresno. *Modern Hospital*, 25 1925, 493 – 496.

130   PLUMB, R. W. Hospital library service in Muskegon. *Michigan Library Bulletin*, 16 (3) 1925, 17 – 19.

131   SCHAUFFLER, R. H. *The poetry cure*. New York, Dodd, 1925.

132   SIOUX CITY, Iowa. Public Library. *Sioux City public library hospital service*. [Sioux City Star Printing Co., 1925.] 15 pp.

133   STOCKETT, J. C. The growth of institution library work. *Wisconsin Library Bulletin*, 21 1925, 2 – 7; abstract in *Libr. J.*, 50 1925, 178.

134   STOCKETT, J. C. Growth of libraries in state hospitals. *South Dakota Library Bulletin*, 11 1925, 29 – 32.

135   STOCKETT, J. C. What is your library doing to help institutions. *Wisconsin Library Bulletin*, 21 1925, 174 – 176.

136   SUMNER, C. W. The public library and hospital library service. *Libr. J.*, 50 1925, 169 – 170.

1926

137 ALETHA, *sister*. How the Fort Wayne public library is serving our hospital. *Michigan Library Bulletin*, 17 1926, 10 – 11.

138 CAREY, M. E. Organized library service in state institutions. *Wisconsin Library Bulletin*, 22 1926, 47 – 52; abstract in *Libr. J.*, 51 1926, 338 – 339.

139 TARTRE, P. E. The child in the hospital [extract]. *ALA Bull.*, 20 1926, 510 – 511.

140 UNITED STATES. VETERANS BUREAU. *First 500 titles for a hospital library*. The Bureau, 1926.

1927

141 BEARD, R. O. Hospital library service. *Minnesota Medicine*, 10 1927, 295 – 296.

142 BIRDSALL, G. H. Training for hospital librarians as carried on in the Western Reserve library school [extract]. *ALA Bull.*, 21 1927, 373.

143 LIND, J. E. Mental patient and the library. *Bookman*, 65 1927, 138 – 141; abstract in *Libr. J.*, 52 1927, 427.

144 POMEROY, Elizabeth. Book therapy in veterans' hospitals. *U.S. Veterans Bureau Medical Bulletin*, 3 March 1927, 231 – 235.

145 STOCKETT, J. C. Hospital libraries in Honolulu County, Oahu, T.H. *ALA Bull.*, 21 1927, 373 – 374.

146 SUMNER, C. W. The hospital of the community and the public library. *ALA Bull.*, 21 1927, 372 – 373.

147 SWEET, Louise. Reading predilections of patients in veterans' hospitals. *U.S. Veterans Bureau Medical Bulletin*, 3 Sept. 1927, 911 – 914.

1928

148 BAYLIS, I. M. Hospital library work in Montreal [extract]. *ALA Bull.*, 22 1928, 420 – 421.

149 BAYLIS, I. M. War time libraries now bring joy to civilian patients. *Modern Hospital*, 31 Nov. 1928, 74 – 78.

150 [Books suitable for hospital libraries.] *Wisconsin Library Bulletin*, 24 1928, 265 – 267.

151 BRADFORD, E. C. The Riley hospital library. *Library Occurrent*, 8 1928, 240 – 241.

152 CREGLOW, E. R. Therapeutic value of library service in a tuberculosis hospital. *U.S. Veterans Bureau Medical Bulletin*, 4 May 1928, 445 – 448.

153 JONES, E. B. Library service in a tuberculosis hospital. *U.S. Veterans Bureau Medical Bulletin*, 4 1928, 941 – 944.

154 LAMB, Sarah D. Five hundred books for a hospital library. *Libr. J.*, 53 (19) Nov. 1 1928, 893 – 900; (20) Nov 15 1928, 937 – 945.

155 MILLER, M. M. Jottings from the library: Harrisburg state hospital, Harrisburg, Pa. *Pennsylvania Library Notes*, 11 1928, 87 – 89.

156 MORRISSEY, M. R. [Purpose and organization of library work in a mental hospital] [extract]. *ALA Bull.*, 22 1928, 421 – 423.

157 OSTENFELD, Elisabeth. Hospitalsbiblioteker. [Hospital libraries.] *Bogens Verden*, 10 (4 – 5) April – May 1928, 51 – 53.

158 RAINEY, Marie. Books in a hospital for crippled children. *Libr. J.*, 53 (16) Sept. 15 1928, 803 – 804.

159 RAINEY, Marie. [A combination hospital – school library.] *ALA Bull.*, 22 1928, 423 – 425.

160 ROCHESTER GENERAL HOSPITAL. Aid Council. How we use volunteer aids at Rochester General Hospital. *Modern Hospital*, 30 1928, 58 – 61.

161 SCOTT, B. L. Pennsylvania state institutional libraries. *Pennsylvania Library Notes*, 11 1928, 52 – 54.

162 SPERRY, R. S. How one hospital provides books for its patients. *Modern Hospital*, 30 1928, 83 – 84.

163 The tuberculous sanatoria libraries. *Pennsylvania Library Notes*, 11 1928, 54 – 55.

1929

164 AMERICAN LIBRARY ASSOCIATION. Hospital Libraries Committee. *Hospital library service*. [Chicago, ALA, 1929.] [8] pp.

165 BOWMAN, D. Library service as therapeutic aid to hospitals. *Modern Hospital*, 33 Oct. 1929, 81 – 83.

166 CRAIGIE, A. L. Cheering stimulus of poetry in Veterans Bureau hospitals. *Modern Hospital*, 33 Nov. 1929, 85 – 88; extract in *ALA Bull.*, 23 1929, 319 – 321.

167 DUBOIS, Isabel. Biography and travel have large place in naval hospital libraries. *ALA Bull.*, 23 1929, 321 – 323; also in *Hospital Management*, 29 1930, 45 – 48.

168 IRELAND, G. O. Bibliotherapy: the use of books as form of treatment in a neuropsychiatric hospital. *U.S. Veterans Bureau Medical Bulletin*, 5 June 1929, 440 – 445; also in *Libr. J.*, 54 Dec. 1 1929, 972 – 974.

169 JONES, P. Hospital libraries in state hospitals of Minnesota. *Bulletin of the American Hospital Association*, 3 1929, 433 – 436.

170 LINDE, I. Büchereien für patienten von Krankenanstalten. [Libraries for patients in hospitals.] *Zeitschrift für das gesamte Krankenhauswesen*, 25 1929, 471 – 476.

171 LITTLE, L. T. The mystery story in the hospital. *Libraries*, 34 1929, 359 – 362.

172 MORRIS, E. F. The selection of modern fiction for hospital use. *Libr. J.*, 54 Dec. 1 1929, 975 – 978.

173 MORRISSEY, M. R. Library in a mental hospital. *American Journal of Nursing*, 29 1929, 139 – 142.

174 O'CONNOR, R. A. Library hospital service in Sioux City. *Libr. J.*, 54 Dec. 1 1929, 978 – 980.

175 SCHULZ, Maximillian. Libraries in tuberculosis sanatoria. *Wilson Bulletin*, 4 (3) 1929, 111 – 112.

176 SEXTON, L. A. Library building serves dual purpose. *Modern Hospital*, 32 1929, 81 – 82.

177 SWEET, Louise. Prescribing books for the sick. *Libr. J.*, 54 Dec. 1 1929, 969 – 971.

1930

178 AMERICAN LIBRARY ASSOCIATION. Institution Libraries Committee. *Aids in book buying for institution librarians.* Chicago, ALA, 1930. 8 pp.

179 ANDERSEN, Johanne Buene. Bibliotekarbeidet ved Vestfold Fylkessykehus. [Library work at Vestfold County Hospital.] *For Folkeoplysning*, 1930, 202 – 203.

180 BEAUSEJOUR, Mary. How the hospital serves the community. *Michigan Library Bulletin*, 21 1930, 117 – 120.

181 Books for the hospitals (leading article). *The Times*, Sept. 25 1930, 13c.

182 BRUCE-PORTER, *Sir* Bruce. The need for libraries in hospitals as part of scheme of curative medicine. [Paper read at the Portsmouth Congress.] *Journal of State Medicine*, 38 1930, 710 – 715.

183 CRAIN, E. R. The treatment value of hospital library. *U.S. Veterans Bureau Medical Bulletin*, 6 June 1930, 515 – 518.

184 [Empire Red Cross conference, 1930.] *The Times*, May 21 1930, 21d.

185 Hospital libraries. *The Times*, Aug. 11 1930, 15d; Sept. 24 1930, 7a.

186 Hospital libraries: Cambridge conference. *Lancet*, ii Oct. 4 1930, 777 – 778.

187 Hospital libraries: [report of Empire Red Cross conference]. *Lancet*, i June 21 1930, 1357.

188 IRELAND, G. O. Bibliotherapy as aid in treating mental cases. *Modern Hospital*, 34 1930, 87 – 91.

189 JONES, Edith Kathleen. Hospital libraries I. The development of hospital libraries. *In*: Library Association. *Year's work in librarianship vol. II, 1929.* London, LA, 1930, 237 – 238.

190 JONES, Perrie. Hospital libraries. II. Hospital libraries in 1929. *In*: Library Association. *Year's work in librarianship vol. II, 1929.* London, LA, 1930, 239 – 242.

191 KURTZ, M. E. Discrimination necessary in the circulation of books to tuberculous patients. *U.S. Veterans Bureau Medical Bulletin*, 6 Oct. 1930, 901 – 903.

192 LIBRARY ASSOCIATION. At home and abroad notes: hospital libraries. *Libr. Ass. Rec.*, 32 (new series 8) Dec. 1930, 289 – 291.

193 LINDE, I. Bücherei für Krankenhaus oder Krankenversorgung mit Büchern. [Books for hospitals . . .] *In: Handbücherei fur das gesamte Krankenhauswesen 1930*, vol. 3, 207 – 218.

194 MACRUM, A. M. How to organize a hospital library. *Modern Hospital*, 35 1930, 69 – 75.

195 MACRUM, A. M. Prescribing books for tuberculous patients. *Modern Hospital*, 35 1930, 77 – 78.

196 OSTENFELD, Elisabeth. Hospitalsbiblioteket. En bogvogn. [The hospital library. A book trolley.] *Bogens Verden*, 12 (3) March 1930, 38 – 40.

197 OSTENFELD, Elisabeth. Hospitals – biblioteksarbejde. [Hospital library work.] *Ugeskrift for Læger*, 42 1930, 437 – 458; also in *Tidsskrift for Danske Sygehuse*, 6 1930, 105 – 106.

198 PETERSON-DELANEY, S. The library as a factor in Veterans' Bureau hospitals. *U.S. Veterans Bureau Medical Bulletin*, 6 April 1930, 331 – 334.

199 Reading in hospital: [report of Public Health Congress]. *Lancet*, ii Nov. 29 1930, 1195.

200 Report of discussion on hospital libraries at Public Health Congress, 1930. *Nursing Mirror*, 52 1930, 1977.

201 ROBERTS, M. E. The hospital library. *Nursing Mirror*, 51 Sept. 27 1930, 526.

202 RUHBERG, G. A. Books as a therapeutic agent. *ALA Bull.*, 24 Sept. 1930, 422 – 423.

203 UNITED STATES. VETERANS' BUREAU. List of new books as an aid to book selection in hospital libraries. *Libr. J.*, 55 1930, 167 – 169 et seq.; also in *Libraries*, 36 1931, 232 – 234.

204 WRIGHT, C. Hagberg. Hospital libraries [correspondence]. *Libr. Ass. Rec.*, 32 Dec. 1930, 300.

1931

205 BACON, Asa *and* LINDEM, Selma. Library service in hospitals. *American Hospital Association Bulletin*, 5 June 1931, 8 – 10.

206 BARBER, E. M. Library activities in a hospital for neuropsychiatric patients. *U.S. Veterans Bureau Medical Bulletin*, 7 1931, 180 – 182.

207 BERGAUS, M. V. The patients' library. *Hospital Progress*, 12 Feb. 1931, 48 – 50.

208 BISHOP, W. J. Hospital libraries and bibliotherapy: a bibliography. *Libr. Ass. Rec.*, third series, 1 June 1931, 198 – 200; July 1931, 231 – 232; Aug. 1931, 274 – 275.

209 Books for the hospitals. *The Times*, March 10 1931, 17c.

210 CABLE, M. If you'd be a hospital librarian. *Hospital Management*, 3 Feb. 1931, 40 – 42.

211 CREGLOW, E. R. Therapeutic value of properly selected reading material with bibliography. *Medical Bulletin of the Veterans Administration,* 7 Nov. 1931, 1086 – 1089.

212 CROSBY, A. A. Selecting books for neuro-psychiatric patients. *U.S. Veterans Bureau Medical Bulletin,* 7 1931, 1214 – 1217; summary in *ALA Bull.,* 25 1931, 541 – 542.

213 FÉDÉRATION INTERNATIONALE DES ASSOCIATIONS DE BIBLIOTHÉCAIRES. Project de création d'une Sous-Commission pour les bibliothèques d'hôpitaux. [Plan to form a sub-committee for libraries in hospitals.] *In: Actes du Comité International des Bibliothèques* III, *4me session Cheltenham, 1931.* Genève, Albert Kundig, 1931, 18 – 19.

214 Hospital libraries. *The Times,* March 10 1931, 15c [leading article]; March 13 1931, 10c [correspondence].

215 JONES, Perrie. What the librarian can and should mean to the hospital. *Modern Hospital,* 37 Nov. 1931, 53 – 56.

216 LIBRARY ASSOCIATION. Proceedings of the 53rd annual conference . . . Cambridge Sept. 22 – 27 1930. Supplement to *Libr. Ass. Rec.,* 33 (third series, 1) Jan. 1931, *IX – *X, *XX.

217 LIBRARY ASSOCIATION. Proceedings of the 54th annual conference [1931]. Supplement to *Libr. Ass. Rec.* 33 (third series, 1) 1931, †IV – †V.

218 LIBRARY ASSOCIATION. Hospital Libraries Committee. *Memorandum and recommendations of the hospital libraries committee.* London, LA, [1931]. 7 pp.

219 LIBRARY ASSOCIATION. Hospital Libraries Committee. *Suggestions for the organising of hospital libraries* [drafted by A. C. Piper]. London, LA, 1931, 4 pp.

220 LINDEM, S. Hospital libraries. *Illinois Libraries,* 13 1931, 215 – 218.

221 MACRUM, A. M. Supplying the reading needs of the tuberculous patient. *Modern Hospital,* 37 Sept. 1931, 52 – 56; summarised in *ALA Bull.,* 25 1931, 542.

222 O'CONNOR, R. A. *Hospital library service: why and how.* Sioux City, Iowa, Public Library, 1931. 11 pp.

223 OSTENFELD, Elisabeth. *Biblioteksarbejde paa sygehuse.* [Library work in hospitals.] København, 1931. 36 pp. (Danmarks biblioteksforenings skrifter, 4.)

224 ÖSTLING, G. Sjukhusbibliotek. [Hospital library.] *Biblioteksbladet,* 16 1931, 231 – 235.

225 P., E. M. The Middlesex Hospital Library. *Nursing Mirror,* 52 Jan. 24 1931, 345.

226 POMEROY, Elizabeth. Hospital libraries. *ALA Bull.,* 25 Sept. 1931, 430 – 435; also in *Bulletin of the American Hospital Association,* 6 Oct 1931, 68 – 77; also in *Medical Bulletin of the Veterans Administration,* 7 Oct. 1931, 986 – 994.

227   RAINEY, Marie. Hospital library work with children: some of its educational, recreational, and therapeutic aspects. *ALA Children's Library Yearbook*, 3 1931, 22 – 27.

228   [ROBERTS, Marjorie E.] *British Red Cross Society and Order of St. John hospital library: its origin aim and development.* London, BRCS, [1931].

229   ROBERTS, Marjorie E. Hospital libraries. *In*: Library Association. *The year's work in librarianship, vol. III, 1930.* London, LA, 1931, 186 – 188.

230   ROBERTS, [Marjorie E.] Memorandum on the need for an international sub-committee for hospital library services. *In*: *Actes du Comité International des Bibliothèques III, 4me session Cheltenham, 1931.* Genève, Albert Kundig, 1931, Annexe VI, 44 – 47.

231   STEWART, H. G. Libraries and hospitals. *Western Hospital Review*, Jan. 1931, 11 – 13.

1932

232   BRUCE-PORTER, *Sir* Bruce. Hospital libraries. [Speech made at Library Association Conference, Cheltenham, 1931.] *Library World*, 34 July 1931 – June 1932, 84, 86, 88.

233   COACHMAN, D. F. Therapeutic value of light fiction in hospital libraries. *U.S. Veterans Bureau Medical Bulletin*, 9 July 1932, 97 – 99.

234   CRAMER, Grace. Selection of books for hospitalized readers. *U.S. Veterans Bureau Medical Bulletin*, 8 1932, 83 – 84.

235   CREGLOW, E. R. Reading for tuberculous patients. *U.S. Veterans Bureau Medical Bulletin*, 8 1932, 321 – 322.

236   DUBOIS, Isabel. Books as a solace for the sick. *Hygeia*, 10 1932, 55 – 58; also in *Modern Librarian*, 2 1932, 149 – 153.

237   FÉDÉRATION INTERNATIONALE DES ASSOCIATIONS DE BIBLIOTHÉCAIRES. Sous – Commission des Bibliothèques d'Hôpitaux. [Report.] *In*: *Actes du Comité International des Bibliothèques IV, 5me session Berne, 1932.* La Haye, Martinus Nijhoff, 1932, 27 – 28; Annexe V, 66 – 87.

238   JONES, Perrie. International hospital group. *ALA Bull.*, 26 1932, 451 – 452.

239   KNOX, Dorothy. Free hospital libraries. *Publishers' Weekly*, 121 1932, 1034 – 1035.

240   LIBRARY ASSOCIATION. *Annual report, 1931.* London, LA, 1932, 16R – 17R Hospital libraries committee.

241   MACRUM, A. M. Pennsylvania hospital library survey. *Pennsylvania Library Notes*, 13 1932, 220 – 230.

242   MINTO, John. *A history of the public library movement in Great Britain and Ireland.* London, Allen & Unwin, 1932, 290 – 293, Hospital libraries.

243   POMEROY, Elizabeth. The librarian and the social worker in the hospital. *Hospital Social Service*, 25 May 1932, 365 – 370.

244   POWELL, M. JOYCE. The patient reader. *Library Review*, 3 1932, 281 – 285.

245   ROBERTS, Marjorie E. Hospital libraries. *In*: Library Association. *The year's work in librarianship, vol. IV, 1931*. London, LA, 1932, 107 – 113.

246   ROBERTS, Marjorie E. Libraries for hospital patients of the world over. *Hospital Management*, 34 Aug. 15 1932, 34 – 36, 41.

247   ROBERTS [Marjorie E.] L'organisation des bibliothèques d'hôpitaux en Grande – Bretagne; transl. by H. and P. Karsakoff. *In*: *Actes du Comité International des Bibliothéques IV, 5me session Berne, 1932*. La Haye, Martinus Nijhoff, 1932, Annexe VI, 88 – 92.

248   SEAMAN, F. H. The hospital hostess: a modern 'Good Samaritan'. *Modern Hospital*, 39 1932, 73 – 76.

249   SUMNER, C. W. Methods of administering hospital libraries to suit the changing times. *ALA Bull.*, 26 1932, 567 – 568.

250   WOODMAN, R. State institution libraries. *Psychiatric Quarterly*, 6 1932, 213 – 225; also in *Libr. J.*, 58 Jan. 15 1933, 62 – 67.

1933

251   BLAKE, F. I. Veterans Administration hospital library, Waco. *News Notes* (Texas Library Association), 9 April 1933, 11 – 12.

252   BROWN, S. J. M. Library service for hospitals. *Leabharlann*, 3 Dec. 1933, 112 – 117.

253   FOLZ, C. Pied piper of the modern hospital. *Library Occurrent*, 11 April/June 1933, 39 – 44.

254   FOREMAN, E. T. Carefully chosen books have therapeutic value. *Modern Hospital*, 41 Nov. 1933, 69 – 70.

255   FORREST, L. B. Books as a line of defense. *Libr. J.*, 58 Jan. 15 1933, 53 – 56.

256   HENRIOT, Gabriel. Des livres pour nos malades. [Books for our sick.] *Revue du Livre et des Bibliothèques*, 1 Dec. 1933, 39 – 40.

257   Hospital library work. [LA, London and Home Counties Branch meeting.] *Libr. Ass. Rec.*, 35 (third series, 3) March 1933, 93 – 97.

258   JONES, P. International hospital conference, Belgium. *Libr. J.*, 58 Oct. 15 1933, 847.

259   LIBRARY ASSOCIATION. *Annual report, 1932*. London, LA, 1933, 13R Hospital libraries committee.

260   LIBRARY ASSOCIATION. Summary of papers and discussions at the Harrogate conference, 1933. Supplement to *Libr. Ass. Rec.*, 35 (third series, 3) Oct. 1933, †iii – †v.

261   MACRUM, A. M. Hospital libraries and public library participation. *Libr. J.*, 58 Jan. 15 1933, 59 – 61.

262   MACRUM, A. M. Hospital libraries for patients (a bibliography). *Libr. J.*, 58 Jan. 15 1933, 78 – 81.

263 ORMEROD, James. Hospital libraries in the United States. *Library World*, 35 Jan. 1933, 155 – 156.

264 POMEROY, Elizabeth. Progress in hospital library work. *Libr. J.*, 58 Oct. 15 1933, 837 – 838.

265 SYTZ, F. Adapting bibliotherapy to the patient's needs in the changing social order. *Libr. J.*, 58 Jan. 15 1933, 57 – 58.

266 WATT-SMITH, M. Hospital library practice. *Library Assistant*, 26 Nov. 1933, 199 – 202.

267 WETLESEN, Johanne Mowinckel. Sykehusbiblioteker i Sverige og Danmark. [Hospital libraries in Sweden and Denmark.] *For Folkeoplysning*, 18 May 1933, 54 – 56.

1934

268 CAPDEVEILLE, J. Les bibliothèques d'hôpitaux en Espagne. [Hospital libraries in Spain.] *In*: *Actes du Comité International des Bibliothèques VI, 7me session Madrid, 1934*. La Haye, Martinus Nijhoff, 1934, Annexe 11, 51 – 56.

269 CLARKE, E. K. Mental hygiene of reading. *New York Libraries*, 14 Aug. 1934, 98 – 101.

270 CREMONESI, G. C. F. Croce rossa italiana e biblioteche degli ospedale. [Italian Red Cross and hospital libraries.] *In*: *Actes du Comité International des Bibliothèques V, 6me session Chicago et Avignon, 1933*. La Haye, Martinus Nijhoff, 1934, Annexe XXII, 163 – 164.

271 FÉDÉRATION INTERNATIONALE DES ASSOCIATIONS DE BIBLIOTHÉCAIRES. Sous – Commission des Bibliothèques d'Hôpitaux. Rapport [par Henri Lemaître]. *In*: *Actes du Comité International des Bibliothèques V, 6me session Chicago et Avignon, 1933*. La Haye, Martinus Nijhoff, 1934, Annexe XX, 155 – 159.

272 FÉDÉRATION INTERNATIONALE DES ASSOCIATIONS DE BIBLIOTHÉCAIRES. Sous – Commission des Bibliothèques d'Hôpitaux [report]. *In*: *Actes du Comité International des Bibliothèques VI, 7me session Madrid, 1934*. La Haye, Martinus Nijhoff, 1934, 19.

273 FISHBEIN, Morris. Libraries and the patient. *ALA Bull.*, 28 March 1934, 129 – 133.

274 GALLIVAN, K. C. Library day for hospital children. *Libr. J.*, 59 Nov. 1 1934, 834 – 835.

275 HENRIOT, Gabriel. La lecture publique et les hôpitaux dans le départment de la Seine. *In*: *Actes du Comité International des Bibliothèques V, 6me session Chicago et Avignon, 1933*. La Haye, Martinus Nijhoff, 1934, Annexe XXI, 160 – 162.

276 JAMESON, M. Book work with blind children. *Librarian & Book World & Curator*, 24 Dec. 1934, 107 – 108.

277 KAMMAN, G. R. The doctor and the patients' library. *American Hospital Association. Transactions*, 36 1934, 374 – 384.

278 LEMAITRE, H. Rapport sur les bibliothèques d'hôpitaux. [Report on hospital libraries.] *In*: *Actes du Comité International des Bibliothèques VI, 7me session Madrid, 1934*. La Haye, Martinus Nijhoff, 1934, Annexe III, 57 – 58.

279 MIRALDA, Maria. *Les biblioteques d'hospital a Catalunya*. [Hospital libraries in Catalonia.] Barcelona, Casa de Caritat, 1934. 40 pp. (Escola de bibliotecàries de la generalitat de Catalunya. Quaderns de treball, 1.)

280 MONTOJO, C. Las bibliotecas de hospitales. [Hospital libraries.] *Boletin de Bibliotecas y Bibliografia*, 1 July/Sept. 1934, 25 – 32.

281 PRITCHARD, Frank Cyril. *The development of hospital libraries in the United Kingdom: including a study of their present and possible future relations with the public libraries*. A thesis submitted for the Honours Diploma of the Library Association, 1934. 174 pp.

282 Sjukhusbiblioteken. [Hospital libraries.] *Biblioteksbladet*, 19 (8) 1934, 309 – 310.

283 STOCKETT, J. C. Convincing librarians that hospital service should be a recognized activity of every fair sized public library. *ALA Bull.*, 28 Sept. 1934, 611 – 612.

1935

284 Biblioteksarbejde paa hospitaler. [Library work in hospitals.] *Bogens Verden*, 17 Oct. 1935, 222 – 223.

285 BROM, A. De Braille – bibliotheek voor organisten. [Braille library for organists.] *Bibliotheekleven*, 20 June 1935, 101 – 106.

286 COMPTON, C. H. Hospital library service – its present status and possible future. *American Hospital Association. Transactions*, 37 1935, 586 – 592; also in *Hospitals*, Chicago, 10 March 1936, 49 – 51.

287 DANIELSON, Ingrid. Något om biblioteksverksamhet vid sjukhus. [About library work in hospital.] *Biblioteksbladet*, 20 1935, 140 – 142.

288 EBAUCH, F. G. Library facilities for mental patients. [Abridged paper given at ALA conference, June 1935.] *ALA Bull.*, 29 Sept. 1935, 619 – 621.

289 GYDE-PEDERSEN, Mette. Hospitalsbiblioteksarbejde: hvad læser patienterne paa vore hospitaler og hvorledes forsynes de med bøger. [Hospital library work: what do the patients in our hospitals read and how are they supplied with books?] *Ugeskrift for Læger*, 47 1935, 760 – 763, 889.

290 LILLY, E. Hospital library service. *Iowa Library Quarterly*, 12 Jan. – March 1935, 140.

291 MILLER, N. Adult education in the hospital library? *Libr. J.*, 60 March 1 1935, 194 – 195.

292 Något om biblioteksverksamhet vid sjukhus. [Library work in hospital.] *Biblioteksbladet*, 20 (4) 1935, 140 – 142.

293 SCHULZ, K. Über Krankenhausbüchereien. [About hospital libraries]. *Zeitschrift für des Gesamte Krankenhauswesen*, 31 1935, 51.

294   SOHON, J. A. Hospital library service in Bridgeport. *Libr. J.*, 60 Dec. 15 1935, 958 – 960.

295   WEBB, G. B. Prescribing books for the tuberculous. *Modern Hospital*, 45 Nov. 1935, 61 – 63.

296   WEBB, G. B. Reading for the tuberculous patient. *ALA Bull.*, 29 Sept. 1935, 621 – 624.

297   WIRTH-STOCKHAUSEN, Julia. Die Bücherei im Städtischen Krankenhaus Frankfurt a. Main – Sachsenhausen. [The library in Frankfurt am Main municipal hospital.] *Zeitschrift für das Gesamte Krankenhauswesen*, (25) 1935, 588 – 590.

1936

298   ACKERKNECHT, Erwin. Krankenhausbüchereien. [Hospital libraries.] *In*: *Lexikon des gesamten Buchwesens*. Leipzig, Hirsemann, 1936, vol. 2.

299   AMERICAN HOSPITAL ASSOCIATION. Committee on Hospital Libraries. Third annual report. *American Hospital Association. Transactions*, 38 1936, 183 – 186.

300   AMERICAN LIBRARY ASSOCIATION. Committee on Hospital Libraries. Annual report 1936. *ALA Bull.*, 30 May 1936, 386 – 387.

301   AMERICAN LIBRARY ASSOCIATION. Committee on Hospital Libraries. Proceedings at ALA conference, 1936. *ALA Bull.*, 30 Aug. 1936, 696.

302   BACHMANN, Ida. Blindebiblioteker. [Libraries for the blind.] *Bogens Verden*, 18 Nov. 1936, 302 – 312.

303   BARTINE, O. H. Library of the Bridgeport hospital. *Hospitals*, Chicago, 10 July 1936, 56 – 59.

304   BEDWELL, Cyril Edward Alfred. Hospital libraries. *Contemporary Review*, 150 Aug. 1936, 224 – 228.

305   BEDWELL, Cyril Edward Alfred. Relations between hospital authorities and municipal library authorities with regard to hospital libraries. *Book Trolley*, 1 (7) Oct. 1936, 114 – 122.

306   Bibliothèques des Hôpitaux. [Hospital libraries.] *Bulletin du Livre Français*, July/Aug. 1936, 102 – 103.

307   Bravo India! *Book Trolley*, 1 (5) April 1936, 38 – 39.

308   BRITISH RED CROSS SOCIETY *and* ORDER OF ST. JOHN. Hospital Library. *How to run a hospital library*. London, [1936]. Reviewed in *Libr. Ass. Rec.* 38 May 1936, 221 – 222.

309   CHIAROMONTE, G. I libri e le biblioteche per i ciechi. [Books and libraries for the blind.] *Accademie e Biblioteche d'Italia*, 10 July/Aug. 1936, 267 – 274.

310   CLOUGH, H. D. Library service in the modern hospital. *Libr. J.*, 61 Oct. 15 1936, 758 – 761.

311 CONDELL, Lucy. Library as a road to re-education in responsibility for neuro-psychiatric patients. *Medical Bulletin of the Veterans' Administration*, 13 July 1936, 77 – 84.

312 FÉDÉRATION INTERNATIONALE DES ASSOCIATIONS DE BIBLIOTHÉCAIRES. Congrès international des bibliothèques d'hôpitaux: rapport par Henri Lemaître. *In*: *Actes du Comité International des Bibliothèques VIII, 9me session Varsovie, 1936*. La Haye, Martinus Nijhoff, 1936, Annexe II, 66 – 68.

313 FÉDÉRATION INTERNATIONALE DES ASSOCIATION DE BIBLIOTHÉCAIRES. Rapport sur bibliothèques d'hôpitaux 1935 – 36. *In*: *Actes du Comité International des Bibliothèques VIII, 9me session Varsovie, 1936*. La Haye, Martinus Nijhoff, 1936, Annexe III, 69 – 72.

314 Det første offentlige Blindebibliotek. [The first public library for the blind.] *Bogens Verden*, 18 1936, 229 – 230.

315 GREENSLADE, L. K. Library service to hospitals. *Libr. J.*, 61 Oct. 15 1936, 761 – 762.

316 GYDE-PEDERSEN, Mette. Biblioteksarbejde blandt patienter og sygeplejersker. [Library work with patients and nurses.] *Tidsskrift for Sygepleje*, 36 1936, 648 – 659.

317 HENRIOT, Gabriel. Le service social a l'hôpital et la bibliothèque des hôpitaux. [Social service in the hospital and the hospital library.] *Book Trolley*, 1 (7) Oct. 1936, 107 – 113.

318 HENSEL, H. Benefits and costs of hospital library service. *American Hospital Association. Transactions*, 38 1936, 623 – 628; also in *Hospitals*, 10 1936, 82 – 84.

319 HERING, L. C. New wine from old bottles: ways of increasing interest in the hospital library without increasing expenditures. *Libr. J.*, 61 Oct. 15 1936, 763 – 764.

320 INTERNATIONAL GUILD OF HOSPITAL LIBRARIANS. Conference, 1936, Paris. *Libr. Ass. Rec.* 38 June 1936, 252 – 253; also in *Archives et Bibliothèques*, (1) 1936, 75 – 77; and in *Accademie e Biblioteche d'Italia*, 11 April 1937, 200.

321 JONES, P. Peg in and look around. *Libr. J.*, 61 March 1 1936, 186 – 187.

322 KINDELSPERGER, B. E. S. Reading ways to health. *Hospitals*, Chicago, 10 Feb. 1936, 30 – 33.

323 KINDELSPERGER, B. E. S. Value of the library in the sanatorium. *American Hospital Association. Transactions*, 38 1936, 430 – 436; also in *Hospital Management*, 42 Dec. 1936, 22 – 23 (with title Reading and recovery).

324 LEMAÎTRE, H. Bibliothèques d'hôpitaux. [Hospital libraries.] *Archives et Bibliothèques*, (2) 1936, 134 – 136.

325 OSTENFELD, Elisabeth. Forening hospitalsbiblioteker. [Association of Danish hospital libraries.] *Bogens Verden*, 18 Aug./Sept. 1936, 236.

326 RAYMOND, H. How the Red Cross hospital libraries are helping the book trade. *Publishers Circular*, 145 Dec. 26 1936, 1036 – 1037.

327 ROSSELL, M. *Les biblioteques per a cecs a Barcelona: notes per a llur historia.* [Library for the blind in Barcelona.] Barcelona, Casa de Caritat, 1936. (Escola de Bibliotecàries de la Generalitat de Catalunya. Quaderns de treball, 4.)

328 SAUER, J. L. Hospital library service in Rochester, New York. *American Hospital Association. Transactions*, 38 1936, 628 – 640; also in *Hospitals*, Chicago, 10 Dec. 1936, 54 – 58.

329 TÜLLMANN, Anni. Krankenhausbüchereien. [Hospital libraries.] *Blätter des Deutschen Roten Kreuzes*, 15 (10) 1936.

330 TYLER, A. S. Pioneer work in hospital libraries. *American Hospital Association. Transactions*, 38 1936, 620 – 623.

331 WETLESEN, Johanne Mowinckel. Hvordan pasientbiblioteket på Ullevål sykehus ble til. [How the patients' library at Ullevål hospital was founded.] *Deichmanbladet,* 1936, 41 – 42.

1937

332 AMERICAN LIBRARY ASSOCIATION. Committee on Hospital Libraries. Annual report 1937. *ALA Bull.*, 31 Sept. 1937, 564.

333 AMERICAN LIBRARY ASSOCIATION. Committee on Hospital Libraries. Proceedings at ALA conference, 1937. *ALA Bull.*, 31 Oct. 15 1937, 776 – 777.

334 BEDDINGTON, Sybil. The Middlesex hospital library. *Book Trolley*, 1 July 1937, 215 – 216.

335 Bibliothèques d'hôpitaux: les resultats de l'expérience de Paris. *Book Trolley*, 1 Oct. 1937, 234 – 237.

336 BINSWANGER, O. [Hospital libraries in Switzerland.] *Book Trolley*, 1 April 1937, 175 – 177. In German with English summary.

337 BLACKLER, E. W. Hill End hospital and clinic, St. Albans, Herts. *Book Trolley*, 1 Nov. 1937, 258 – 259.

338 Books to shut-ins. *Kansas Library Bulletin*, 6 Sept. 1937, 6 – 7.

339 BROCK, Laurence. Mental hospital libraries. *Book Trolley*, 1 (9) April 1937, 172 – 174.

340 BROWN, G. Shut-in's library. *Colorado Libraries*, (2) June 1937, 6.

341 CLARKE, E. K. Books for the convalescent. *Libr. J.*, 62 Dec. 1 1937, 893 – 895.

342 CROSLEY, C. E. Books for shut-ins. *Libr. J.*, 62 Jan. 15 1937, 81; also in *Kansas Library Bull.*, 6 March 1937, 12 – 13.

343 DISTEL, H. Büchereien für Kranke. [Libraries for the sick.] *Book Trolley*, 1 April 1937, 178 – 183. Summary in English and French.

344 DUHAMEL, G. Le chariot de consolation. [The book trolley.] *Book Trolley*, 1 Nov. 1937, 253 – 256.

345 EASTMAN, L. A. Substitutes for life. *Journal of Adult Education*, 9 April 1937, 189 – 190.

346 FORBES, H. A. We call it bibliotherapy. *Modern Hospital*, 49 July 1937, 45 – 46.

347   From a bookseller's point of view. *Book Trolley*, 1 Jan. 1937, 148 – 151.

348   FULLER, K. H. Books for hospital libraries. *Hygeia*, 15 May 1937, 409 – 412.

349   GASKELL, Helen Mary. Hospital libraries, past and present. *Book Trolley*, 1 (10) July 1937, 203 – 207.

350   GYDE-PEDERSEN, Mette. Sociale og kulturelle særopgaver. [Social and cultural extension work.] Danske Folkebiblioteker, *Festskrift til Th. Døssing*, 1937, 132 – 152.

351   HODGE, H. A. Books and librarians for the mentally sick. *Book Trolley*, 1 July 1937, 217 – 219.

352   HOFRÉN, M. Sjukhusbibliotek i Kalmar. [Kalmar hospital library.] *Biblioteksbladet*, 22 (8) 1937, 312.

353   Hospital libraries in Ireland. *Librarian & Book World*, 27 Nov. 1937, 67.

354   Hospital libraries section of the CLA formed at St. Louis. *Catholic Library World*, 8 April 1937, 58 – 59.

355   Hospital library council [Irish Republic]. *Leabharlann*, 6 June 1937, 15.

356   INTERNATIONAL GUILD OF HOSPITAL LIBRARIANS. British Section. Annual report, 1936 – 37. *Book Trolley*, 1 April 1937, 195 – 199.

357   Irish hospital library service. *Book Trolley*, 1 Dec. 1937, 268.

358   JONES, Perrie. Mental patients can read. *Modern Hospital*, 49 Sept. 1937, 72 – 75.

359   KAYSER, F. Der Bücherwagen in Krankenhaus. [The book trolley in the hospital.] *Zeitschrift für das Gesamte Krankenhauswesen*, (22) Oct. 26 1937, 492 – 493; abstract in *Zweiter Internationaler Kongress für Krankenhausbibliotheken, Bern 1938, Bericht* . . . 142 – 143; also in *Veska – Zeitschrift*, 2 (10) Oct. 1938, 306.

360   KING, F. A. Suggesting books for invalids to read. *Librarian & Book World*, 27 Sept. 1937, 4 – 5.

361   Københavns kommunebiblioteker udvider. [Copenhagen's public library expands.] *Bogens Verden*, 19 Nov. 1937, 295 – 296.

362   LIBRARY ASSOCIATION. Papers and discussions at the Scarborough conference, June 1 – 4 1937. *Libr. Ass. Rec.*, 39 (fourth series, 4) June 1937, 365 – 370.

363   LINDER, G. *and* SÖDERBERGH, M. L. *Sjukhusbibliotek*. [Hospital libraries.] Stockholm, Sveriges Allmänna Biblioteksforening, 1937. (SAB småskrifter, 3.)
      Review by G. Stenersen. *Bok og Bibliotek*, 5 Sept. 1938, 338 – 339.

364   LYELL, L. Hospital libraries in North America. *Book Trolley*, 1 Jan. 1937, 153 – 156.

365   MENNINGER, W. C. Bibliotherapy. *Bulletin of the Menninger Clinic*, 1 Nov. 1937, 263 – 274.

366 NOWELL, Charles. Hospital libraries as a public service. *Libr. Ass. Rec.*, 39 (6) June 1937, conference suppl., 365 – 369.

367 PLENGE, Jørgen. Centralisation eller decentralisation af dansk blinde-biblioteksvæsen. *Bogens Verden*, 19 Oct. 1937, 250 – 257.

368 POMEROY, Elizabeth. Bibliotherapy: a study in results of hospital library service. *Medical Bulletin of the Veterans' Administration*, 13 April 1937, 360 – 364.

369 POWERS, R. K. Library goes to the shut-in. *Journal of Adult Education*, 9 June 1937, 305 – 307.

370 RAYMOND, Vera. St. Bartholomew's hospital library. *Book Trolley*, 1 Oct. 1937, 243 – 245.

371 ROBERTS, M. E. Les bibliothèques d'hôpitaux. [Hospital libraries.] *In*: International Institute of Intellectual Co-operation. *Mission sociale et intellectuelle des bibliothèques populaires: son organisation, ses moyens d'action*. Paris, The Institute, 1937, 307 – 322.

372 ROBERTS, M. E. Hospital libraries, alternative suggestions for their development. *Book Trolley*, 1 July 1937, 222 – 224.

373 ROBERTS, M. E. Hospital library movement. *World Association Adult Education Bulletin*, second series, 8, Feb. 1937, 26 – 31.

374 ROBERTS, M. E. Meeting on hospital libraries. *Book Trolley*, 1 Oct. 1937, 229 – 233.

375 ROBERTS, M. E. Pre-natal history of the Guild. *Book Trolley*, 1 Jan. 1937, 164 – 167.

376 SCHÜLLER, Maria. A German hospital library. *Libr. Ass. Rec.*, 39 (3) March 1937, 116 – 117.

377 Session on the mental hospital library. *Book Trolley*, 1 Dec. 1937, 269 – 283.

378 SHOREY, K. Hospital library. *Libr. J.*, 62 Dec. 1 1937, 895 – 897.

379 Sjukhusbiblioteken. [Hospital libraries.] *Biblioteksbladet*, 22 (6) 1937, 246.

380 Stockholm får moderna sjukhusbibliotek. [Stockholm to get modern hospital library.] *Biblioteksbladet*, 22 (2) 1937, 60 – 62.

381 WOODMAN, E. State hospital libraries. *Occupational Therapy and Rehabilitation*, 16 Aug. 1937, 253 – 261.

382 WRIGHT, Z. Bibliotherapy in a children's hospital. *Libr. J.*, 62 Dec. 1 1937, 898 – 900.

1938

383 AMERICAN LIBRARY ASSOCIATION. Committee on Hospital Libraries. Annual report, 1938. *ALA Bull.*, 32 Sept. 1938, 641 – 642.

384 AMERICAN LIBRARY ASSOCIATION. Committee on Hospital Libraries. Proceedings at ALA conference, 1938. *ALA Bull.*, 32 Oct. 15 1938, 878.

385 As a mental patient sees the library. *Minnesota Library Notes & News*, 12 June 1938, 183 – 184.

386 BEDDINGTON, Sybil. Die Spitalbibliothekarin ihre Gewinnung und ihre Stellung. [The hospital librarian: her recruitment and status.] *In*: *Zweiter Internationaler Kongress für Krankenhausbibliotheken, Bern 1938, Bericht . . .* 59 – 61; also in *Veska – Zeitschrift*, 2 Oct. 1938, 275; and paper in full, in English, in *Book Trolley*, 2 Jan. 1939, 83 – 85; Feb. 1939, 107 – 111.

387 Bibliothèques des hôpitaux: appareil pour la désinfection des livres. [Hospital libraries: apparatus for disinfecting the books.] *L'Architecture d'Aujourd'hui*, 9 March 1938, 96.

388 BOLDERO, H. E. A. Ladies' association and the hospital library. *Book Trolley*, 1 May 1938, 356 – 358.

389 BRITISH RED CROSS SOCIETY *and* ORDER OF ST. JOHN. Hospital Library, London. *How to run a hospital library service*; [rev. edition]. London, The Library, 1938.

390 CALAME, Lily. Bücherausleihe im Berner Inselspital. [Book loans in the Berne sanitorium.] *In*: *Zweiter Internationaler Kongress für Krankenhausbibliotheken, Bern 1938, Bericht . . .* 51 – 54.

391 CLEMMESEN, C. *and* OSTENFELD, E. Foredrag om biblioteksarbejde paa sindssygehospitaler og nerveafdelinger. [Lecture on library work in mental hospitals and neurological departments.] *Bogens Verden*, 20 Nov. 1938, 311 – 318.

392 COOKE, A. S. The problem of hospital library service for the county library authority. *Libr. Ass. Rec.*, 40 (6) June 1938, conference suppl., 345 – 347.

393 DOPF, K. Wesen, einrichtung und verwaltung von Krankenhausbüchereien. [Organization and administration of hospital libraries.] *Zeitschrift für das Gesamte Krankenhauswesen*, (7) March 29 1938, 139 – 140; abstract in *Zweiter Internationaler Kongress für Krankenhausbibliotheken, Bern 1938, Bericht . . .* 143 – 144; also in *Veska – Zeitschrift*, 2 (10) Oct. 1938, 306 – 307.

394 DUCKITT, D. Dulwich hospital library. *Book Trolley*, 2 Nov. 1938, 57 – 59.

395 FÉDÉRATION INTERNATIONALE DES ASSOCIATIONS DE BIBLIOTHÉCAIRES. Sous – Commission des Bibliothèques d'Hôpitaux. [Rapport]. *In*: *Actes du Comité International des Bibliothèques IX, 10me session Paris, 1937*. La Haye, Martinus Nijhoff, 1938, 32 – 33; Annexe II, 54 – 58.

396 FÉDÉRATION INTERNATIONALE DES ASSOCIATIONS DE BIBLIOTHÉCAIRES. Commission des Bibliothèques d'Hôpitaux. Rapport et discussion. *In*: *Actes du Comité International des Bibliothèques X, 11me session Bruxelles, 1938*. La Haye, Martinus Nijhoff, 1938, 29 – 30.

397 FÉDÉRATION INTERNATIONALE DES ASSOCIATIONS DE BIBLIOTHÉCAIRES. Commission des Bibliothèques d'Hôpitaux. Rapport par Henri Lemaître. *In*: *Actes du Comité International des Bibliothèques X, 11me session Bruxelles, 1938*. La Haye, Martinus Nijhoff, 1938, Annexe XXXVI, 183.

398 First general report, Hospital Library Council (editorial). *Leabharlann*, 6 April 1938, 65.

399   FOLEY, M. R. Patients' library. *American Hospital Association. Transactions,* 40 1938, 668 – 670.

400   FOLEY, M. R. School library in a children's hospital. *Minnesota Library Notes & News,* 12 June 1938, 184 – 185.

401   FRIEDENTHAL, Robert. Sanatoriumsbibliotheken in Leysin. [The library of the Leysin sanatorium.] *In*: *Zweiter Internationaler Kongress für Krankenhausbibliotheken, Bern 1938, Bericht* . . . 86 – 98; also in *Veska – Zeitschrift,* 2 (10) Oct. 1938, 288 – 291; English abstract in *Book Trolley,* 2 March 1939, 126 – 127.

402   GARDNER, W. P. Psychiatric hospital library. *Minnesota Library Notes & News,* 12 June 1938, 179 – 181.

403   GAREVSKIĬ, V. Bibliotechnaĭa rabota v domakh otdykha i na kurortakh. [Library work in 'homes of rest' and health resorts.] *Krasnyi Bibliotekar,* Moscow, (5) 1938, 51 – 53.

404   GAUSSEN, Ivan. L'organisation des bibliothèques hospitalières de l'Administration générale de l'Assistance Publique à Paris et les resultats obtenus. [Organization of hospital libraries . . .] *In*: *Zweiter Internationaler Kongress für Krankenhausbibliotheken, Bern 1938, Bericht* . . . 70 – 77; also in *Veska – Zeitschrift,* 2 (10) Oct. 1938, 283 – 285.

405   GERARD, Ethel. Hospitals and the smaller libraries. *Libr. Ass. Rec.,* 40 (6) June 1938, conference suppl., 347 – 349.

406   GODET, M. Discours. *In*: *Zweiter Internationaler Kongress für Krankenhausbibliotheken, Bern, 1938, Bericht* . . . 55 – 59; also in *Veska – Zeitschrift,* 2 (10) Oct. 1938, 273 – 275; English abstract in *Book Trolley,* 2 Feb. 1939, 106.

407   GUEX, Suzanne. Une bibliothèque pour malades à l'Hôpital Cantonal Vaudois. [Library service to patients at the cantonal hospital in Lausanne.] *In*: *Zweiter Internationaler Kongress für Krankenhausbibliotheken, Bern 1938, Bericht* . . . 46 – 51; also in *Veska – Zeitschrift,* 2 (10) Oct. 1938, 272 – 273.

408   GUT, Walter. Der Kranke und das Buch. [The sick and the book.] *In*: *Zweiter Internationaler Kongress für Krankenhausbibliotheken, Bern 1938, Bericht* . . . 115 – 124; also in *Veska – Zeitschrift,* 2 (10) Oct. 1938, 297 – 300.

409   GYDE-PEDERSEN, Mette. Hospitalsbiblioteksarbejde. [Hospital library work.] *Tidsskrift for Danske Sygehuse,* 14 1938, 225 – 227.

410   Head librarian's dream. *Book Trolley,* 1 Jan. 1938, 292 – 294.

411   Hospital libraries. [U.S.A.] *Book Trolley,* 1 Feb. 1938, 313 – 315; March 1938, 327; April 1938, 346 – 347; 2 June 1939, 173 – 174.

412   HOUËL, *Mme* Hubert. Création de comités nationaux. [Formation of national hospital library committees.] *In*: *Zweiter Internationaler Kongress für Krankenhausbibliotheken, Bern 1938, Bericht* . . . 21 – 29; also in *Veska – Zeitschrift,* 2 (10) Oct. 1938, 264 – 266; abstract in *Book Trolley,* 2 April 1939, 142 – 143.

413   HULMANN, M. Une nouvelle tendance de l'assistance hospitalière; l'aide morale, les bibliothèques d'hôpitaux. [A new trend in hospitals to raise the morale, hospital libraries.] *Presse Médicale,* 46 Nov. 16 1938, 1699 – 1701.

414 INTERNATIONAL GUILD OF HOSPITAL LIBRARIANS. Report, 1936 – 1937, presented by M. E. Roberts, honorary secretary. *In: Actes du Comité International des Bibliothèques IX, 10me session Paris, 1937.* La Haye, Martinus Nijhoff, 1938, 59 – 60.

415 INTERNATIONAL GUILD OF HOSPITAL LIBRARIANS. Report 1937 – 1938; Hospital libraries: brief summary of international position [by M. E. Roberts]. *In: Actes du Comité International des Bibliothèques X, 11me session Bruxelles, 1938.* La Haye, Martinus Nijhoff, 1938, Annexe XXXVI, 183 – 184.

416 INTERNATIONAL GUILD OF HOSPITAL LIBRARIANS. Report of two years' work. *Book Trolley*, 2 July 1938, 27 – 28; also (with title Präsidialbericht der International Guild of Hospital Librarians) in: *Zweiter Internationaler Kongress für Krankenausbibliotheken, Bern 1938, Bericht* ... 30 – 31; and in *Veska – Zeitschrift*, 2 (10) Oct. 1938, 267.

417 [INTERNATIONAL GUILD OF HOSPITAL LIBRARIANS.] *Zweiter Internationaler Kongress für Krankenhausbibliotheken, Bern, 7 – 10 Juni 1938. Bericht erstattet vom Präsidenten des Organisationskomitees Dr. Hans Georg Wirz.* Bern, Hans Huber [1939]. 147 pp. (Vereinigung Schweizerischer Bibliothekare. Publikationen XVIII.) Reprinted from *Veska – Zeitschrift*, 2 (10) Oct. 1938 and 3 (5) May 1939. Summary of proceedings in *Book Trolley*, 2 July 1938, 21 – 26. Brief report in *Archives et Bibliothèques*, (4) 1937 – 1938, 312 – 313; and in *International Institute of Documentation Quarterly Communications*, 5 (2) 1938, 81.
For papers presented *see* nos. 359, 386, 390, 393, 401, 404, 406, 407, 408, 412, 416, 420, 424, 432, 441, 442, 451, 452.

418 INTERNATIONAL GUILD OF HOSPITAL LIBRARIANS. British Section. Annual report, 1937 – 1938. *Book Trolley*, 1 May 1938, 362 – 367.

419 IRISH REPUBLIC. HOSPITAL LIBRARIES COUNCIL. First annual report. *Book Trolley*, 2 Nov. 1938, 63.

420 JEANNERET, René. Les livres et la lecture dans les établissements de cure pour les tuberculeux. [Books and reading in TB Sanatoria.] *In: Zweiter Internationaler Kongress für Krankenhausbibliotheken, Bern 1938, Bericht* ... 78 – 86; also in *Veska – Zeitschrift*, 2 (10) Oct. 1938, 285 – 288; English abstract in *Book Trolley*, 2 Oct. 1938, 40 – 41.

421 KAMMAN, G. R. Future aims of the hospital library. *Minnesota Medicine*, 21 Aug. 1938, 559 – 561.

422 KELLAWAY, H. Out of school: extracts. *Book Trolley*, 2 Oct. 1938, 36 – 38.

423 KENNEDY, M. E. These students have two libraries. *American Journal of Nursing*, 38 Feb. 1938, 137 – 138.

424 Kurze Berichte aus verschiedenen Ländern. [Short reports from various countries.] *In: Zweiter Internationaler Kongress für Krankenhausbibliotheken, Bern 1938, Bericht* ... 31 – 36; also in *Veska – Zeitschrift*, 2 (10) Oct. 1938, 267 – 268.

425 Länslasarettets i Halmstad bibliotek. [The library of the public hospital in Halmstad.] *Biblioteksbladet*, 23 (3) 1938, 115.

426 Lasarettsbibliotek i Falun. [Library in Falun hospital.] *Biblioteksbladet*, 23 (1) 1938, 23.

427 LEMAÎTRE, H. Les bibliothèques d'hôpitaux pour maladies mentales. [Hospital libraries for the mentally ill.] *Archives et Bibliothèques*, (2) 1937 – 1938, 110 – 115.

428 LEMAÎTRE, H. Bibliothèque nationale pour les aveugles. [National library for the blind, London.] *Archives et Bibliothèques*, (3) 1937 – 1938, 205 – 209.

429 LEMKE, [   ]. Die Krankenhausbücherei. [The hospital library.] *Zeitschrift für das Gesamte Krankenhauswesen*, (18) 1938, 361.

430 LEWIS, C. Sheffield hospital library service. *Book Trolley*, 1 Jan. 1938, 295 – 296.

431 LIBRARY ASSOCIATION. *Papers and discussions at the Portsmouth and Southsea conference, 13 – 17 June, 1938.* London, LA [1938]; also supplement to *Libr. Ass. Rec.*, 40 June 1938, 345 – 350.

432 LIEBRICH-LAUR, Gertrud. Erfahrungen aus der Bibliothek des Bürgerspitals Basel. [Experiences in the library of the Bürgerspital, Basel.] *In: Zweiter Internationaler Kongress für Krankenhausbibliotheken, Bern 1938, Bericht* . . . 64 – 70; also in *Veska – Zeitschrift*, 2 (10) Oct. 1938, 277 – 278; English abstract in *Book Trolley*, 2 Dec. 1938, 75 – 76.

433 MCFARLANE, D. M. Hospital libraries now assume important role: books acknowledged to have therapeutic value. *Ontario Library Review*, 22 Feb. 1938, 19 – 20.

434 MOISIO, A. H. Library service in the University Hospital. *Libr. Ass. Rec.*, 40 Jan. 1938, 9 – 12.

435 OSTENFELD, Elisabeth. Hospitalsbibliotekerne. [Hospital libraries.] *Bogens Verden*, 20 March 1938, 78 – 79.

436 Patientbiblioteket paa Ortopædisk Hospital. [The patients' library in the Orthopaedic hospital, Copenhagen.] *Fremad. Maanedsblad for Foreningen "Fremad" paa "Samfundet og Hjemmet for Vanføre"*, I – II (4) 1937 – 1938, 5.

437 PÉRIER, G. D. La bibliothérapie. [Bibliotherapy.] *Archives Bibliothèques et Musées de Belgique*, 15 (2) 1938, 109 – 110.

438 PETERSEN, M. C. Psychiatric research and the library. *Minnesota Library Notes & News*, 12 June 1938, 182 – 183.

439 PETERSON-DELANEY, S. Place of bibliotherapy in a hospital. *Libr. J.*, 63 April 15, 1938, 305 – 308; also in *Opportunity – a journal of Negro Life*, 16 Feb. 1938, 53 – 56.

440 PLESKIĬ, G. Bibliotechnoe obsluzhivanie bol'nykh i otdykhaiushchikh. [Hospital libraries.] *Krasnyĭ Bibliotekar*, Moscow, (11) 1938, 18 – 22.

441 RAYMOND, Vera. Methods of collecting books. *Book Trolley*, 2 Oct. 1938, 41 – 44; also in French translation, Les moyens d'acquérir des livres pour une bibliothèque d'hôpital *In: Zweiter Internationaler Kongress für Krankenhausbibliotheken, Bern 1938, Bericht* . . . 62 – 64; and in *Veska – Zeitschrift*, 2 Oct. 1938, 276.

442 ROBERTS, M. E. Methods of establishing hospital libraries. *Book Trolley*, 2 Nov. 1938, 51 – 56; Dec. 1938, 72 – 75; also German abstract, Methoden zur einrichtung von Krankenhausbibliotheken *In: Zweiter Internationaler Kongress für Krankenhausbibliotheken, Bern 1938, Bericht* . . . 18 – 20; and in *Veska – Zeitschrift*, 2 (10) 1938, 263 – 264.

443 Sjukhusbiblioteken. [Hospital libraries.] *Biblioteksbladet*, 23 (5) 1938, 169 – 174.

444 SOHON, J. A. Hospital library publicity: a factual report. *ALA Bull.*, 32 Sept. 1938, 608 – 609.

445 STEWART, Nathaniel. Library service and the old. *Libr. J.*, 63 (6) March 15 1938, 218 – 222.

446 TALBOYS, R. ST. C. Sanatorium library. *School Librarian & School Library Review*, 2 (2) Christmas term 1938, 54 – 55.

447 TURNER, P. B., *compiler*. Bibliography [based on bibliography appended to F. C. Pritchard's thesis 1934 *see* nos. 281 and 485]. *Book Trolley*, 1 Dec. 1937, 286 – 287; Jan. 1938, 303; Feb. 1938, 318 – 319; March 1938, 335; April 1938, 351; May 1938, 361; 2 June 1938, 15; July 1938, 31.

448 WALTER, F. K. Training for hospital librarianship. *Libr. J.*, 63 Aug. 1938, 579 – 583.

449 WATSON, H. E. Libraries in sanatoria and tuberculosis hospitals. Library Authorities in Wales, and Monmouthshire. *Conference proceedings, Aberystwyth 1938*, 12 – 17.

450 WETLESEN, Johanne Mowinckel. Foredrag om hospitals – biblioteker i U.S.A. *Bogens Verden*, 20 Nov. 1938, 306 – 311.

451 WIRZ, Hans Georg. Volksbibliotheken und Krankenhausbibliotheken in der Schweiz. [Public libraries and hospital libraries in Switzerland.] *In: Zweiter Internationaler Kongress für Krankenhausbibliotheken, Bern 1938, Bericht* . . . 37 – 45; also in *Veska – Zeitschrift*, 2 (10) Oct. 1938, 269 – 271; English abstract in *Book Trolley*, 2 Oct. 1939, 205 – 207.

452 WYRSCH, Jacob. Bücher in anstalten für Geisteskranke. [Books in mental hospitals.] *In: Zweiter Internationaler Kongress für Krankenhausbibliotheken, Bern 1938, Bericht* . . . 98 – 114; also in *Veska – Zeitschrift*, 2 (10) Oct. 1938, 292 – 297; English abstract in *Book Trolley*, 2 Nov. 1938, 60 – 61.

1939

453 ÅHLIN, G. Hur ett sjukhusbibliotek arbetar. [How a hospital library works.] *Biblioteksbladet*, 24 (3) 1939, 86 – 88.

454 AMERICAN LIBRARY ASSOCIATION. Committee on Hospital Libraries. Annual report, 1939. *ALA Bull.*, 33 Sept. 1939, 618 – 619.

455 AMERICAN LIBRARY ASSOCIATION. Committee on Hospital Libraries. Proceedings at ALA conference 1939. *ALA Bull.*, 33 Oct. 15 1939, P129 – 130.

456 ANET, *Mme.* Pierre. Hospital libraries no. 13. La bibliothèque Reine Astrid, Brussels. *Book Trolley*, 2 (30) July 1939, 184 – 186.

457 BELKIN, N. *and* GLAZYKIN, I. Organisatsiia i postanovka bibliotechnogo dela dlia slepykh. [Organization of libraries for the blind.] *Krasnyĭ Bibliotekari*, (4) 1939, 59 – 69.

458 BRODMAN, E. Patients' libraries; abridged. *Special Libraries Association Proceedings*, 2 1939, 57 – 58.

459 BRYAN, A. I. Can there be a science of bibliotherapy? *Libr. J.*, 64 Oct. 15 1939, 773 – 776.

460 CHAPMAN, M. T. Johns Hopkins hospital library [abridged conference paper]. *Special Library Association Proceedings*, 2 1939, 61 – 62.

461 DEVEREUX, R. Reflections on four years' library work at St. George's hospital. *Book Trolley*, 2 March 1939, 120 – 121.

462 Editorial [hospital libraries in war-time]. *Book Trolley*, 2 Oct. 1939, 195 – 196.

463 HAFFENDEN, J. W. Book collecting. *Book Trolley*, 2 Jan. 1939, 92 – 93.

464 Hospital libraries in Cardiff. *Book Trolley*, 2 March 1939, 122 – 123.

465 Hospital libraries, no. 11. The Toronto General Hospital. *Book Trolley*, 2 (28) May 1939, 148 – 151.

466 HOUËL, H. Comité de lecture & service de documentation. [Reading committee and documentation service.] *Book Trolley*, 2 Oct. 1939, 200 – 202.

467 INTERNATIONAL GUILD OF HOSPITAL LIBRARIANS. British Section. Annual report, 1938 – 1939. *Book Trolley*, 2 May 1939, 152 – 157.

468 JONES, E[dith] Kathleen. *Hospital libraries*. Chicago, Ill., American Library Association, 1939. 208 pp.

469 KAMMAN, G. R. The role of bibliotherapy in the care of the patient. *Bulletin of the American College of Surgeons*, 24 June 1939, 183 – 184.

470 Kent and Canterbury hospital library. *Book Trolley*, 2 Jan. 1939, 90 – 91.

471 Leeds General Infirmary library. *Book Trolley*, 2 April 1939, 140 – 142.

472 LEMAÎTRE, H. Bibliothèque centrale des aveugles, Association Valentin Haüy. [Central library for the blind.] *Archives et Bibliothèques*, 4 (1) 1939, 29 – 40.

473 MAAS, Georg. Neugestaltung der Krankenhaus – Büchereien für Kranke und Personal. Richtlinien der Deutschen Krankenhausgesellschaft. [Reorganisation of hospital libraries for patients and staff: guidelines.] *Zeitschrift für das Gesamte Krankenhauswesen*, 19 (18) Aug. 1939, 402.

474 MORRISSEY, M. R. Hospital library interneship; abridged. *Special Libraries Association Proceedings*, 2 1939, 60 – 61.

475 PAINE, M. M. Hospital library work in an American city; by M. Paine, G. Grant and P. M. Paine. *Book Trolley*, 2 Feb. 1939, 102 – 103.

476 PALIVEC, V. Nemocnični knihovny a knihovnici. [Hospital library service.] *Časopis Čes Knihovniku*, 18 (5) 1939, 62 – 66.

477 Patients' libraries in hospitals. *Journal of the Royal Institute of British Architects*, 46 Jan. 9 1939, 232 – 235.

478 PHILBROOK, L. F. Value of the hospital library. *Libr. J.*, 64 Nov. 15 1939, 890 – 891.

479 POMEROY, Elizabeth. Selected reading an aid to the recovery of the patient [abridged conference paper]. *Special Libraries Association Proceedings*, 2 1939, 58 – 60.

480 RANGANATHAN, S. R. Indian report for the International conference in Berne. *Book Trolley*, 2 June 1939, 172.

481 Report on questionnaires, 1937 – 38. *Book Trolley*, 2 March 1939, 119.

482 *Richtlinien für den Auf – und Ausbau von Krankenhausbüchereien.* [Guidelines for establishment and development of hospital libraries.] hrsg. v. d. Deutschen Krankenhausgesellschaft in Verbindung mit der Reichstelle f. d. Volks-büchereiwesen, 14 Nov. 1939.

483 ROSE MARY, *sister*. Hospital library for patients. *Hospital Progress*, 20 March 1939, 82 – 83.

484 SCHENSTRÖM, B. Hur ett sjukhusbibliotek arbetar. [How a hospital library works.] *Sveriges Landstings Tidskrift*, 26 (3) 1939, 86 – 90.

485 TURNER, P. B., *compiler*. Bibliography [based on bibliography appended to F. C. Pritchard's thesis 1934 *see* nos. 281 and 447]. *Book Trolley*, 2 Jan. 1939, 96; March 1939, 128; April 1939, 137; June 1939, 176; Oct. 1939, 208.

486 TYNELL, K. O. L. Sjukhusens biblioteksfråga. [Hospital library questions.] *Sveriges Landstings Tidskrift*, 26 (3) 1939, 84 – 86.

487 Value of the hospital library [editorial]. *Libr. J.*, 64 Nov. 15 1939, 890 – 891.

1940

488 ALDERSON, C. I. Library and the blind. *Libr. J.*, 65 March 1940, 193 – 195.

489 AMERICAN LIBRARY ASSOCIATION. Committee on Hospital Libraries. Annual report, 1940. *ALA Bull.*, 34 Sept. 15 1940, 583 – 584.

490 AMERICAN LIBRARY ASSOCIATION. Hospital Libraries Round Table. Proceedings at ALA conference, 1940. *ALA Bull.*, 34 Aug. 1940, P120 – 121.

491 British Red Cross Society and Order of St. John hospital library. *Publishers Circular*, 152 Feb. 24 1940, 133 – 134.

492 BROWN, M. Hospital library service. *New Zealand Libraries*, 3 June 1940, 126.

493 BULLOCK, M. Hospital library war organisation and the B.E.F. *Book Trolley*, 3 April 1940, 3 – 4.

494 BULLOCK, M. Year's retrospect. *Book Trolley*, 3 Sept./Oct. 1940, 67 – 70.

495 County depôts. *Book Trolley*, 2 Feb. 1940, 256 – 261; March 1940, 268 – 270.

496 CREGLOW, E. R. Hospital library service in the District of Columbia. *D.C. Libraries*, 12 Oct. 1940, 6 – 7.

497 DAVIE, Lou. The function of a patients' library in a psychiatric hospital. *Bulletin of the Menninger Clinic*, 4 July 1940, 124 – 129.

498   From an outside point of view. *Book Trolley*, 3 June 1940, 39 – 42.

499   Hospital librarianship. *ALA Bull.*, 34 Feb. 1940, 104 – 105; also in *Minnesota Libraries*, 13 March 1940, 23.

500   Hospital libraries in Oxfordshire and Hampshire. *Book Trolley*, 3 Nov./Dec. 1940, 84 – 85.

501   Hospital libraries. (South Africa). *Book Trolley*, 3 May 1940, 27 – 29.

502   HYATT, R. Book service in a general hospital. *Libr. J.*, 65 Sept. 1 1940, 684 – 687.

503   INTERNATIONAL GUILD OF HOSPITAL LIBRARIANS. British Section. Annual report, 1939 – 1940. *Book Trolley*, 3 May 1940, 21 – 26.

504   IRISH REPUBLIC. HOSPITAL LIBRARY COUNCIL. Fourth annual report, 1940. *Leabharlann*, 7 June 1941, 108.

505   JEFFREYS, G. L. O. Bibliotherapy. *New Zealand Libraries*, 3 June 1940, 128 – 129.

506   LEMAÎTRE, H. Rapport sur les bibliothèques d'hôpitaux en 1938 – 39. *In*: *Actes du Comité International des Bibliothèques XI, 12me session Amsterdam, 1939.* La Haye, Martinus Nijhoff, 1940, Annexe XII, 91 – 93.

507   PETERSON-DELANEY, S. Library activities at Tuskegee. *U.S. Medical Bulletin of the Veterans Administration*, 17 Oct. 1940, 163 – 169.

508   POMERANZ, E. B. Aims of bibliotherapy in tuberculosis sanatoria. *Libr. J.*, 65 Sept. 1 1940, 687 – 689.

509   Die Reichsliste für Krankenhausbüchereien. [Official book list for hospital libraries.] *Bücherei*, 7 July/Aug. 1940, 221 – 223.

510   REICHSSTELLE FÜR DAS VOLKSBÜCHEREIWESEN. *Reichsliste für Krankenhausbüchereien, gemeinsam mit der Deutschen Krankenhausgesellschaft zusammengestellt.* [Book list for hospital libraries. . .] Leipzig, Einkaufshaus für Büchereien, 1940.

511   Richtlinien für den Auf und Ausbau der deutschen Krankenhausbüchereien. [Guidelines for the establishing and developing of German hospital libraries.] *Bücherei*, 7 Jan./Feb. 1940, 40 – 42.

512   RIDDELL, M. A. Survey of the reading interests of the blind. *Libr. J.*, 65 March 1 1940, 189 – 192.

513   ROBERTS, M. E. Guild in war-time. *Book Trolley*, 2 Jan. 1940, 236 – 238; Feb. 1940, 251 – 254; 3 May 1940, 30 – 31.

514   ROBERTS, M. E. Report of hospital libraries, 1938 – 39. *In*: *Actes du Comité International des Bibliothèques XI, 12me session Amsterdam, 1939.* La Haye, Martinus Nijhoff, 1940, Annexe XI, 90.

1941

515   ALEXANDER, L. Hospital library venture at the Toronto hospital for incurables. *Ontario Library Review*, 25 Nov. 1941, 359 – 361.

516   AMERICAN LIBRARY ASSOCIATION. Committee on Hospital Libraries. Annual report, 1941. *ALA Bull.*, 35 Oct. 15 1941, 621 – 622.

517   AMERICAN LIBRARY ASSOCIATION. Hospital Libraries Round Table. Proceedings at ALA conference, 1941. *ALA Bull.*, 35 Sept. 1941, P105 – 108.

518   CHADWICK, B. Needs of hospital library service in Massachusetts sanatoria. *Massachusetts Health Journal*, 22 Oct./Dec. 1941, 5 – 6.

519   First annual report of the hospital library of an R.A.F. station sick quarters. *Book Trolley*, 3 Oct. 1941, 167 – 169.

520   Hospital libraries and the war [editorial]. *Libr. Ass. Rec.*, 43 June 1941, 99.

521   HUSSEY, E. R. J. Experiences of a county organiser. *Book Trolley*, 3 Jan. 1941, 97 – 100.

522   LINDEM, S. M. Can I afford hospital library service? [abridged conference paper]. *Illinois Libraries*, 23 Jan. 1941, 14 – 15; also in *Ontario Library Review*, 25 May 1941, 118.

523   MAAS, Georg. Die Neugestaltung der Krankenhausbüchereien: Kriegs – und Friedensaufgaben. [Reorganisation of hospital libraries: tasks in war and peace.] *Zeitschrift für das Gesamte Krankenhauswesen*, 37 (12) June 1941, 225 – 228.

524   MAAS, Georg. Die Zentralisation der Krankenhausbüchereien in Paris verglichen mit der Neugestaltung der Büchereien in deutschen Krankenhäusern. [The centralisation of hospital libraries in Paris compared with the reorganisation of German hospital libraries.] *Zeitschrift für das Gesamte Krankenhauswesen*, 37 (10) May 1941, 185 – 188.

525   MASON, M. F. Training of volunteers for patients libraries [abridged conference paper]. *Spec. Libr.*, 32 Sept. 1941, 238 – 239.

526   METHVEN, M. L. Hospital library internships. *ALA Bull.*, 35 June 1941, 379 – 381.

527   PAYNE, K. Librarian goes to the hospital. *Wilson Libr. Bull.*, 15 Feb. 1941, 504 – 507.

528   ROBERTS, M. E. Improvisation. *Book Trolley*, 3 April 1941, 116 – 119.

529   ROURKE, H. L. Reading is sound therapy. *Modern Hospital*, 57 Dec. 1941, 64.

530   SCHUMACHER, M. Patients' libraries. *Spec. Libr.*, 32 Sept. 1941, 235 – 237.

531   Statistik over hospitalsbiblioteksarbejdet i 1940 – 41. [Hospital library statistics, 1940 – 1941.] *Bogens Verden*, 23 June/July 1941, 143 – 144.

532   TURK, H. M. Psychiatrist evaluates the hospital library. *Hospitals,* Chicago, 15 Feb. 1941, 45 – 46.

533   Visit to Red Cross hospital libraries in East End hospitals during May, 1941. *Book Trolley*, 3 Oct. 1941, 159 – 162.

534   WALLACE, M. L. Bibliotherapy of tomorrow. *Library Occurrent*, 13 Jan./March 1941, 252 – 255.

535 Year's working of a Royal naval hospital library. *Book Trolley*, 3 April 1941, 120 – 123.

1942

536 AMERICAN LIBRARY ASSOCIATION. Hospital Libraries Round Table. Proceedings at ALA conference 1942. *ALA Bull.*, 36 Sept. 5 1942, P96 – 98.

537 Birmingham is making big strides. *Book Trolley*, 4 Jan. 1942, 14 – 15.

538 BRADLEY, C. E. Sending libraries overseas. *Library World*, 44 April 1942, 140 – 141.

539 BRODMAN, E. Patients do read [abridged address]. *Spec. Libr.*, 33 Nov. 1942, 329 – 331.

540 BULLOCK, M. Visit to west country hospitals. *Book Trolley*, 4 Jan. 1942, 8 – 9.

541 CHAPMAN, M. T. Patients' free library Johns Hopkins hospital, Baltimore, Maryland. *Spec. Libr.*, 33 Nov. 1942, 332 – 334.

542 CHESSHIRE, K. Library at Mosten Hall. *Book Trolley*, 4 July 1942, 82 – 83.

543 Collecting centres in London are urgently needed. *Book Trolley*, 4 Jan. 1942, 16 – 18.

544 DAVIES-BROADHOUSE, D. Royal National Orthopaedic hospital. *Book Trolley*, 4 July 1942, 76 – 77.

545 DELEON, M. Hospital library. *Hygeia*, 20 Jan. 1942, 24 – 25.

546 DE LISLE, M. M. You, the nurse, and I, the hospital librarian. *Cath. Libr. Wld.*, 13 April 1942, 208 – 213.

547 FAULDS, E. From Parkwood convalescent home. *Book Trolley*, 4 July 1942, 78 – 80.

548 FREEMAN, M. W. Hospital library service and the home front. *Libr. J.*, 67 March 1 1942, 207 – 210.

549 GAGNON, Salomon. Is reading therapy? *Diseases of the Nervous System*, 3 July 1942, 206 – 212.

550 GAGNON, Salomon. Organization and physical set-up of the mental hospital library. *Diseases of the Nervous System*, 3 May 1942, 149 – 157.

551 HOLM, Anna Dorthea. Hospitalsbiblioteksarbejde. [Hospital library work.] *Bibliotekaren*, 4 April 1942, 21 – 30.

552 Hospital libraries in wartime. *ALA Bull.*, 36 April 1942, 250 – 252.

553 Hospital library progress in the Middle East. *Book Trolley*, 4 April 1942, 45 – 47.

554 INTERNATIONAL GUILD OF HOSPITAL LIBRARIANS. British Section. Annual general meeting, 1941 – 1942. *Book Trolley*, 4 Dec. 1942, 105 – 106.

555 KING, E. A. Oldchurch county hospital library service. *Book Trolley*, 4 Dec. 1942, 111 – 112.

556 MAAS, Georg. Auf – und Ausbau der Krankenhausbüchereien. [The estab-lishment and building-up of hospital libraries.] *Zeitschrift für das Gesamte Krankenhauswesen*, 21 (17) Sept. 1942, 265.

557 MASON, Mary Frank. *Patients' library: a guide book for volunteer hospital library service*. New York, H. W. Wilson, 1942. 111 pp.

558 MINNESOTA ASSOCIATION OF HOSPITAL, MEDICAL AND INSTITUTION LIBRARIANS. Book Committee. *Patients speaking: a list of books circulated in the hospitals of Minnesota, with comments by the patients who read them*. St. Paul, Minn., The Association, 1942? [mimeographed].

559 Opening of the East Surrey hospital library depot at Croydon. *Book Trolley*, 4 April 1942, 58 – 59.

560 SILCOCK, G. M. Lancashire proves the value of book depots. *Book Trolley*, 4 Jan. 1942, 10 – 12.

561 SMITH, B. A. Creative therapy. *Wilson Libr. Bull.*, 16 March 1942, 529 – 531.

562 STRAGER, Henny. Nogle indtryk fra en rejse til hospitalsbiblioteker. [Impressions from a visit to hospital libraries.] *Bogens Verden*, 24 Nov. 1942, 317 – 324.

563 STÜRUP, G. K. Bibliotekernes sindshygiejniske opgaver. [Libraries and mental hygiene.] *Bogens Verden*, 24 Nov. 1942, 317 – 324.

564 TOMLINSON, J. A. Books and boredom in hospitals: report of an address to an Otago branch meeting on hospital libraries. *New Zealand Libraries*, 6 (1) Aug. 1942, 16.

1943

565 ALEXANDER, L. Hospital libraries. *Ontario Library Review*, 27 (3) Aug. 1943, 329 – 330.

566 AMBERG, R. M. Patients' libraries. *Libr. J.*, 68 March 1 1943, 195 – 197.

567 CROUCHER, L. Report from the Surrey hospital library service. *Book Trolley*, 4 Nov. 1943, 182 – 184.

568 DE LISLE, M. M., *sister*. Catholic books in Catholic hospitals. *Cath. Libr. Wld.*, 14 Jan. 1943, 110 – 117+.

569 DICK, J. Mystery bar assumes new role. *Libr. J.*, 68 June 15 1943, 520 – 521.

570 FARRINGTON, A. Hospital library volunteers? No! *ALA Bull.*, 37 Sept. 1943, 261 – 263.

571 FRYER, C. Problem – and a suggestion. *Book Trolley*, 4 July 1943, 156 – 157.

572 HARVEY, M. L. Morning in the library at a naval hospital. *Book Trolley*, 4 Nov. 1943, 175 – 177.

573 JONES, A. F. Read and get well. *ALA Bull.*, 37 July 1943, 224 – 226.

574 MOORE, T. V. Bibliotherapy. *Cath. Libr. Wld.*, 15 Oct. 1943, 11 – 20+.

575   NAND, M. Plea for a hospital library in India. *Modern Librarian*, 13 July/Sept. 1943, 145 – 148.

576   POMEROY, Elizabeth. *A B Cs for hospital librarians*. Chicago, ALA, 1943. 18 pp.

577   SCHMIDT, Barbro. Lasarettsbiblioteket i Lund. [The hospital library in Lund.] *Biblioteksbladet*, 28 1943, 56 – 59.

578   SCHULZE, [   ]. Die Krankenhausbücherei der Reichsmessestadt Leipzig. [Leipzig hospital library.] *Zeitschrift für das Gesamte Krankenhauswesen*, 39 (9/10) May 1943, 118+.

579   SCHUMACHER, M. Hospital library volunteers? Yes! *ALA Bull.*, 37 Sept. 1943, 258 – 260.

580   SMITH, X. P. Army hospital libraries. *School Library Association of California. Bulletin*, 14 May 1943, 16 – 17+.

581   Southern hospital library. *Book Trolley*, 4 March 1943, 127 – 130.

582   STRONG, T. Hospital library service at Newton. *Massachusetts Library Association. Bulletin*, 33 Oct. 1943, 48 – 50.

583   TÜLLMANN, Anni. Aufbau und Ausbau der Krankenbüchereien. [Establishment and development of hospital libraries.] *Zeitschrift für das Gesamte Krankenhauswesen*, 39 (9/10) May 1943, 117.

1944

584   ALEXANDER, L. Hospital library service and the public libraries. *Book Trolley*, 4 June 1944, 238 – 240.

585   ALEXANDER, L. Public library branch at the Toronto hospital for incurables. *Book Trolley*, 4 Feb. 1944, 214 – 217.

586   AMERICAN LIBRARY ASSOCIATION. Hospital Libraries Round Table. Report. *ALA Bull.*, 38 Oct. 1 1944, 377 – 378.

587   AMERICAN LIBRARY ASSOCIATION. Hospital Libraries Round Table. *A statement of objectives and standards for hospital libraries and librarians* [1944]. 5 pp. (for ALA Council meeting Oct. 13 – 14 1944).

588   ANDERSEN, Johanne M. Centralbiblioteket for tuberkulosepatienter. [The Central library for tuberculous patients.] *Bogens Verden*, 26 April/May 1944, 105 – 108.

589   BOLDT, Barbro. Biblioteksarbete vid sjukhus. [Library work in hospitals.] *Svenskbygden*, 1944, 142 – 146.

590   COWLES, R. L. Books, beards, and bathrobes. *News Notes*, 20 Feb. 1944, 9 – 11.

591   CURTIUS, F. Die ärztliche Bedeutung der Krankenhausbücherei. [The medical value of the hospital library.] *Die Medizinische Welt,* 18 (13/14) 1944, 191.

592   GRIESON, V. E. Veterans are not forgotten. *Libr. J.*, 69 June 1 1944, 481 – 484.

593   HEINZE, L. Hospital libraries. *Spec. Libr.*, 35 July/Aug. 1944, 315 – 317.

594 HERVEY, G. S. Forces' library at Alexandria. *Book Trolley*, 4 June 1944, 229 – 231.

595 Hospital library work in the Veterans' Administration. *ALA Bull.*, 38 Oct. 15 1944, 427 – 428.

596 HOWARD, A. L. Mental hospital library. *Spec. Libr.*, 35 Nov. 1944, 444 – 448.

597 HUTCHINSON, L. C. Hospital librarianship. *News Notes*, 20 Feb. 1944, 5 – 7+.

598 INTERNATIONAL GUILD OF HOSPITAL LIBRARIANS. British Section. [Conference, 9th, 1943, London.] *Book Trolley*, 4 Feb. 1944, 198 – 199.

599 JONES, Perrie. Hospital libraries – today and tomorrow. *Bull. Med. Libr. Ass.*, 32 (4) Oct. 1944, 467 – 478.

600 JONES, Perrie, *comp. One thousand books for hospital libraries: an annotated bibliography*. Minneapolis, University of Minnesota Press, 1944. 58 pp.

601 KANNINEN, Mauno *and* NOHRSTRÖM, Kyllikki. *Sairaalakirjastot*. [Hospital libraries.] Helsingfors, 1944.

602 KINOS, Hilppa. Sairaalakirjastotyön pskologinen perusta. [Hospital library work – psychological element.] *Kansanvalistus – ja Kirjastolehti*, 1944, 161 – 170.

603 Library as part of a rehabilitation scheme. *Book Trolley*, 4 Sept. 1944, 270 – 272.

604 PIETERS, E. Library on wheels. *Spec. Libr.*, 35 Nov. 1944, 448 – 451.

605 QUINT, M. D. The mental hospital library. *Mental Hygiene*, 28 April 1944, 263 – 272.

606 REB, C. L. How one G.I. hospital library grew. *Kansas Library Bulletin*, 13 Dec. 1944, 8 – 11.

607 ROGAN, O. F. World War II veteran's hospital. *News Notes*, 20 Feb. 1944, 12 – 14.

608 SMITH, J. W. Army hospital library. *Missouri Library Association Quarterly*, 5 March 1944, 13 – 15.

609 SPORE, V. Patients library. *News Notes*, 20 Feb. 1944, 17 – 21.

610 STANDLEE, M. W. American military hospital. *Book Trolley*, 4 Dec. 1944, 288 – 289.

611 TEWS, Ruth M. Case histories of patients' reading. *Libr. J.*, 69 June 1 1944, 484 – 487.

612 Training syllabus. *Book Trolley*, 4 June 1944, 226 – 228.

613 What shall I do all day? *Book Trolley*, 4 Sept. 1944, 273 – 275.

1945

614 AMERICAN LIBRARY ASSOCIATION. Hospital Libraries Division. Report. *ALA Bull.*, 39 Oct. 15 1945, 396 – 397.

615 AMERICAN LIBRARY ASSOCIATION. Hospital Libraries Round Table. Standards for Libraries and Librarians Committee. Objectives and standards for hospital libraries and librarians. *Illinois Libraries*, 27 March 1945, 172 – 175.

616 BAKER, M. C. Library service at the United States naval hospital, Oakland. *Spec. Libr.*, 36 Oct. 1945, 332 – 339.

617 BEDWELL, Cyril Edward Alfred. Hospital library accommodation. *In*: Aslib. *Report of proceedings of the 20th annual conference 1945*. London, Aslib, 1945, 77 – 81; also in *Book Trolley*, 5 (4) Winter 1945/1946, 97 – 100.

618 CLIFF, B. Books à la carte. *California Library Association. Bulletin*, 7 Dec. 1945, 57 – 58+.

619 CONDELL, Lucy. Story hour in a neuropsychiatric hospital; with list of picture books used. *Libr. J.*, 70 Sept. 15 1945, 805 – 807.

620 ELLER, C. S. No ivory tower. *Libr. J.*, 70 Dec. 1 1945, 1126 – 1127.

621 GOULD, E. C. Hospital library service. *Pacific Northwest Library Association Quarterly*, 9 April 1945, 116 – 117.

622 HEINZE, L. Training volunteer aides for patients' libraries. *Libr. J.*, 70 Jan. 1 1945, 25 – 26.

623 HOLM, Anna Dorthea. Hospitalsbiblioteker. [Hospital libraries.] *Bibliotekaren*, 7 Jan. 1945, 12 – 16.

624 Hospital library activities in Belgium, 1940 – 45. *Book Trolley*, 5 Summer 1945, 50 – 51.

625 Hospital library work: proposed scheme of training of librarians of the British Red Cross Society, and Order of St. John of Jerusalem. *Libr. Ass. Rec.*, 47 (6) June 1945, 108 – 111.

626 INTERNATIONAL GUILD OF HOSPITAL LIBRARIANS. British Section. [Conference, 1945, London.] *Book Trolley*, 5 Spring 1945, 3 – 4.

627 JUDGE, Anne. Read-habilitation, day in a tuberculosis hospital. *Wilson Libr. Bull.*, 19 June 1945, 686 – 687.

628 KAPPES, M. L. Plan for a small hospital library. *Spec. Libr.*, 36 Oct. 1945, 340 – 343.

629 KOLMODIN, T. Ny bokvagn för sjukhusbibliotek. [New trolley for hospital library.] *Biblioteksbladet*, 30 1945, 159 – 160.

630 Library at the London. *Book Trolley*, 5 Spring 1945, 16 – 18.

631 Library service for tuberculosis patients. (Letter from the Director, Division of Tuberculosis, Department of Health.) *New Zealand Libraries*, 8 (8) Sept. 1945, 138 – 141.

632 LUND, E. Biblioteksarbejde paa hospitaler. [Library work in hospitals.] *Bibliotekaren*, 7 April 1945, 36 – 40.

633 LUNDEEN, A. *and* HOWARD, V. St. John's sanitarium library. *Illinois Libraries*, 27 Feb. 1945, 103 – 104.

634   MACKENZIE, C. Books in illness. *Book Trolley*, 5 Autumn 1945, 71 – 72.

635   MASON, Mary Frank. *Patients library: a guide book for volunteer hospital library service*. New York, H. W. Wilson, 1945. 117 pp.

636   O'CONNELL, J. A. Chaplain looks at the hospital library. *Illinois Catholic Librarian*, 1 May/Aug. 1945, 46 – 47.

637   OLIVER, B. *and others*. Training of the librarians of the British Red Cross Society and Order of St. John of Jerusalem. *Book Trolley*, 5 (3) Autumn 1945, 59 – 67.

638   PLEASANTS, M. G. At Olive View sanatorium. *California Library Association Bulletin*, 7 Dec. 1945, 63 – 64.

639   Proposed scheme of training of librarians of the British Red Cross Society and Order of St. John of Jerusalem. *Book Trolley*, 5 Summer 1945, 27 – 31.

640   SCHILLER, M. B. Books are good medicine. *Trained Nurse and Hospital Review*, 115 July 1945, 37 – 40.

641   SCHNECK, Jerome M. A bibliography on bibliotherapy and hospital library activities. *Bull. Med. Libr. Ass.*, 33 July 1945, 341 – 356.

642   SCHNECK, Jerome M. A bibliography on bibliotherapy and libraries in mental hospitals. *Bulletin of the Menninger Clinic*, 9 Sept. 1945, 170 – 174.

643   SCHNECK, Jerome M. Bibliotherapy and hospital library activities for neuro-psychiatric patients: a review of the literature with comments on trends. *Psychiatry*, 8 May 1945, 207 – 228.

644   SHIELS, *Sir* D. Therapeutic value of reading. *Book Trolley*, 5 Autumn 1945, 67 – 70.

645   SOUTHERDEN, M. G. H. Hospital librarians: professional or voluntary? *Library World*, 48 Aug./Sept. 1945, 23 – 26.

646   SWINNERTON, F. A. How to grade your patient. *Book Trolley*, 5 Autumn 1945, 73 – 74.

647   Tubercular patients need a specialized library service. *Book Trolley*, 5 Summer 1945, 43 – 45.

648   UNITED STATES. WAR DEPARTMENT. *Hospital library service*. Washington DC, U.S. G.P.O., 1945. 32 pp. (War Department technical manual, TM 28 – 306.)

1946

649   ALLEN, E. B. Books help neuropsychiatric patients. *Libr. J.*, 71 Dec. 1 1946, 1671 – 1675+.

650   AMERICAN LIBRARY ASSOCIATION. Hospital Libraries Division. Report. *ALA Bull.*, 40 Oct. 15 1946, 382 – 383.

651   AMERICAN LIBRARY ASSOCIATION. Hospital Libraries Division. Summary of proceedings at ALA conference, 1946. *ALA Bull.*, 40 Sept. 15 1946, P62 – 65.

652   BALME, H. Future of hospital libraries. *Book Trolley*, 5 Summer 1946, 140 – 142.

653 BRUCE, L. R. What, why and when is a hospital librarian. *Spec. Libr.*, 37 July/Aug. 1946, 171 – 175.

654 BRYANT, A. Reading and the sick. *Book Trolley*, 5 Spring 1946, 128 – 130.

655 CRIST, E. Book collection in hospital libraries. *Cath. Libr. Wld.*, 18 Nov. 1946, 49 – 51.

656 FELLIN, O. A. Even a cheerful workroom in Bruns general hospital. *Libr. J.*, 71 Feb. 1 1946, 170 – 171.

657 GUILD OF HOSPITAL LIBRARIANS. Constitution. *Book Trolley*, 5 Summer 1946, 137 – 138.

658 GYDE-PEDERSEN, Mette. Hospital libraries in Denmark. *Book Trolley*, 5 Spring 1946, 125 – 126.

659 HOPKINS, T. W. General infirmary, Leeds. *Book Trolley*, 5 Summer 1946, 148 – 151.

660 INTERNATIONAL GUILD OF HOSPITAL LIBRARIANS. British Section. Annual meeting of the international guild of hospital librarians. *Book Trolley*, 5 Spring 1946, 112 – 113.

661 JONES, P. What hospital librarianship offers. *Libr. J.*, 71 Dec. 1 1946, 1667 – 1670.

662 KINNEY, M. M. Bibliotherapy and the librarian. *Spec. Libr.*, 37 July/Aug. 1946, 175 – 180.

663 Komitéen for sykehusbibliotekar reorganisert. [Committee for hospital libraries reorganised.] *Bok og Bibliotek,* 13 Feb. 1946, 45 – 46.

664 LUCIOLI, Clara E. The library enters the home. *Wilson Libr. Bull.*, 21 (4) Dec. 1946, 293 – 295, 298.

665 MASON, M. F. What shall the patient read? *Modern Hospital*, 66 Feb. 1946, 75 – 76.

666 METHVEN, M. L. Books on wheels: the hospital libraries division and how it will travel. *ALA Bull.*, 40 Dec. 1 1946, 467 – 469.

667 MICHAELS, J. J. Approach of the librarian to the neuropsychiatric in an army general hospital. *Spec. Libr.*, 37 July/Aug. 1946, 180 – 183.

668 PREBLE, M. C. Volunteers in hospital libraries. *Bull. Med. Libr. Ass.*, 34 Jan. 1946, 26 – 28.

669 RAYMOND, Vera. Important news. *Book Trolley*, 5 (4) Winter 1945/1946, 84 – 85.

670 ROBERTS, M. E. Hospital library activities in England. *Spec. Libr.*, 37 (3) March 1946, 87 – 91.

671 SKINNER, M. E. Personnel in hospital libraries. *Cath. Libr. Wld.*, 18 Nov. 1946, 47 – 49.

672 SMITH, M. S. Budget for hospital libraries. *Cath. Libr. Wld.,* 18 Nov. 1946, 51 – 53+.

673 Therapeutic value of reading (editorial). *Medical Journal of Australia*, 2 Nov. 2 1946, 637 – 638; also in *Occupational Therapy and Rehabilitation*, 26 Oct. 1947, 299 – 301.

674 WELCH, H. F. Hospital library. *Massachusetts Library Association Bulletin*, 36 April 1946, 25 – 26.

1947

675 AMERICAN LIBRARY ASSOCIATION. Hospital Libraries Division. Report. *ALA Bull.*, 41 Oct. 15 1947, 398.

676 AMERICAN LIBRARY ASSOCIATION. Hospital Libraries Division. Summary of proceedings at ALA conference, 1947. *ALA Bull.*, 41 Sept. 15 1947, P31 – 32.

677 ASKWITH, *Mrs.* Howard. Enlistment of voluntary service. *In*: Bedwell, C.E.A. *Manual for hospital librarians*. London, Library Association, 1947, 62 – 68.

678 BARLOW, E. Book selection and library service in a children's hospital. *Illinois Catholic Librarian*, 3 May/Aug. 1947, 45 – 47.

679 BEDWELL, Cyril Edward Alfred, *editor. Manual for hospital librarians*. London, Library Association, 1947. 120 pp.
For contents *see* nos. 677, 681, 683, 697, 700, 703, 711, 714.

680 BRYANT, A. St. John and Red Cross hospital library department. *Libr. Ass. Rec.*, 49 Dec. 1947, 306 – 307.

681 BUCHANAN, *Mrs.* Co-operation between public and hospital libraries (ii) Public libraries with voluntary librarians. *In*: Bedwell, C.E.A. *Manual for hospital librarians*. London, Library Association, 1947, 88 – 89.

682 [BUTCHART, R.] Edinburgh public libraries hospital service. *Book Trolley*, 5 (9) April 1947, 195 – 199.

683 CARTLEDGE, J. A. Co-operation between public and hospital libraries. (1) Volunteers with public libraries. *In*: Bedwell, C.E.A. *Manual for hospital librarians*. London, Library Association, 1947, 85 – 87.

684 CONNELL, S. M. Library service in a veterans administration general hospital. *Spec. Libr.*, 38 July/Aug. 1947, 176 – 178.

685 CORSON, H. F. Libraries in mental hospitals. *In*: South-Eastern Library Association. *Twelfth biennial conference papers and proceedings*. The Association, 1947, 132 – 139.

686 DUNNINGHAM, A. G. W. Hospital service in Dunedin. *In*: New Zealand Library Association. *Proceedings of the sixteenth conference and report of the nineteenth annual meeting held at Christchurch, 20 – 23 May 1947*, 75 – 77.

687 FÉDÉRATION INTERNATIONALE DES ASSOCIATIONS DE BIBLIOTHÉCAIRES. Sous – Commission des Bibliothèques d'Hôpitaux. [Rapport]. *In*: *Actes du Comité International des Bibliothèques XII, 13me session Oslo, 1947*. La Haye, Martinus Nijhoff, 1947, 37 – 38.

688 FÉDÉRATION INTERNATIONALE DES ASSOCIATIONS DE BIBLIOTHÉCAIRES. Sous –
Commission des Bibliothèques d'Hôpitaux. Rapport présénte par P.
Poindron. *In*: *Actes du Comité International des Bibliothèques XII, 13me session
Oslo, 1947*. La Haye, Martinus Nijhoff, 1947, Annexe XXIX, 159 – 164.

689 FORSYTH, M. H. Hospital library in action. *Library Review*, (84) Winter 1947,
322 – 324.

690 FORSYTH, M. H. Hospital library readers. *Library Review*, (83) Autumn 1947,
290 – 292.

691 How to run a hospital library. *Book Trolley*, 5 Jan. 1947, 179 – 180.

692 KENT, M. L. Veterans are looking up. *Libr. J.*, 72 Jan. 1 1947, 26 – 30.

693 KENT, M. L. *and* KINNEY, M. M. Medical care second to none. *Spec. Libr.*, 38
July/Aug. 1947, 172 – 176.

694 KINGSLAND, G. S. Village library serves its hospital. *Vermont. Free Public
Library Commission and State Library. Bulletin*, 42 March 1947, 59 – 61.

695 KIRCHER, C. J. Bibliotherapy: the librarian acts. *Cath. Libr. Wld.*, 19 Dec.
1947, 95 – 98+.

696 MACASKILL, H. Patients' needs. *In*: New Zealand Library Association. *Proceedings of the sixteenth conference and report of the nineteenth annual meeting held at
Christchurch, 20 – 23 May 1947*, 77 – 79.

697 MACKENZIE, N. Psychology. *In*: Bedwell, C. E. A. *Manual for hospital librarians*.
London, Library Association, 1947, 23 – 33.

698 MUSHAKE, K. Library service in a veterans administration neuropsychiatric
hospital. *Spec. Libr.*, 38 July/Aug. 1947, 179 – 181.

699 NORRIE, J. Hospital library service. *In:* New Zealand Library Association.
*Proceedings of the sixteenth conference and report of the nineteenth annual meeting
held at Christchurch, 20 – 23 May 1947*, 67 – 75.

700 PAGET-COOKE, *Mrs*. The approach to the patient. *In*: Bedwell, C. E. A.
Manual for hospital librarians. London, Library Association, 1947, 34 – 37.

701 PALIVEC, V. Rapport de la délégation Tchécoslovaque sur les bibliothèques
d'hôpitaux. *In*: *Actes du Comité International des Bibliothèques XII, 13e session
Oslo, 1947*. La Haye, Martinus Nijhoff, 1947, Annexe XXXI, 167 – 168.

702 ROBERTS, M. E. My post-war visit to Denmark, including comparative
impressions of Danish and British hospital libraries. *Book Trolley*, 5 Jan. 1947,
174 – 177.

703 ROBERTS, O. W. Hospital patients. *In*: Bedwell, C. E. A. *Manual for hospital
librarians*. London, Library Association, 1947, 5 – 22.

704 ROBINSON, C. E. *and* FLINN, G. H. We like veterans administration work.
Libr. J., 72 Jan. 1 1947, 21 – 23.

705 ROOME, W. H. Some veterans must read in bed. *Libr. J.*, 72 Jan. 1 1947,
23 – 26.

706 ST. JOHN, F. R. *and* HAYS, D. O. Veterans Administration library service. *Wilson Libr. Bull.*, 22 Nov. 1947, 262 – 266.

707 SHAPLEIGH, D. R. General library administration in a Veterans Administration tuberculosis hospital. *Spec. Libr.*, 38 July/Aug. 1947, 181 – 187.

708 SHAPLEIGH, D. R. [Hospital library work.] *In*: Southeastern Library Association. *Twelfth biennial conference, papers and proceedings.* The Association, 1947, 121 – 123.

709 STANDLEE, M. W. Lady, what you need is a horse! *Wilson Libr. Bull.*, 22 Sept. 1947, 43 – 45.

710 STANISZEWSKI, I. Bibliotherapy and the child who has problems. *Illinois Catholic Librarian*, 3 Jan./April 1947, 26 – 28.

711 STOKES, Roy. The features of a hospital library. *In*: Bedwell, C. E. A. *Manual for hospital librarians.* London, Library Association, 1947, 69 – 84.

712 Training for hospital librarianship for professional librarians. *Book Trolley*, 5 July 1947, 220 – 222.

713 TURNER, G. Report on the present position of hospital libraries in Great Britain. *In*: *Actes du Comité International des Bibliothèques XII, 13me session Oslo, 1947.* La Haye, Martinus Nijhoff, 1947, Annexe XXX, 165 – 166.

714 VOLLANS, R. F. Book selection for hospital patients. *In*: Bedwell, C. E. A. *Manual for hospital librarians.* London, Library Association, 1947, 90 – 109.

1948

715 AMERICAN LIBRARY ASSOCIATION. Hospital Libraries Division. Report. *ALA Bull.*, 42 Oct. 15 1948, 460 – 461.

716 AMERICAN LIBRARY ASSOCIATION. Hospital Libraries Division. Summary of proceedings at ALA conference, 1948. *ALA Bull.*, 42 Sept. 15 1948, P34 – 36.

717 ANDERSEN, Johanne M. Tuberkulosebiblioteksarbejde i Danmark. [TB library work in Denmark.] *In*: Gyde-Pedersen, M. *and others. Folkebibliotekernes sociale særopgaver.* København, Folkebibliotekernes Bibliografiske Kontor, 1948, 118 – 122.

718 BERSET, I. V. Sykehusbibliotekarbeid i Norge. [Hospital library work in Norway.] *In*: Gyde-Pedersen, M. *and others. Folkebibliotekernes sociale særopgaver.* København, Folkebibliotekernes Bibliografiske Kontor, 1948, 23 – 28.

719 BERTELSEN, Eli. Biblioteksarbejde paa sindssygehospitaler i Danmark. [Library work in mental hospitals in Denmark.] *In*: Gyde-Pedersen, M. *and others. Folkebibliotekernes sociale særopgaver.* København, Folkebibliotekernes Bibliografiske Kontor, 1948, 72 – 76.

720 BRIGGS, A. D. The value of the hospital library. [Conference paper, Paisley, May 1947.] *In*: Scottish Library Association. *Annual report, 1947.* Hamilton, printed by the Hamilton Advertiser Ltd. [1948], 60 – 64.

721 BUTCHART, R. Hospital libraries. [Conference paper, Paisley, May 1947.] *In*: Scottish Library Association. *Annual report, 1947.* Hamilton, printed by The Hamilton Advertiser Ltd. [1948], 51 – 59.

722 Censorship of books for hospital patients. *Book Trolley*, 5 March 1948, 253 – 256.

723 COWERN, A. G. Library service, Veterans Administration, branch no. 8. *Minnesota Libraries*, 15 March 1948, 272 – 274.

724 EATON, E. S. Patients' library, Unit one, Veterans Administration hospital, Hines, Illinois. *Illinois Libraries*, 30 Jan. 1948, 64 – 66.

725 FÉDÉRATION INTERNATIONALE DES ASSOCIATIONS DE BIBLIOTHÉCAIRES. Sous – Commission des Bibliothèques d'Hôpitaux. Rapports [par P. Poindron]. *In*: *Actes du Comité International des Bibliothèques XIII, 14e session London, 1948*. La Haye, Martinus Nijhoff, 1948, Annexe XVI a. Rapport préliminaire sur le matériel, 108 – 109; b. Des machines à lire au plafond pour malades, 109 – 110; c. Rapport préliminaire sur la formation professionnelle des bibliothécaires ... 111 – 117; d. Rapport préliminaire sur les relations entre les bibliothèques d'hôpitaux et les bibliothèques publiques, 118; e. Rapport préliminaire sur les bibliothèques centrales de prêt pour malades tuberculeux, 120 – 123; g. Projet d'une bibliographie internationale, 128 – 129; h. Rapport préliminaire sur la propagande, 129 – 130.

726 GADE, E. Biblioteksarbejde for døvstumme i Danmark. [Library work with the deaf and dumb in Denmark.] *In*: Gyde-Pedersen, M. *and others. Folke-bibliotekernes sociale særopgaver.* København, Folkebibliotekernes Bibliografiske Kontor, 1948, 47 – 48.

727 GOTTSCHALK, L. A. Bibliotherapy as an adjuvant in psychotherapy. *American Journal of Psychiatry*, 104 April 1948, 632 – 637.

728 GYDE-PEDERSEN, Mette *and others. Folkebibliotekernes sociale særopgaver.* [Social problems of public libraries.] København, Folkebibliotekernes Bibliografiske Kontor, 1948.
For contents *see* nos. 717, 718, 719, 726, 729, 731, 733, 734, 735, 738, 740, 744, 755, 756.

729 GYDE-PEDERSEN, Mette *and* OSTENFELD, Elisabeth. Biblioteksarbejde blandt blinde i Danmark. [Library work with the blind in Denmark.] *In*: Gyde-Pedersen, M. *and others. Folkebibliotekernes sociale særopgaver.* København, Folkebibliotekernes Bibliografiske Kontor, 1948, 38 – 40.

730 HENDERSON, Jemima Millar. Books in hospital. *Book Trolley*, 5 (13) March 1948, 267 – 268.

731 HÖK-LUNDIN, Elin. Biblioteksarbete bland blinda i Sverige. [Library work with the blind in Sweden.] *In*: Gyde-Pedersen, M. *and others. Folkebiblio-tekernes sociale særopgaver.* København, Folkebibliotekernes Bibliografiske Kontor, 1948, 43 – 46.

732 HOLLWAY, Marion *and* EILOLA, Rebecca. The ceiling reflects new hope for the handicapped. *Book Trolley*, 5 (14) July 1948, 287 – 291.

733 HOLM, Anna Dorthea. Hospitalsbiblioteksarbejde i Danmark. [Hospital library work in Denmark.] *In*: Gyde-Pedersen, M. *and others. Folkebiblio-tekernes sociale særopgaver,* København. Folkebibliotekernes Bibliografiske Kontor, 1948, 9 – 19.

734 HOLMSTEN, Ulrikke. Biblioteksarbete på sinnessjukhus i Finland. [Library work in mental hospitals in Finland.] *In*: Gyde-Pedersen, M. *and others. Folkebibliotekernes sociale særopgaver.* København, Folkebibliotekernes Bibliografiske Kontor, 1948, 69 – 72.

735 IGNATIUS, Elsa. Biblioteksarbete bland blinda i Finland. [Library work with the blind in Finland.] *In*: Gyde-Pedersen, M. *and others. Folkebibliotekernes sociale særopgaver.* København, Folkebibliotekernes Bibliografiske Kontor, 1948, 41 – 43.

736 IL'INSKAÎA, O. Bibliotechnoe obsluzhivanie invalidov Velikoĭ Otechestvennoĭ voĭny. [Library service to invalids of the Great Fatherland war.] *Bibliotekar'*, May 1948, 40.

737 JONES, P. Public library and the hospital. *Public Libraries,* 2 Jan. 1948, 32 – 34.

738 KANNINEN, Mauno. Sjukhusbiblioteksarbete i Finland. [Hospital library work in Finland.] *In*: Gyde-Pedersen, M. *and others. Folkebibliotekernes sociale særopgaver.* København, Folkebibliotekernes Bibliografiske Kontor, 1948, 19 – 23.

739 Library furnishings and fittings. *Book Trolley,* 5 March 1948, 271 – 273.

740 LYNGEN, Gunlaug. Bibliotekarbeid blandt blinde i Norge. [Library work with the blind in Norway.] *In*: Gyde-Pedersen, M. *and others. Folkebibliotekernes sociale særopgaver.* København, Folkebibliotekernes Bibliografiske Kontor, 1948, 35 – 38.

741 MACKOWN, M. *and* DIXEY, E. Library service as a treatment for mental sickness. *Bulletin of the New Hampshire Public Libraries,* 44 Sept. 1948, 73 – 75.

742 MATHEWS, K. R. *Public library service to hospitals in Canada.* Thesis (M.S.) Columbia University, 1948. 57 pp. typewritten.

743 MILKOVICH, M. Relationship of hospital libraries to physical medicine rehabilitation. *In*: Southeastern Library Association. [*Conference, 13th 1948, Louisville, proceedings*], 40 – 45.

744 MUNCK AF ROSENSCHÖLD, Kerstin. Sjukhusbiblioteksarbete i Sverige. [Hospital library work in Sweden.] *In*: Gyde-Pedersen, M. *and others. Folkebibliotekernes sociale særopgaver.* København, Folkebibliotekernes Bibliografiske Kontor, 1948, 29 – 33.

745 NOE, B. Hospital library service. *In*: South-Western Library Association. [*Conference 12th 1948, New Orleans; proceedings*], 40 – 45.

746 NORRIE, Jean. Hospital libraries in New Zealand: a survey. *New Zealand Libraries,* 11 (8) Sept. 1948, 201 – 207.

747 OŜTENFELD, E. Library for the tuberculous patients in Denmark. *In*: *Actes du Comité International des Bibliothèques XIII, 14me session, London, 1948.* La Haye, Martinus Nijhoff, 1948, Annexe XVIf, 124 – 127.

748 PEPINO, Jan. Büchereiarbeit im Krankenhaus. (Entwicklung d. Patientenbibliothek in Dresden vor und nach 1945.) [Library work in hospital: development of the patients' library in Dresden before and since 1945.] *Der Volksbibliothekar,* 2 (5) 1948, 298.

749 PHILLIPS, E. Problems in book selection for physical and mental balance. *Public Libraries*, 2 Jan. 1948, 28 – 31.

750 ROBERTS, M. E. Hospital libraries in Sweden. *Book Trolley*, 5 March 1948, 280 – 281.

751 ROBERTS, M. E. Libraries in mental hospitals. *Mental Health*, 7 Feb. 1948, 70 – 71.

752 ROBERTS, M. E. Objectives and standards for hospital libraries. *Book Trolley*, 5 (14) July 1948, 294 – 295.

753 SIMON, B. V. Training of medical, hospital and nursing librarians. *Spec. Libr.*, 39 March 1948, 71 – 76.

754 TRAMMEL, G. R. Sick men only: Veterans Administration hospital library service Fayetteville, Arkansas. *Arkansas Libraries*, 4 Jan./April 1948, 7 – 10.

755 TYRIHJELL, Marta. Bibliotekarbeid på sinnsykehospitaler i Norge. [Library work in mental hospitals in Norway.] *In*: Gyde-Pedersen, M. *and others*. *Folkebibliotekernes sociale særopgaver*. København, Folkebibliotekernes Bibliografiske Kontor, 1948, 77 – 79.

756 TYRIHJELL, Marta. Tuberkulosebibliotekarbeid i Norge. [TB library work in Norway.] *In*: Gyde-Pedersen, M. *and others*. *Folkebibliotekernes sociale særopgaver*. København, Folkebibliotekernes Bibliografiske Kontor, 1948, 122 – 124.

757 VOORTHUYSEN, R. L. van *and* KOUMANS, F. P. Hospital libraries in the Netherlands. *Book Trolley*, 5 July 1948, 292 – 294.

758 WEBSTER, H. E. Patients' library. *Pacific Northwest Library Association Quarterly*, 12 Jan. 1948, 74 – 77.

759 WILSON, B. K. This job stimulates and satisfies. *Illinois Libraries*, 30 June 1948, 251 – 253.

1949

760 ALLSOP, Kathleen M. Mental hospital library work. *Book Trolley*, 5 Jan. 1949, 334 – 339.

761 BAATZ, W. H. Library service in the Veterans Administration. *Library Quarterly*, 19 July 1949, 166 – 177.

762 BERGMANN, G. Die Krankenlektüre. [Reading for patients.] *Grenzgebiete der Medizin*, 2 1949, 204 – 205.

763 BERSET, I. V. Et pasientbibliotek blir til. [A patients' library is established.] *Bok og Bibliotek*, 16 April 1949, 105 – 107.

764 Les bibliothèques pour malades en Belgique. [Libraries for the sick in Belgium.] *In*: *Actes du Comité International des Bibliothèques XIV, 15me session Bâle, 1949*. La Haye, Martinus Nijhoff, 1949, Annexe XII, 80 – 82. LSA 1950/50.

765 BIERMANN, W. *and* FINCKH, G. Von der Bücherei des Krankenhauses. [The hospital library.] *Anstalts – Umschau*, 18 (5) Oct. 1949, 6 – 7.

766   BRACE, E. A. Hospital libraries and hospital librarians. *Book Trolley*, 5 Dec. 1949, 389 – 392.

767   CONNELL, S. M. Hospital library experiments with special programmes. *Book Trolley*, 5 Aug. 1949, 373 – 375.

768   CONNELL, S. M. Publicity for a hospital library. *Wilson Libr. Bull.*, 23 March 1949, 520 – 521.

769   CONNELL, S. M. Some misconceptions about hospital librarianship. *Libr. J.*, 74 Oct. 1 1949, 1354+.

770   CONNELL, S. M. Working combination: professionals and volunteers. *Wilson Libr. Bull.*, 24 Nov. 1949, 234 – 235.

771   DELISLE, M. M., *sister*. Annotated readings for hospital librarians. *Cath. Libr. Wld.*, 20 May 1949, 247 – 250.

772   Editorial. [Library work with children in hospital.] *Book Trolley*, 5 Aug. 1949, 365 – 367.

773   FÉDÉRATION INTERNATIONALE DES ASSOCIATIONS DE BIBLIOTHÉCAIRES. Sous – Commission des Bibliothèques d'Hôpitaux. [Rapport]. *In*: *Actes du Comité International des Bibliothèques XIV, 15me session Bâle, 1949*. La Haye, Martinus Nijhoff, 1949, 29 – 31.

774   GRILLS, M. A. *Selective bibliography of audio-visual materials suitable for the hospitalized child*. Thesis (A.M.) University of Denver, 1949. 72 pp. typewritten.

775   GUILD OF HOSPITAL LIBRARIANS (GREAT BRITAIN). Annual report. *In*: *Actes du Comité International des Bibliothèques XIV, 15me session Bâle, 1949*. La Haye, Martinus Nijhoff, 1949, Annexe XIX, 104 – 105.

776   HANKAR, [   ]. Hospital libraries in Belgium. *Spec. Libr.*, 40 July/Aug. 1949, 216 – 218.

777   HORCASITAS, C. *Special library service to the bilingual patients in the Veterans Administration hospital, Albuquerque, New Mexico, March 1949*. Thesis (A.M.) University of Denver, 1949. 55 pp. typewritten.

778   Hospital librarian in the children's ward: the needs of the child patient. *Book Trolley*, 5 Dec. 1949, 387 – 389.

779   Hospital libraries in Paris. *Book Trolley*, 5 Jan. 1949, 340 – 342.

780   International congress on mental health: cultural activities with mental hospital patients. *Book Trolley*, 5 Jan. 1949, 346 – 347.

781   KERSLAKE, J. F. Patient looks at the library trolley. *Book Trolley*, 5 Aug. 1949, 377 – 378.

782   LATINI, L. A. Cooperative library service for the hospital. *Cath. Libr. Wld.*, 20 April 1949, 206 – 208.

783   LIBRARY ASSOCIATION. Council notes [memorandum to the Ministry of Health on hospital library services]. *Libr. Ass. Rec.*, 51 (1) Jan. 1949, 16 – 17.

784   LIBRARY ASSOCIATION. Council notes [report of the deputation to the Ministry of Health on the provision of hospital libraries]. *Libr. Ass. Rec.*, 51 (3) March 1949, 79.

785   LIBRARY ASSOCIATION. *Papers and summaries of discussions at the Eastbourne conference, 23rd to 27th May, 1949.* London, LA, 1949, 55 – 63.

786   Michigan cares for her children. *Book Trolley*, 5 Dec. 1949, 394 – 396.

787   NIELSEN, Helga. På kursus for hospitalsbibliotekarer i Minnesota. [Courses for hospital librarians in Minnesota.] *Bibliotekaren*, 11 (4/5) 1949, 73 – 76.

788   PETERSON, M. V. *Use of books in the rehabilitation of amputees in military and veterans administration hospitals.* Thesis (A.M.) University of Denver, 1949. 106 pp.

789   ROSS, James. Southmead hospital library, Bristol. *Libr. Ass. Rec.*, 51 (11) Nov. 1949, 345 – 347.

790   ST. JOHN, F. R. Personality of library service. *Bull. Med. Libr. Ass.*, 37 April 1949, 164 – 167.

791   La situation des bibliothèques d'hôpitaux en Suisse en 1949. [Hospital libraries in Switzerland in 1949.] *In*: *Actes du Comité International des Bibliothèques XIV, 15me session Bâle, 1949.* La Haye, Martinus Nijhoff, 1949, Annexe XXVI, 125.

792   SOUTHERDEN, M. G. H. Public libraries and the provision of libraries in hospitals. *In*: Library Association. *Papers and summaries of discussions at the Eastbourne conference, 23rd to 27th May 1949.* London, LA, 1949, 55 – 63.

793   Southmead hospital library, Bristol. *Publishers Circular*, 163 June 18 1949, 621 – 622.

794   SULLIVAN, Margaret R. The lovely lady and the red basket. *Wilson Libr. Bull.*, 23 (10) June 1949, 780 – 781, 783.

795   Syke kan bli friskere av å lese. [Reading makes sick people better.] *Bok og Bibliotek*, 16 Dec. 1949, 338 – 340.

796   THORNTON, John L. Libraries in the hospital. *Library World*, 51 March 1949, 175 – 176.

797   YAST, H. T. Illinois hospital libraries. *Illinois Library Association Record*, 3 Sept. 1949, 11 – 14.

798   YOCKEY, R. M. *Winged bequest: an account of the Cleveland public library's service to the incapacitated.* Thesis (M.S.L.S.) Western Reserve University, 1949. 83 pp.

195?

799   ST. JOHN AND RED CROSS HOSPITAL LIBRARY DEPARTMENT. *A handbook for hospital librarians.* [London.] St. John & Red Cross [195 ?]. 16 pp.

1950

800 BAATZ, Wilmer H. Hospital library administration in neuropsychiatric hospitals of the Veterans Administration. *Spec. Libr.*, 41 (8) Oct. 1950, 284 – 288.

801 BIERMANN, W. Verwaltung einer Krankenhausbüchereie. [The administration of a hospital library.] *Anstalts – Umschau*, 19 (2) Feb. 1950, 24 – 26.

802 BISHOP, W. J. The future of the hospital library. *Hospital and Social Service Journal*, 60 June 23 1950, 695 – 696.

803 Books for the blind. *Book Trolley*, 6 (1) Spring 1950, 19 – 24.

804 BROWN, S. J. M. Hospital library service. *Irish Library Bulletin*, 11 Dec. 1950, 208 – 210.

805 CARDINAL, J. Ziekenhuisbibliotheken in Belgie. [Hospital libraries in Belgium.] *Bibliotheekgids*, 26 Jan./Feb. 1950, 4 – 6.

806 CLARK, Robert S. *Books and reading for the blind.* London, LA, 1950. 40 pp. (LA pamphlet, 1).

807 COATES, Joyce L. Books and mental health. *Libr. Ass. Rec.*, 52 (1) Jan. 1950, 8 – 10.

808 COATES, Joyce [L.] Books in mental illness. *Book Trolley*, 6 (3) Autumn 1950, 50 – 55.

809 CONNELL, S. M. Magic carpets; or escape through travel books. *Book Trolley*, 6 Spring 1950, 15 – 17.

810 CONNELL, S. M. The reading interests of hospitalized veterans. *Spec. Libr.*, 41 (8) Oct. 1950, 289 – 290, 302 – 303.
LSA 1950/510

811 DELISLE, M. M., *sister. Analysis of some of the problems of book selection for the Catholic hospital library, with a classified and annotated bibliography.* Thesis (M.S.L.S.) Catholic University of America, 1950. 126 pp. typewritten.

812 DOUGLASS, H. Library service in a mental hospital. *Book Trolley*, 6 (3) Autumn 1950, 55 – 56.
LSA 1951/722

813 GREAT BRITAIN. MINISTRY OF HEALTH. *Hospital libraries for patients.* London, The Ministry, 1950. (R.H.B. (50) 32.)

814 GUILD OF HOSPITAL LIBRARIANS. [Conference, 1950, London.] *Book Trolley*, 6 Summer 1950, 40 – 42.

815 HILL, William. Books and infectious diseases. *Libr. Ass. Rec.*, 52 (5) May 1950, 144 – 146.
LSA 1950/139

816 HILLSON, Norman. Curing through reading. *Wilson Libr. Bull.*, 25 (4) Dec. 1950, 316 – 317.
LSA 1950/508

817 HILLSON, Norman. The kinder world of books assists in rehabilitation [for iron lung patients]. *Canadian Hospital*, 27 Sept. 1950, 60+.

818 HIRSCH, Lore. How a doctor uses books. *Libr. J.*, 75 Dec. 1 1950, 2046 – 2049.

819 Hospital libraries for patients. *Libr. Ass. Rec.*, 52 (7) July 1950, 237 – 238.

820 HOUNSOME, J. Mental hospital libraries. *Book Trolley*, 6 (3) Autumn 1950, 56 – 59.

821 IRVING, Jean S. Bibliotherapy at Essondale. *Pacific Northwest Library Association Quarterly*, 14 April 1950, 105 – 106.

822 IRVING, Jean S. New library for the provincial mental hospital. [Essondale BC.] *British Columbia Library Association Bulletin*, Jan. 1950; also in *Book Trolley*, 6 (1) Spring 1950, 17 – 19.
     LSA 1950/289

823 JAMIESON, John. *Books for the army: the army library service in the second world war.* New York, Columbia U.P., 1950, 80 – 88.

824 JENSEN, K. M. Sygehusbibliotekarernes uddannelse. [Training of hospital librarians.] *In: Biblioteket och vi.* Svenska Folkebibliotekarieföreningen, 1950, 103 – 108.

825 LONG, D. E. But this job has everything. *Wilson Libr. Bull.*, 25 Sept. 1950, 73 – 74.

826 MCALISTER, Clifton. Bibliotherapy: the nurse and the librarian working together can make the library a valuable therapeutic tool. *American Journal of Nursing*, 50 June 1950, 356 – 357.

827 MCCORKLE, Ruth. Bedside bookcase. *American Journal of Nursing*, 50 Sept. 1950, 630.

828 MCNUTT, Ruth J. Librarians bring projected books to rescue of patients. *Hospital Management*, 69 March 1950, 74.

829 POINDRON, P. Bibliothèques de malades. [Libraries for the sick.] *Education Nationale*, Dec. 1950, 39.

830 POWELL, J. W. Group reading in mental hospitals. *Psychiatry*, 13 May 1950, 213 – 226.

831 PRZYBYLSKI, F., *father.* Reading: an aid to psychosomatic medicine. *Cath. Libr. Wld.*, 22 Dec. 1950, 72 – 73.

832 SPOHN, A. J. *Crile Veterans Administration hospital library: its past and present activities.* Thesis (M.S.L.S.) Western Reserve University, 1950. 82 pp. typescript.

833 STEIN, E. A. *Bibliotherapy: a discussion of the literature and an annotated bibliography for the librarian.* Thesis (M.S.L.S.) Western Reserve University, 1950. 53 pp. typescript.

834 STUCKEY, Elizabeth C. Librarian in the children's ward. *Book Trolley*, 6 Spring 1950, 2 – 4.

835 SUMNER, J. J. An aid for supine bed patients. *Lancet,* ii Dec. 2 1950, 698.

836 Svenska sjukhusbibliotek, 1948. [Swedish hospital libraries 1948.] *Biblio-teksbladet,* 35 (1) 1950, 4.

837 Svenska sjukhusbibliotek 1949. [Swedish hospital libraries 1949.] *Biblio-teksbladet,* 35 (7) 1950, 347 – 350.

1951

838 ALLSOP, Kathleen M. *A mental hospital library: report of an experiment at Lancaster Moor hospital in 1947 – 49.* London, LA, 1951. 44 pp. (LA pamphlet, 6).

839 ARNOT, Jean F. Institutional library service in New South Wales. *Aust. Libr. J.,* 1 (1) July 1951, 18 – 20. LSA 1951/1155

840 BERGMANN, G. Eigenart und Aufgaben der Krankenhausbücherei. [Origin and purpose of the hospital library.] *Bücherei und Bildung,* 3 1951, 1028 – 1030.

841 BERSET, I. V. The hospital library work in Norway. *In: Actes du Comité International des Bibliothèques XV, 16me session London, 1950.* La Haye, Martinus Nijhoff, 1951, Annexe IX, 68; also in *Book Trolley,* 6 (4 and 5) Winter 1950 and Spring 1951, 74 – 77. LSA 1951/1007

842 BURKET, Rose, R. The patient approach. *Wilson Libr. Bull.,* 25 (6) Feb. 1951, 437 – 439. LSA 1951/724

843 CHANCE, B. Books for the blind. *American Journal of Ophthalmology,* 34 1951, 452 – 453.

844 CONNELL, S. M. On the other side of the trolley: a hospital librarian's experiences as a patient. *Book Trolley,* 6 Winter 1950/Spring 1951, 82 – 84.

845 COOKE, Marian. Children's library in the Hospital for Sick Children (Toronto). *Ontario Library Review,* 35 (3) Aug. 1951, 230 – 231.

846 DUNKEL, Beatrice. Bibliotherapy and the nurse [in a psychiatric hospital]. *Nursing World,* 125 April 1951, 146 – 147.

847 FÉDÉRATION INTERNATIONALE DES ASSOCIATIONS DE BIBLIOTHÉCAIRES. Sous – Commission des Bibliothèques d'Hôpitaux. [Rapport]. *In: Actes du Comité International des Bibliothèques XV, 16me session, London 1950.* La Haye, Martinus Nijhoff, 1951, 31 – 32.

848 FORBES, A. P. *Importance of bibliotherapy in book selection and readers' advisory service in hospital libraries.* Thesis (A.M.L.S.) University of Michigan, 1951. 39 pp.

849 FORSDYKE, John. Microfilms for the disabled. *Book Trolley,* 6 (4 and 5) Winter 1950 and Spring 1951, 67 – 68. LSA 1951/1005

850 GREAT BRITAIN. DEPARTMENT OF HEALTH FOR SCOTLAND. Scottish Health Services Council. *The reception and welfare of in-patients in hospitals.* Edinburgh, HMSO, 1951, paras 34 – 37, supply of books and newspapers.

851   GUILD OF HOSPITAL LIBRARIANS. [Conference, 1951, London.] *Book Trolley*, 6 Summer 1951, 95 – 98.

852   GUNNESS, Virginia. The children's library in the hospital. *American Journal of Nursing*, 51 May 1951, 318 – 319.

853   GYDE-PEDERSEN, Mette. Hospitalsbiblioteksarbejdet jubilerer. [Hospital library work celebrates a jubilee.] *Bogens Verden,* 33 (8) Nov. 15 1951, 400 – 402.

854   HOWARD, A. L. *Evaluation of hospital library service by volunteers.* Thesis (M.S.) Columbia University, 1951. 86 pp. typewritten.

855   KERWIN, P. F. Hospital volunteer. *Cath Libr. Wld.*, 22 May 1951, 246 – 248.

856   LANGE, [   ]. Aus der Arbeit einer Krankenhausbücherei (Köln). [Some of the work of a hospital library.] *Bücherei und Bildung*, 3 (10) Dec. 1951, 1030 – 1031.

857   LORD, E. Bibliotherapy. *Arizona Librarian*, 8 Jan. 1951, 12 – 16.

858   MCFARLAND, John H. Indirect reading guidance. *Wilson Libr. Bull.*, 25 (6) Feb. 1951, 440 – 444.
LSA 1951/725

859   MAHON, S. H. Recent developments in school and hospital libraries. *Library Assistant,* 44 (6) June/July 1951, 85 – 87.
LSA 1951/1209

860   MAHONEY, Anna. Adult education for the ill. *Libr. J.*, 76 (14) Aug. 1951, 1177 – 1180.
LSA 1951/1220

861   MANUCHAROVA, E. V. [A book for the patients.] *Meditsinskaya Sestra*, (5) 1951, 24 – 26. (In Russian.)

862   MOHRHARDT, F. E. Veterans Administration libraries reach from ocean to ocean. *Libr. J.*, 76 July 1951, 1098 – 1103.

863   MOODY, E. P. Books can build a bridge. *ALA Bull.*, 45 Nov. 1951, 344 – 345.

864   MUNCK AF ROSENSCHÖLD, Kerstin. Hospital libraries in Sweden. *In*: *Actes du Comité International des Bibliothèques XV, 16me session London, 1950.* La Haye, Martinus Nijhoff, 1951, Annexe X, 69 – 71; also in *Book Trolley*, 6 (4 and 5) Winter 1950 and Spring 1951, 74 – 77.
LSA 1951/1008

865   NIELSEN, Helga. Hospital libraries in Denmark. *In*: *Actes du Comité International des Bibliothèques XV, 16me session London, 1950.* La Haye, Martinus Nijhoff, 1951, Annexe VIII, 65 – 67; also in *Book Trolley*, 6 (4 and 5) Winter 1950 and Spring 1951, 68 – 72.
LSA 1951/1006

866   NYQUIST, Roy H. *and* CLIFTON, E. Over-bed reading device. *Archives of Physical Medicine*, 32 Sept. 1951, 595 – 597.

867   PATTERSON, Donald. National conference on library service for the blind. *Library of Congress Information Bulletin*, 10 (48) Nov. 26 1951, 6 – 8.
LSA 1952/2181

868 PETERS, I. Krankenhausbüchereien. [Hospital libraries.] *Kulturarbeit,* 3 (5) 1951, 110 – 112.

869 SEVERIN, V. Bibliotechnaîa rabota sredi slepykh. [Library work among the blind.] *Bibliotekar'*, Sept. 1951, 36 – 38.
LSA 1952/2391

870 Sykehusbiblioteker. [Hospital libraries.] *Bok og Bibliotek,* 18 Feb. 1951, 27 – 28.

871 TAYLOR, Nettie B. *and* ROBINSON, G. Canby. How a library service grew. *Bulletin of the National Tuberculosis Association,* 37 July 1951, 103 – 104.

872 THORNTON, John L. Hospital libraries. *Libr. Ass. Rec.,* 53 (9) Sept. 1951, 284 – 288.

873 VALLERY-RODOT, P. Avec les Goncourt dans les hôpitaux de Paris. *Presse Médicale,* 59 1951, 1138 – 1139.

874 WALLACE, Margaret L. Hospital library service by public library. *Book Trolley,* 6 (4 and 5) Winter 1950 and Spring 1951, 77 – 81.
LSA 1951/1010

875 WILLIAMS, M. J. Storyland on the ceiling (projected books for children). *Crippled Child,* 29 Aug. 1951, 8+.

876 WITH, Torben K. Periskopbriller: en hjælp til læsning i liggende stilling. [Periscope glasses a help for reading while lying on one's back.] *Ugeskrift for Læger,* 113 1951, 1705 – 1706.

1952

877 ARBORELIUS, Brita. Verksamhet vid sjukhusbibliotek. [Hospital library work.] *Biblioteksbladet,* 37 (7), 1952, 300 – 306; English summary, 320.
LSA 1952/2179

878 BAILEY, D. H. Hospital libraries in Britain under the National Health Service scheme. *Cath. Libr. Wld.,* 23 Jan. 1952, 111 – 113.

879 BARRY, James, Presidential address. *Leabharlann,* 10 (6) Dec. 1952, 169 – 173.
LSA 1953/2479

880 BERTELSEN, Eli. Biblioteks – og studiekredsarbejde på sindssygehospitalet. [Library and study circle work at the mental hospital.] *Bibliotekaren,* 14 (1) 1952, 9 –14.

881 Books infected by scarlet-fever patients (note). *Lancet,* ii Oct. 18 1952, 783 – 784; correspondence, Nov. 8 1952, 936; Nov. 29 1952, 1085.

882 CLOKE, Joan. Hospital library service. *Hospital,* London, 48 (4) April 1952, 269 – 274.

883 FENWICK, Helen. Hospital library service in a King country town. *New Zealand Libraries,* 15 (2) March 1952, 38 – 41.

884 FORSDYKE, J. Microfilms for the disabled. *Aslib. Proc.,* 4 (1) Feb. 1952, 39 – 40.
LSA 1952/1995

885 GILKISON, E. E. Salesmanship with a book cart. *ALA Hospital Book Guide*, 13 Nov. 1952, 111 – 113.

886 GUILD OF HOSPITAL LIBRARIANS. Conference on mental hospital libraries, 23 Jan. 1952. *Book Trolley*, 6 Spring/Summer 1952, 128 – 132.

887 HANDEL, R. S. *Library service to the blind.* Thesis (M.L.S.) Pratt Institute Library School, 1952. 55 pp.

888 JENSEN, Frode. Et biblioteksarbejde blandt psykopater. [Library work amongst psychopaths.] *Bogens Verden*, 34 (3) April 1 1952, 126 – 130.

889 JONES, L. E. Veterans Administration hospital library. *Missouri Library Association Quarterly*, 13 Sept. 1952, 67 – 70.

890 KILDAL, Arne. Pasientbiblioteker ved sykehusene. [Libraries for patients in hospital.] *Bok og Bibliotek*, 19 (3) June 1952, 176 – 183.
LSA 1952/1963

891 LOCKETT, W. J. Optical and other aids for recumbent patients. *BRA Review, Journal of the British Rheumatic Association*, 1 (6) May 1952, 178 – 179.
LSA 1952/1964

892 MCFARLAND, John H. A method of bibliotherapy. *American Journal of Occupational Therapy*, 6 March/April 1952, 66+.

893 MARKUS, Florence. *Analysis of reading interests of tuberculous veterans at Wood, Wisconsin, for the period Oct. 1 1950 to Oct. 1 1951.* Thesis (M.S.L.S.) Western Reserve University, 1952, 60 pp.

894 MAYDEN, Priscilla M. What shall the psychiatric patient read? *American Journal of Nursing*, 52 Feb. 1952, 192 – 193.

895 MERI, Sirkka-Liisa. Kokemuksia sairaalakirjastotyösta. [Experiences of hospital library work.] *Kirjastolehti*, 45 (4) April 1952, 74 – 76; 45 (5) May/June 1952, 102 – 104.
LSA 1952/2392

896 MOODY, E. P. Books bring hope for mental patients . . . *Libr. J.*, 77 March 1 1952, 387 – 392.

897 NÄRHI, Mauri K. Kirjat ja virkailijat. [Books and library staff.] *Kirjastolehti*, 45 (1) Jan. 1952, 13 – 14.
LSA 1952/1925

898 NEELAMEGHAN, A. Adequate library service in Indian hospitals; a very real necessity. *Indian Librarian*, 7 Dec. 1952, 77 – 81.

899 NEUMAN, S. Hospital's cinderella (patients' library). *Southern Hospitals*, 20 Feb. 1952, 40 – 42.

900 NIEUWENBORGH, P. van. Lectuur voor de blinden. [Reading matter for the blind.] *Bibliotheekgids*, 28 Nov./Dec. 1952, 113 – 115.

901 NISTRI, M. [Elements of bibliotherapy.] *Rassegna di Studi Psichiatrici* (Ospedale Psichiatrico di S. Niccolo, Siena), 41 1952, 209 – 216.

902 Objectives and standards for patients' libraries. *Bull. Med. Libr. Ass.*, 40 Oct. 1952, 389 – 394.

903 SEVRĪUGINA, E. Zaochnyĭ abonament dlĭa slepykh. [Non-resident borrowing for blind people.] *Bibliotekar'*, Aug. 1952, 43 – 44.

904 SOUTHERDEN, Mildred G. H. Libraries in mental hospitals. *Book Trolley*, 6 (8) Spring/Summer 1952, 133 – 140.
LSA 1952/2180

905 STONE, J. E. Picture libraries in hospitals. *Canadian Hospital*, 29 June 1952, 74.

906 THOMPSON, V. A. *Library service to children hospitalized in Philadelphia during 1952*. Thesis (M.S.L.S.) Drexel Institute of Technology, 1952. 49 pp. typewritten.

907 TIGHE, Joan. Advice to readers and bibliotherapy. *Aust. Libr. J.*, 1 July 1952, 112 – 115.

908 UNITED STATES. VETERANS ADMINISTRATION. *The librarian in the Veterans Administration*. Washington DC, U.S. G.P.O., 1952. (VA pamphlet, 5 – 14.)

909 UNITED STATES. VETERANS ADMINISTRATION. Medical and General Reference Library. *Bibliotherapy: a bibliography 1900 – 1952*. Washington DC, VA, 1952. 18 pp.

910 WOOD, J. E. The South African Library for the Blind, Grahamstown, C.P. *S. Afr. Lib.*, 20 (1) July 1952, 15 – 17.
LSA 1952/2183

1953

911 AMERICAN LIBRARY ASSOCIATION. Hospital Libraries Division. *Hospital libraries objectives and standards*. Chicago, *ALA*, 1953. 19 pp.

912 CROIX ROUGE DE BELGIQUE. Conseil National des Bibliothèques d'Hôpitaux et de Sanatoriums. Rapport général des activités pendant l'exercice 1952. *In*: *Actes du Conseil de la Fiab XVIII, 19me session Vienne, 1953*. La Haye, Martinus Nijhoff, 1953, Annexe XVI, 138 – 141.

913 EATON, E. S. *Free-reading use of the library by patients in a veterans hospital*. Thesis (M.A.) University of Chicago, 1953. 85 pp. typewritten.

914 EATON, E. S. Library program furthers adjustment of blind patients. *Hospitals*, Chicago, 27 Jan. 1953, 65 – 66.

915 FÉDÉRATION INTERNATIONALE DES ASSOCIATIONS DE BIBLIOTHÉCAIRES. Sous – Commission Jumelée de Bibliothèques d'Hôpitaux. [Rapport par Mme. Schmid-Schädelin.] *In*: *Actes du Comité International des Bibliothèques, XVII, 18me session Copenhagen, 1952*. La Haye, Martinus Nijhoff, 1953, 42.

916 FÉDÉRATION INTERNATIONALE DES ASSOCIATIONS DE BIBLIOTHÉCAIRES. Sous – Commission des Bibliothèques d'Hôpitaux. Rapport par P. Poindron. *In*: *Actes du Comité International des Bibliothèques XVII, 18me session Copenhagen, 1952*. La Haye, Martinus Nijhoff, 1953, Annexe IV, 79.

917 FÉDÉRATION INTERNATIONALE DES ASSOCIATIONS DE BIBLIOTHÉCAIRES. Commission Jumelée des Bibliothèques d'Hôpitaux. Report of joint Committee, presented by Mme. Schmid-Schädelin. *In*: *Actes du Conseil de la Fiab XVIII, 19me session Vienne, 1953*. La Haye, Martinus Nijhoff, 1953, 45 – 47.

918 FLANDORF, Vera S. Getting well with books. *Libr. J.*, 78 (8) April 15 1953, 651 – 655.

919 GATLIFF, J. W. *Study of library service in a selected group of general hospitals in the United States.* Thesis, Atlanta University, 1953. 66 pp. typewritten.

920 HIRSCH, Lore. Book service to patients. *Wilson Libr. Bull.*, 27 April 1953, 634 – 639.

921 Hospital libraries: report of a meeting of LA Medical Section [discussion of patients' libraries]. *Lancet,* i Jan. 3 1953, 49 – 50.

922 MCKENNA, C. E. *Patients' libraries in Pittsburgh hospitals.* Thesis (M.L.S.) Carnegie Institute of Technology, 1953. 63 pp. typewritten.

923 MARTIN, W. A. *Devices to encourage the use of the library in the Veterans Administration hospital.* Thesis (M.S.) Kansas State Teachers College, 1953. 48 pp. typewritten.

924 MOHRHARDT, F. E. Service to those who served. *Wilson Libr. Bull.*, 27 June 1953, 833 – 835.

925 MOORE, Sheila. The therapy of books: library service at St. Thomas' Hospital. *Hospital,* London, 49 (10) Oct. 1953, 559 – 563.

926 NEELAMEGHAN, A. Book selection for patients. *Abgila,* 3 June 1953, B67 – 72.

927 PRESAR, M. A. *Methods of service to hospitals by public libraries in Indiana, Michigan and Ohio.* Thesis (M.S.L.S.) Drexel Institute of Technology, 1953. 68 pp.

928 St. John and Red Cross hospital libraries. *In: Actes du Conseil de la Fiab XVIII, 19me session Vienne, 1953.* La Haye, Martinus Nijhoff, 1953, Annexe XXVII, 175.

929 SCHMID-SCHÄDELIN, I. Bericht der Vereinigung Schweizerischer Krankenhaus Bibliotheken, 1952. [Report of the Association of Swiss Hospital Libraries, 1952.] *In: Actes du Comité International des Bibliothèques XVII, 18me session Copenhagen, 1952.* La Haye, Martinus Nijhoff, 1953, Annexe XXXVII, 196 – 197.

930 STEFFENS, Magda. En bibliotekars arbeide ved et dansk sinnsykehospital. [A librarian's work in a Danish psychiatric hospital viewed by a Norwegian librarian.] *Bok og Bibliotek,* 20 July 1953, 182 – 184.

931 Sykehusbibliotekene. [Hospital libraries.] *Bok og Bibliotek,* 20 Sept. 1953, 222 – 224.

932 THOMPSON, Alice M. C. *The patients' library, past, present and future.* Essay no. 259 accepted for the Library Association final exam. 1953, typescript.

933 TREUTWEIN, I. Die Einrichtung einer Krankenbücherei. [Setting up a hospital library.] *Anstalts – Umschau,* 22 (5) May 1953, 143 – 145.

1954

934 BAKER, M. C. Role of volunteer hospital librarian. *Libr. J.*, 79 May 15 1954, 870 – 872.

935 BARKER, Gilbert W. The St. John and British Red Cross hospital library. [Proceedings of the first international congress on medical librarianship, London, 20 – 25 July 1953.] *Libri*, 3 1954, 393 – 400.

936 BURSINGER, Bess C. *and* KENYON, Xena. Neuro-psychiatric hospital library. *Libr. J.*, 79 (20) Nov. 15 1954, 2153 – 2155.
LSA 1955/4283

937 Det første kurs for pasientbibliotekarer. [The first course for patients' librarians.] *Bok og Bibliotek*, 21 July 1954, 189 – 190.

938 GERMAINE. M. Hospital library service. *Cath. Libr. Wld.*, 25 April 1954, 218 – 222.

939 GREAT BRITAIN. MINISTRY OF HEALTH. *Hospital libraries for patients*. London, The Ministry, 1954. (H.M. (54) 96.)

940 HANNIGAN, M. C. Hospital-wide group bibliotherapy program. *Bookmark*, 13 June 1954, 203 – 210.

941 JOHNS, Helen. Readers without sight. *Libr. J.*, 79 (17) Oct. 1 1954, 1715 – 1718.
LSA 1955/4375

942 JORDAN, D. Work in a hospital library. *Wessex Bookman*, 4 (2) Winter 1954, 8 – 9.

943 KAUPPI, Hilkka. Kirjastoterapiaa mielisairaalassa. [Bibliotherapy in a mental hospital.] *Kirjastolehti*, 47 (1 – 3) Jan. – March 1954, 2 – 8, 30 – 32, 54 – 57; English summary, (4) April, 93.
LSA 1954/3880

944 KNIBBE, Werner. Noch einmal Patientenbücherei. [The patients' library once more.] *Bibliothekar*, 8 (23/24) 1954, 714 – 715.

945 KNOX, J. B. City hospital library service. *Massachusetts Library Association Bulletin*, 44 Jan. 1954, 23 – 25.

946 MERI, Sirkka-Liisa. Krankenhausbüchereiarbeit in Helsinki. [Hospital library work in Helsinki.] *Bücherei und Bildung*, 6 (7/8) July/Aug. 1954, 675 – 678.

947 MOHRHARDT, F. E. Standards of performance for hospital libraries. *Library Trends*, 2 (3) Jan. 1954, 452 – 462.
LSA 1954/3472

948 NEVERMANN, Charlotte. Mehr Aufmerksamkeit den Heim und Anstaltsbibliotheken. [Further observation on the home and institutional library.] *Bibliothekar*, 8 (7) April 1954, 211 – 212.

949 OATHOUT, Melvin C. Books and mental patients. *Libr. J.*, 79 (5) March 1 1954, 405 – 409.
LSA 1954/3879

950 OATHOUT, Melvin C. Censorship and mental patients. *Library Quarterly*, 24 (1) Jan. 1954, 47 – 53.
LSA 1954/3878

951   RICHARDS, John S. Newest Seattle branch library is also centre for the blind. *Pioneer*, 17 (6) Nov./Dec. 1954, 2 – 5.
LSA 1955/4371

952   ROZENBLUM, S. E. [Bibliotherapy.] *Meditsinskaya Sestra*, (7) 1954, 20 – 24. (In Russian.)

953   SCULLIN, V. Bibliotherapy in mental hospitals. *New York Library Association Bulletin*, 2 June 1954, 42 – 43.

954   SEVERIN, Erik. Läsapparat för sängliggande. [Reading apparatus for bedfast patients.] *Nordisk Medicin*, 52 (49) Dec. 2 1954, 1701 – 1702.

955   SJÖGREN, Hakon. Patients and books: some personal considerations. *Libr. Ass. Rec.*, 56 (9) Sept. 1954, 342 – 346.
LSA 1954/4089

956   SMITH, Elsie P. Without the walls. *Manchester Review*, 7 Winter 1954, 136 – 138.
LSA 1955/4990

957   THOMPSON, Alice M. C. Libraries for patients. *Nursing Times*, 50 March 13 1954, 292 – 293.

958   TONE, M. Hospital story hour. *Libr. J.*, 79 Dec. 15 1954, 7 – 8.

959   ZEMIS, S. Czytelnictwo niedwidomych. [Reading of the blind.] *Bibliotekarz*, 21 Jan. – Feb. 1954, 30 – 31.

1955

960   ANDREASSEN, Johs. Patienter og bøger (Foredrag). [Patients and books (Lecture).] *Bibliotekaren*, 17 (5) 1955, 128 – 134.

961   ANDREWS, Joseph L. *and* STERN, William B. Law books for the blind. *Law Libr. J.*, 48 (2) May 1955, 150 – 154.

962   BARLOW, Vernon. Books for the blind. *British Book News*, (177) May 1955, 959 – 963.
LSA 1955/4502.

963   BASSET, *Mlle. and* HURI, *Mme.* Les bibliothèques d'hôpitaux et la bibliothèque universitaire centrale des étudiants malades. *In*: *Congrès International des Bibliothèques et des Centres de Documentation, Bruxelles, 11 – 18 Sept. 1955* . . . La Haye, Martinus Nijhoff, 1955, vol. IIA Communications, 270 – 273.

964   Bibliothèques d'hôpitaux. Hospital libraries. *In*: *Congrès International des Bibliothèques et des Centres de Documentation, Bruxelles, 11 – 18 Sept. 1955* . . . La Haye, Martinus Nijhoff, 1955, vol. III Proceedings, 116 – 120.

965   BLOMQUIST, H. Patient libraries in our state hospitals and special schools. *Texas Libraries*, 17 Jan. 1955, 3 – 8+.

966   BURKET, R. R. When books are therapy. *Wilson Libr. Bull.*, 29 Feb. 1955, 450 – 452.

967   CROIX ROUGE DE BELGIQUE. Conseil National des Bibliothèques d'Hôpitaux et
de Sanatoriums. Activités pendant l'exercice 1952. *In: Actes du Conseil de la
Fiab XIX, 20me session Zagreb, 1954.* La Haye, Martinus Nijhoff, 1955, Annexe
XIX, 144 – 145.

968   ELY, V. Right book for the right patient. *Wilson Libr. Bull.*, 29 Feb. 1955,
453 – 458.

969   ENGELHARDT, Dora. Zum Thema Krankenhausbücherei. [On the subject of
the hospital library.] *Das Krankenhaus*, 47 (1) Jan. 1955, 18 – 19.

970   FÉDÉRATION INTERNATIONALE DES ASSOCIATIONS DE BIBLIOTHÉCAIRES. Commission Jumelée des Bibliothèques d'Hôpitaux. [Report]. *In: Actes du Conseil
de la Fiab XIX, 20me session Zagreb, 1954.* La Haye, Martinus Nijhoff, 1955,
64 – 65.

971   FRASER, Alex W. A mental hospital library. *North Western Newsletter* (Library
Assoc. N.W. Branch), (32) March 1955, 1 – 2.

972   FRÖHLICH, Herta. Aus der Arbeit der Deutschen Zentralbücherei für Blinde.
[The work of the German Central Library for the Blind.] *Bibliothekar*, 9 (8)
Aug. 1955, 488 – 489.
LSA 1955/4890

973   HAGGERTY, Charles E. Our responsibility to older people. *Illinois Libraries*,
37 (5) May 1955, 132 – 136.
LSA 1955/4992

974   HANNAH, R. G. Navy bibliotherapy: experiments in the use of books carried
out at the naval hospital, Portsmouth, Virginia. 1. Library programs. *Libr. J.*,
80 (10) May 15 1955, 1171 – 1173.

975   HANNIGAN, M. C. Library service to neuropsychiatric patients. *In: Congrès
International des Bibliothèques et des Centres de Documentation, Bruxelles, 11 – 18
Sept. 1955* . . . La Haye, Martinus Nijhoff, 1955, vol. IIA Communications,
275 – 280.

976   JANSSEN, C. E. Bibliothèques d'hôpitaux: communication du CNBHS. *In:
Congrès International des Bibliothèques et des Centres de Documentation, Bruxelles,
11 – 18 Sept. 1955* . . . La Haye, Martinus Nijhoff, 1955, vol. IIA Communications, 273 – 275.

977   KEYES, A. W. Volunteers serve the patients' library. (University Hospital, Ann
Arbor.) *Hospitals*, Chicago, 29 (10) Oct. 1955, 97 – 100.

978   KING, J. E. Library service for shut-ins. *Ontario Library Review*, 39 (3) Aug.
1955, 175.

979   MCCUAIG, Margaret E. Patients and books. *Canadian Hospital*, 32 Jan. 1955,
37 – 39.

980   MURISON, W. J. *The public library* . . . London, Harrap, 1955, 191 – 195.

981   New Swedish reading apparatus: biblioscope. *Hospital*, London, 51 Aug.
1955, 576 – 577; also in *Canadian Medical Association Journal*, 73 Aug. 15 1955,
292.

982 RIEMSDIJK, G. A. van. De bemolienissen van de O.L.B. met de lectuurvoorziening voor de blinden en de problemen met betrekking tot het 'gesproken boek'. [The difficulties of the public library in providing reading matter for the blind and the problems concerning the 'talking book'.] *Bibliotheekgids*, 31 (2) March/April 1955, 23 – 30.
LSA 1955/4963

983 ROCHE, M. W. My patrons are patients. *California Librarian*, 16 Jan. 1955, 108 – 110+.

984 SCHMID-SCHÄDELIN, I. Bericht der Vereinigung Schweizerischer Krankenhausbibliotheken, 1953 – 1954. [Report of the Association of Swiss Hospital Libraries, 1953 – 1954.] *In: Actes du Conseil de la Fiab XIX, 20me session Zagreb, 1954.* La Haye, Martinus Nijhoff, 1955, Annexe XXXVI, 192.

985 SCHMID-SCHÄDELIN, I. Bibliothèques d'hôpitaux. *In: Congrès International des Bibliothèques et des Centres de Documentation, Bruxelles, 11 – 18 Sept. 1955 . . .* La Haye, Martinus Nijhoff, 1955, vol. I Rapports préliminaires, 141 – 143.

986 SHAW, Leonard J. The hospital library service in the borough of Leyton. *Hospital*, London, 51 (12) Dec. 1955, 819 – 824.

987 SIROVS, J. Red Cross hospital libraries in Queensland. *Aust. Libr. J.*, 4 (2) April 1955, 66 – 70.
LSA 1955/4908

988 SPÅNGBERG, M. Göteborgs sjukhusbibliotek. [Gothenburg hospital library.] *Biblioteksbladet*, 40 (3) 1955, 116 – 119.

989 Synpunkter på sjukhusbiblioteksarbete. [Views on hospital libraries.] *Biblioteksbladet*, 40 (10) 1955, 502 – 503.

990 TEWS, R. M. Organizing the hospital library II. The patients' library. *In: Congrès International des Bibliothèques et des Centres de Documentation, Bruxelles, 11 – 18 Sept. 1955 . . .* La Haye, Martinus Nijhoff, 1955, vol. IIA Communications, 286 – 292.

991 UNDERWOOD, Mary Beth. Navy bibliotherapy: experiments in the use of books carried out at the naval hospital, Portsmouth, Virginia. 2. Experiment in group reading. *Libr. J.*, 80 (10) May 15, 1955, 1173 – 1176.

992 UNITED STATES. VETERANS ADMINISTRATION. Medical and General Reference Library. *Bibliotherapy: a bibliography. Supplemental list, 1955.* Washington, Veterans Administration, 1955.

993 WAHROW, L. A. Hospital library service to psychiatric patients. *American Journal of Occupational Therapy*, 9 Nov./Dec. 1955, 268 – 269.

994 WALZ, Hans. Die Krankenhausbücherei. [The hospital library.] *Der Krankenhausarzt*, 28 (12) Dec. 1955, 286 – 288; 29 1956, 10 – 15.

1956

995 AMERICAN LIBRARY ASSOCIATION. Association of Hospital and Institution Libraries. Bibliotherapy Committee. Survey of hospital library activities in reading guidance and bibliotherapy. *ALA Hospital Book Guide*, 17 April 1956, 65 – 66.

996   ARNOT, J. F. Healing through reading. *Royal Prince Alfred Hospital Journal*, Sydney, 55 March 1956, 16 – 17.

997   BAGGELARR, A. Cultureel werk voor bejaarden. [Cultural work for the aged.] *Volksopvoeding*, 5 (6) Dec. 1956, 371 – 373.

998   BLACKSHEAR, Orilla T. Public library serves the aging. *Wisconsin Library Bulletin*, 52 (2) March/April 1956, 60 – 65.

999   Books for the bedside. *Mississippi Library News*, 20 June 1956, 71 – 72.

1000 Books for the sick. *Nursing Times*, 52 Dec. 28 1956, 1343 – 1347.

1001 CANTRELL, C. H. Sadie P. Delaney: bibliotherapist and librarian. *Southeastern Librarian*, 6 Fall 1956, 105 – 109.
      LSA 1956/6545

1002 CROIX ROUGE DE BELGIQUE. Conseil National des Bibliothèques d'Hôpitaux et de Sanatoriums. Activités pendant l'exercice 1954. *In*: *Actes du Conseil de la Fiab XX, 21e session Bruxelles, 1955*. La Haye, Martinus Nijhoff, 1956, Annexe VIII, 95.

1003 EUREN, H. R. Saint Angsvar hospital service. *Minnesota Libraries*, 18 June 1956, 175 – 176.

1004 FLANDORF, Vera S. Books to help children adjust to a hospital situation. *ALA Hospital Book Guide*, 17 Feb. 1956, 24 – 29.

1005 FLANDORF, Vera S. Reading for the hospitalized child. *Hospital Management*, Chicago, 81 (1) Jan. 1956, 45 +.

1006 GRANNIS, Florence. Statewide financial support for Seattle's regional library for the blind. *Wilson Libr. Bull.*, 30 (9) May 1956, 700 – 701.
      LSA 1956/6149

1007 HANNIGAN, Margaret C. Bibliotherapy: its part in library service. *Bookmark*, 15 March 1956, 127 – 133.

1008 HIRSCH, Lore. Bibliotherapy with neuropsychiatric patients. (Individual and group therapy.) *ALA Hospital Book Guide*, 17 (5) May 1956, 87 – 93; 17 (6) June 1956, 111 – 117.
      LSA 1956/6061

1009 JANSSEN, C. E. Belgian Red Cross hospital libraries. *Unesco Bull. Libr.*, 10 (4) April 1956, 76 – 79.
      LSA 1956/6048

1010 JENSEN, Karen Margrethe. Samarbejde mellem læge beskæftigelsesterapeut og bibliotekar. [Co-operation between doctor, occupational therapist and librarian.] *Bibliothekaren*, 18 (5) 1956, 133 – 135.
      LSA 1957/6619

1011 JOHNSON, C. W. *Study of library service in a selected group of medium-sized general hospitals in the United States*. Thesis (M.S.L.S.) Atlanta University, 1956. 50 pp.

1012 LATTANZI, Angela Daneu. Le biblioteche ospedaliere nella Sicilia occidentale. [Hospital libraries in Western Sicily.] *Accademie e Biblioteche d'Italia*, 24 July/Dec. 1956, 293 – 295.

1013 LATTANZI, Angela Daneu. Per una organizzazione delle biblioteche ospedaliere in Sicilia. [Hospital libraries in Sicily.] *In*: *1 Convegno regionale delle biblioteche, Palermo, 1955*. Palermo, 1956, 37 – 38.

1014 LESZCZYŃSKI, J. Książka wśród chorych. [Books for the sick.] *Bibliotekarz*, 33 Jan. 1956, 7 – 17.

1015 MCDANIEL, W. B. Bibliotherapy some historical and contemporary aspects. *ALA Bull.*, 50 Oct. 1956, 584 – 589.

1016 MCPEAKE, J. G. Chester hospitals library service: an experiment in co-operation. *North Western Newsletter*, (42) Nov. 1956, 1 – 2. LSA 1956/6444

1017 MAHOUT, *Mme*. Les bibliothèques pour aveugles. [Libraries for the blind.] *Bull. Bib. Fr.*, 1 (1) Jan. 1956, 27 – 37. LSA 1956/5750

1018 MERI, Sirkka-Liisa. Parantava kirja. [The book as a remedy.] *Kirjastolehti*, 49 (1) Jan. 1956, 13 – 15. LSA 1956/5753

1019 METHVEN, M. L. Fingers and ears to see. *Minnesota Libraries*, 18 (7) Sept. 1956, 209 – 210. LSA 1956/6449

1020 MUNFORD, W. A. Library services for the physically handicapped. *Libr. Ass. Rec.*, 58 (7) July 1956, 251 – 259. LSA 1956/6148

1021 NUNN, M. L. *The library as a therapeutic agency in the Veterans Administration Hospital at West Los Angeles and Sepulveda: a report presented to the School of Library Science, University of Southern California*, typescript, 1956. 63 pp.

1022 Obrazovanje pokretnih bolničkih biblioteka u N R Srbiji. [Organisation of travelling hospital libraries in the National Serbian Republic.] *Bibliotekar* (Belgrade) 8 Jan./May 1956, 112 – 116.

1023 RUBBENS-FRANKEN, E. Boeken, bejaarden, bibliotheken II. De betekenis van het brailleschrift voor slechtziende bejaarden. [Books, old people, libraries. II. The significance of braille for old people with bad sight.] *Onze Bejaarden*, 11 (6) June 1956, 80 – 81.

1024 RYDBERG, B. Det 2. nordiske sykehusbibliotekarkurs i Stockholm. [The second Scandinavian hospital library course in Stockholm.] *Bok og Bibliotek*, 23 Sept. 1956, 218 – 222.

1025 SAARNIO, Lauri. Sairaalakirjastojen psykiatrisesta merkityksestä. [The psychiatric role played by hospital libraries.] *Kirjastolehti*, 49 (10) Dec. 1956, 230 – 233; English summary, 254. LSA 1957/6928

1026 SCHUELLER, H. Wirkungsmöglichkeit der Krankenhausbücherei. [Potentialities for the smooth-running of the hospital library.] *Anstalts – Umschau*, 25 (3) March 1956, 130 – 133.

1027 SHOWELL, G. F. G. A new hospital library. (Saxondale Hospital, Radcliffe, Nottinghamshire.) *Hospital*, London, 56 (6) June 1956, 319 – 322.

1028 STUBKJAER, Myrtle. Institutions and their libraries . . . how they grew. *Minnesota Libraries*, 18 (7) Sept. 1956, 197 – 203.
LSA 1956/6448

1029 THIEKÖTTER, Hans. 'Das sprechende Buch' hilft den Blinden: zur Errichtung der Blindenhörbücherei Nordrhein-Westfalen e.v. zu Münster. [The talking-book helps the blind: the establishment of the talking book library for the blind in North Rhine, Westphalia.] *Kulturarbeit*, 8 (6) 1956, 118 – 119.
LSA 1956/6147

1030 TICKNOR, William E. Books in the fight against tuberculosis. *Libr. J.*, 81 (19) Nov. 1 1956, 2499 – 2502.
LSA 1956/6445

1031 TUCKER, W. B. How reading contributes to the treatment of the TB patient. *ALA Hospital Book Guide*, 17 Jan. 1956, 3 – 4.

1032 YAST, Helen. Co-operation with hospital libraries. *Illinois Libraries*, 38 (2) Feb. 1956, 35 – 37.
LSA 1956/5754

1957

1033 AMERICAN LIBRARY ASSOCIATION. Association of Hospital and Institution Libraries. Bibliotherapy Committee. [Bibliotherapy questionnaire.] *ALA Hospital Book Guide*, 18 May 1957, 94 – 95.

1034 BURKET, R. R. Choosing books for the ill. *Today's Health*, 35 May 1957, 34 – 36.

1035 COPENHAVER, Margaret Sue. The school library and the handicapped in Richmond, Virginia elementary schools. *School Libraries*, 6 (4) May 1957, 14 – 16.
LSA 1957/7267

1036 CORY, Patricia B. Library work with deaf children. *Top of the News*, 13 (3) March 1957, 33 – 36.
LSA 1957/6999

1037 CROIX ROUGE DE BELGIQUE. Conseil National des Bibliothèques d'Hôpitaux et de Sanatoriums. Activités pendant l'exercice 1955. *In*: *Actes du Conseil de la Fiab XXI, 22e session Munich, 1956*. La Haye, Martinus Nijhoff, 1957, Annexe IX, 95.

1038 DARLING, Richard L. Mental hygiene and books: bibliotherapy as used with children and adolescents. *Wilson Libr. Bull.*, 32 (4) Dec. 1957, 293 – 296.
LSA 1958/7830

1039 DARR, F. Die Krankenbücherei. [The hospital library.] *Das Krankenhaus*, 49 (6) June 1957, 251.

1040 DEPOPOLO, Muriel. The integrated library in a community hospital. *Spec. Libr.*, 48 (10) Dec. 1957, 457 – 459.

1041 FÉDÉRATION INTERNATIONALE DES ASSOCIATIONS DE BIBLIOTHÉCAIRES. Bibliothèques d'Hôpitaux. [Rapport présenté par Mlle. Trog.] *In*: *Actes du Conseil de la Fiab XXI, 22e session Munich, 1956*. La Haye, Martinus Nijhoff, 1957, 27 – 28.

1042 FLANAGÁN, J. J., *father*. Import of hospital libraries to the hospital as a whole. *In*: Catholic Library Association. [*Conference, 33rd, 1957, Louisville*; *proceedings*], 137 – 138+.

1043 FRARY, Mildred P. Libraries for physically handicapped children. *School Libraries*, 6 (4) May 1957, 5.
LSA 1957/7264

1044 GARTLAND, Henry J. How to make the most of the library service. *In*: Pattison, H. A., *editor*. *The handicapped and their rehabilitation*. Springfield, Ill., Thomas, 1957, 619 – 627.

1045 GOING, Mona E. Hospital libraries in Scandinavia. *Libr. Ass. Rec.*, 59 (5) May 1957, 164 – 166.
LSA 1957/6929

1046 GROSS, R. *and* GITTLEMAN, F. C. Books for children about hospitals. *Child Study*, 34 1956 – 1957, 40 – 41.

1047 HARRIS, Joan D. Service to blind children in an elementary school library. *School Libraries*, 6 (4) May 1957, 17 – 18.
LSA 1957/7268

1048 HOLMSTRÖM, Bengt. Boken kommer: Shut-in service vid Malmö stadsbibliotek. [The book is coming: Malmö city library housebound service.] *Biblioteksbladet*, 42 (2) 1957, 99 – 102.

1049 HURI, N. La bibliothèque universitaire centrale des étudiants malades (B.U.C.E.M.) et les bibliothèques des sanatoriums universitaires en France. [Library provision for invalid students.] *Bull Bib. Fr.*, 2 (1) 1957, 15 – 31.
LSA 1957/6930

1050 KEARNS, M. M. Bibliotherapy in the V.A. hospital. *In*: Catholic Library Association. [*Conference, 33rd, 1957, Louisville: proceedings*], 139 – 142+.

1051 KŘIVINKOVÁ, Julie. Three types of hospital libraries in the tuberculosis institutions in Czechoslovakia. *ALA Hospital Book Guide*, 18 Feb. 1957, 24 – 28.

1052 Lectuurvoorziening voor bejaarden; gegevens welwillend verstrekt door F.L. Berdenis van Berlekom – Beltman. [Reading matter: provision for the aged.] *Volksontwikkeling*, 32 (2) Feb. 1957, 22 – 25.

1053 LEWIS, M. Joy. On being a hospital librarian. *Libr. Ass. Rec.*, 59 (9) Sept. 1957, 301 – 303.
LSA 1957/7473

1054 LIPCHAK, Amelia C. Use of children's books in a pediatric hospital. *Top of the News*, 14 (2) Dec. 1957, 36 – 39.

1055 LOZANO, C. D. R. Patients' library: periodicals and publicity. *In*: Catholic Library Association. [*Conference, 33rd, 1957, Louisville, proceedings*], 159 – 160.

1056 MCNAMARA, M. E. Hospital librarian promotes hospital. *Libr. J.*, 82 May 1 1957, 1174 – 1175.

1057 PHINNEY, Eleanor. Library service to an aging population: report on a post-card survey. *ALA Bull.*, 51 (8) Sept. 1957, 607 – 609.

1058 Reading periscope for 'iron lung' patients. *British Medical Journal*, ii Nov. 23 1957, 1237.

1059 RICHTER, K. H. Übertragungsmöglichkeit insbesondere der Tuberkülose durch das Leihbuch. [Risks of transmission particularly of tuberculosis by means of the library book.] *Zeitschrift für Ärztliche Fortbildung*, 51 (4) 1957, 164 – 171.

1060 RICKER, Eleanor L. The hospital librarian in a large organization. *Spec. Libr.*, 48 (10) Dec. 1957, 455 – 457.
LSA 1958/7763

1061 RIEMSDIJK, G. A. van. Het gesproken boek in Nederland. [The talking book for the blind in the Netherlands.] *Bibliotheekleven*, 42 (2) Feb. 1957, 33 – 36.
LSA 1957/6727

1062 RIEMSDIJK, G. A. van. The talking book in Holland. *Unesco Bull. Libr.*, 11 (11 – 12) Nov./Dec. 1957, 281 – 282.
LSA 1958/8117

1063 RYAN, Mary Jane. Bibliotherapy and psychiatry: changing concepts, 1937 – 1957. *Spec. Libr.*, 48 May/June 1957, 197 – 199.

1064 SALUM, I. *and* BÖRJESON, O. Om biblioterapi och dess betydelse inom men-talsjukvården. [Bibliotherapy and its value in care of the mentally ill.] *Socialmedicinsk Tidskrift*, 34 1957, 7 – 12.

1065 SIROVS, J. Do you practise bibliotherapy? *Hospital Administration*, Sydney, 5 May 1957, 33+.

1066 SKREFSRUD, Gunhild. Pasientbibliotekene. [Patients' libraries.] *In*: Norsk Bibliotekarlag og Norske Forskningsbibliotekarers Forening. *Bibliotek og forskning årbok, 1957*, 52 – 63.
LSA 1957/7482

1067 TALBOT, Geraldine. Library program at the Spalding High School, Chicago, Ill. *School Libraries*, 6 (4) May 1957, 8 – 9.
LSA 1957/7265

1068 UNITED HOSPITAL FUND OF NEW YORK. Committee on Hospital Library Architecture. *Planning the hospital library: a report*. New York, The Fund, 1957. 6 pp.

1069 Utdeling av statstilskott til pasientbiblioteker. [Government aid to patients' libraries.] *Bok og Bibliotek*, 24 May 1957, 140.

1070 YAST, H. T. Librarian on the hospital team. *ALA Hospital Book Guide*, 18 March 1957, 51 – 55.

1958

1071 AMERICAN LIBRARY ASSOCIATION. Association of Hospital and Institution Libraries. Bibliotherapy Committee. Summary of research project. *ALA Hospital Book Guide*, 19 April 1958, 50 – 51.

1072 Bibliography: hospital libraries. *Illinois Libraries*, 40 (5) May 1958, 459 – 460.

1073 *Bibliotheekwerk voor bejaarden.* [Library work for the aged.] 's Gravenhage, Centr. Verg. voor Openbare Leeszalen en Bibliotheken, 1958. 11 pp.

1074 BLAU, S. A. *Study of the live long and like it library club of the Cleveland Public Library.* Thesis (M.S.L.S.) Western Reserve University, 1958. 61 pp.

1075 CARDWELL, Margaret. Books for the blind. *Books*, (320) Nov./Dec. 1958, 177 – 179.
LSA 1958/8549

1076 CHASTEL, Guy. The Valentin Haüy Association's Braille library. *Unesco Bull. Libr.*, 12 (5 – 6) 1958, 105 – 108.
LSA 1958/8288

1077 CROIX ROUGE DE BELGIQUE. Conseil National des Bibliothèques d'Hôpitaux et de Sanatoriums. [Report]. *In*: *Actes du Conseil de la Fiab XXII, 23e session Paris, 1957.* La Haye, Martinus Nijhoff, 1958, Annexe XV, 119 – 120.

1078 DOOLEY, Kathleen. Library service international style. *Hospital Progress*, 39 (12) Dec. 1958, 69 passim.

1079 EDWARDS, M. Library for the mentally retarded. *Illinois Libraries*, 40 (5) May 1958, 467 – 468.

1080 EULER, Karl Friedrich. Der Wert einer Krankenhausbücherei. [The value of a hospital library.] *Der Krankenhausarzt*, 31 (2) Feb. 1958, 25 – 28.

1081 EULER, Karl Friedrich *and* KUNTZ, E. *Zusammenstellung empfehlenswerter Krankenlektüre.* Aus der Beratungsstelle für Krankenlektüre und Krankenbücherei an der Medizin. Klinik der Justus Liebig – Universität Giessen. [Collection of recommended literature for patients . . .] Dietzenbach, Evang. Gemeindebüchereien in Hessen und Nassau, 1958. 20 pp.

1082 FÉDÉRATION INTERNATIONALE DES ASSOCIATIONS DE BIBLIOTHÉCAIRES. Commission Bibliothèques d'Hôpitaux. [Report]. *In*: *Actes du Conseil de la Fiab XXII, 23e session Paris, 1957.* La Haye, Martinus Nijhoff, 1958, 44 – 45.

1083 FISHER, M. Alton state hospital library. *Illinois Libraries*, 40 Nov. 1958, 757 – 758.

1084 FLANDORF, Vera S. Administration of the reading program in the pediatric department of a hospital. *Cath. Libr. Wld.*, 30 Dec. 1958, 171 – 172.

1085 FLANDORF, Vera S. Recent books for young patients. *ALA Hospital and Institution Book Guide*, 1 Nov. 1958, 36 – 46.

1086 FLANDORF, Vera S. Recent books to help children adjust to a hospital situation. *Top of the News*, 14 March 1958, 35 – 38.

1087 FLOCH, Maurice. Bibliotherapy and the library. *Bookmark*, 18 Dec. 1958, 57 – 59.

1088 FLOCH, Maurice. The use of fiction or drama in psychotherapy and social education. *A.L.A. Hospital and Institution Book Guide*, 1 (4) Dec. 1958, 57 – 64. LSA 1959/9085

1089 FREIBERGER, A. Peoria state hospital libraries. *Illinois Libraries*, 40 (5) May 1958, 452 – 454.

1090 GALLAGHER, Janet. Chicago state hospital patients' library. *Illinois Libraries*, 40 (5) May 1958, 443 – 445.

1091 GARTLAND, Henry J. The how and why: hospital library service. *Hospital Management*, Chicago, 85 Feb. 1958, 51, 99, 102; March 1958, 56 – 57, 130.

1092 GELDERBLOM, Gertrud. Büchereiarbeit im Krankenhäusern. [Library work in hospitals.] *Kulturarbeit*, 10 (12) 1958, 238 – 240. LSA 1959/8820

1093 GRONSETH, O. A. Jacksonville state hospital. *Illinois Libraries*, 40 (5) May 1958, 457 – 458.

1094 HASLER, D. Story book for your littlest patient. *Practical Nursing*, 8 Dec. 1958, 11 – 12.

1095 HEINTZE, Ingeborg. Shut-in service at the Malmö City Library. *Unesco Bull. Libr.*, 12 (10) Oct. 1958, 235 – 236. LSA 1958/8664

1096 HIMWICH, W. A. *and others*. Galesburg state research hospital. *Illinois Libraries*, 40 (5) May 1958, 455 – 456.

1097 Hospitalsbibliotekarernes gruppemøde. [Hospital librarians' meeting.] *Bibliotekaren*, 20 (5) 1958, 155 – 158.

1098 Infection from books. (Any questions?) *British Medical Journal*, ii July 5 1958, 61.

1099 KERWIN, Philomena F. The volunteer in the hospital library. *Hospital Progress*, 39 (10) Oct. 1958, 87 – 138.

1100 KRUZAN, R. East Moline state hospital library. *Illinois Libraries*, 40 (5) May 1958, 446 – 447.

1101 KUNTZ, E. *and* EULER, K. F. Betrachtungen über die psychische Situation tuberkulöser Patienten, den bibliotherapeutischen Wert des Buches und die Einrichtung einer Krankenbücherei. [A look at the mental well-being of TB patients, the bibliotherapeutical value of books and the setting up of a hospital library.] *Münchener Medizinische Wochenschrift*, 100 July 1958, 1077 – 1081.

1102 LEPALCZYK, I. Biblioteki dla chorych w Belgii. [Libraries for patients in Belgium.] *Bibliotekarz*, 25 July 1958, 226 – 229.

1103 LUNDEEN, Alma. Books and rehabilitation. *Illinois Libraries*, 40 (5) May 1958, 403 – 405.

1104 LUNDEEN, Alma, *editor*. Institutional library service. *Illinois Libraries*, 40 (5) May 1958, 401 – 493.
LSA 1958/8301
For contents *see* nos. 1072, 1079, 1089, 1090, 1093, 1096, 1100, 1103, 1119

1105 Microfilmed books for the paralysed. [News and information.] *Unesco Bull. Libr.*, 12 (11 – 12) Nov. – Dec. 1958, 291.

1106 MUNFORD, W. A. The reconstructed building of the National Library for the Blind in Manchester. *Libr. Ass. Rec.*, 60 (8) Aug. 1958, 249 – 251.
LSA 1958/8362

1107 MUNFORD, W. A. *A short history of the National Library for the Blind, 1882 – 1957.* Reprinted from the 75th annual report of the Library (1957 – 1958). London National Library for the Blind [1958]. 8 pp.

1108 The National Library for the Blind. *Bookseller*, (2756) Oct. 18 1958, 1568 – 1570.
LSA 1958/8548

1109 NEPUSTIL, B. Sekce zdravotnických knihoven. [Health administration libraries in Czechoslovakia.] *Knihovnik*, 3 (9/10) 1958, 328 – 329.
LSA 1959/9065

1110 *Rewarding career is waiting for you: its in hospital librarianship.* Chicago, Ill., American Library Association, 1958. 6 pp.

1111 RUBBENS-FRANKEN, E. Het bejaardenvraagstuk. 6. De bejaarden en cultuur. [The problem of the aged. 6. The aged and culture.] *Sociale Zorg,* 20 (19) Oct. 1958, 292 – 297.

1112 SCHENK ZU SCHWEINSBERG, C. Das Märchenbuch im Kinderkrankenhaus. [The fairy tale in the children's hospital.] *Jugendliteratur*, (7) July 1958, 297 – 300.

1113 *Sjukhusbiblioteket.* [The hospital library.] Lund, Bibliotekstjänst, 1958. 47 pp. For English translation *see* no. 1291

1114 TEWS, Ruth M. The patients' library. *In*: Keys, Thomas E. *Applied medical library practice.* Springfield, Ill., Thomas, 1958, 97 – 134.

1115 THIEKÖTTER, Hans. Volksbüchereien für die Blinden. [Public libraries for the blind.] *Bücherei und Bildung*, 10 July 1958, 341 – 344.

1116 UNITED STATES. VETERANS ADMINISTRATION. Medical and General Reference Library. *Bibliotherapy in hospitals: an annotated bibliography 1900 – 1957*; compiled by Rosemary Dolan, June Donnelly [and] June Mitchell. Washington DC, Veterans Administration, 1958, 46 pp.

1117 VANDERBURG, M. A. Indiana hospital libraries versus standards – a survey. *Special Libraries Association Indiana Chapter Slant*, 20 March 1958, 8 – 10+.

1118 WINGBORG, Olle. Kan biblioteken göra något för de psykiskt efterblivna? [Can public libraries do anything for the mentally retarded?] *Biblioteksbladet*, 43 (1) 1958, 8 – 12.
LSA 1958/7805

1119 WROBEL, A. M. Elgin state hospital activities therapy department. *Illinois Libraries*, 40 (5) May 1958, 448 – 451.

1959

1120 AMERICAN LIBRARY ASSOCIATION. Association of Hospital and Institution Libraries. *Reading aids for the handicapped.* Chicago, Ill., The Association, 1959; also in *Rehabilitation Literature*, 20 Nov. 1959, 330 – 334.

1121 BARBOUR, Jane Marie. The handicapped find new horizons through reading guidance. *Hospital Progress*, 40 (1) Jan. 1959, 66 – 69.

1122 BASSET, R. S. Bibliothèques des hôpitaux et sanatoriums de l'Assistance Publique. [Hospital libraries.] *Bull. Bib. Fr.*, 4 (10) Oct. 1959, 437 – 442. LSA 1960/9933

1123 BICKEL, Ruth *and others.* The library as a therapeutic experience. *Bull. Med. Libr. Assoc.*, 47 (3) July 1959, 305 – 311. LSA 1959/9348

1124 BOŽOVIĆ, Z. Osvrt na dosadašnji rad stalnih pokretnih bolničkih biblioteka Crvenog Križa Srbije. [Survey of the present activities of package libraries of the Serbian Red Cross.] *Bibliotekar* (Belgrade), 11 July 1959, 179 – 184.

1125 BRANSON, W. C. *and others.* Twenty-five tried and true favorite titles for use with patients. *ALA Hospital and Institution Book Guide,* 1 May – June 1959, 161 – 164, 182 – 184.

1126 Bringing words to the aged and infirm: public libraries find new ways to serve elderly patrons. *Journal of the American Medical Association,* 170 May 23 1959, 459 – 460.

1127 BRINK, C. J. van den. *Naar een lichtend verschiet: werk en streven der Nederlandse blindebibliotheek.* [To a new vista: work and aims of the Dutch library for the blind.] Den Haag, 1959, 20 pp.

1128 BRUUN, Elsa. Sokeainkirjasto. [Library for the blind.] *Kirjastolehti*, 52 (9) Nov. 1959, 230 – 232; (10) Dec. 1959, 264 – 266; English Summary, 286. LSA 1959/9663

1129 CROIX ROUGE DE BELGIQUE. Conseil National des Bibliothèques d'Hôpitaux. Activités pendant l'exercice 1957. *In: Actes du Conseil de la Fiab XXIII, 24e session Madrid, Oct. 1958.* La Haye, Martinus Nijhoff, 1959, Annexe XII, 103.

1130 DARRIN, R., *editor.* Library as a therapeutic experience. *Bull. Med. Libr. Ass.,* 47 July 1959, 305 – 311.

1131 ELLIOTT, P. G. Bibliotherapy: patients in hospital and sanatorium situations. *Illinois Libraries*, 41 (6) June 1959, 477 – 482.

1132 EULER, Karl Friedrich. Bildbände und lichtbilder als Betreuungsmittel psychiatrisch Kranker. [Illustrated books and photographs as a means of caring for psychiatric patients.] *Das Krankenhaus,* 51 (6) June 1959, 231 – 233.

1133 EULER, Karl Friedrich. Die Stationsbücherei. [The ward library.] *Das Krankenhaus,* 51 (2) Feb. 1959, 48 – 49.

1134 FÉDÉRATION INTERNATIONALE DES ASSOCIATIONS DE BIBLIOTHÉCAIRES. Commission Bibliothèques d'Hôpitaux. [Report]. *In*: *Actes du Conseil de la Fiab XXIII, 24e session Madrid, Oct. 1958*. La Haye, Martinus Nijhoff, 1959, 39 – 40.

1135 FITZGERALD, Mary E. Readers' choice among the blind. *Libr. J.*, 84 (17) Oct. 1 1959, 2885 – 2886.
LSA 1959/9748

1136 FRYE, D. Mentally handicapped children. *Illinois Libraries*, 41 Jan. 1959, 16 – 21.

1137 Huomiota sairaalakirjastotoimintaan. [Attention to hospital library activity.] *Kirjastolehti*, 52 (9) Nov. 1959, 235 – 236; English summary (10) Dec. 1959, 286.
LSA 1959/9664

1138 JUNIER, A. J. *A subject index to the literature of bibliotherapy, 1900 – 1958*. Thesis (M.S. in L.S.) Atlanta University, 1959. 100 pp.

1139 KAUPPI, Hilkka. [Bibliotherapy and library work in hospitals.] *Suomen Laakarilehti*, Helsinki, 14 Nov. 20 1959, 1445 – 1452. (In Finnish.)

1140 KING EDWARD'S HOSPITAL FUND FOR LONDON. *Hospital library services: a pilot survey*. London, The Fund, 1959. 56 pp.

1141 KINNEY, M. M. Hospital librarianship: standards, accreditation, problems. *Cath. Libr. Wld.*, 30 May/June 1959, 492 – 494.

1142 LANGE, K. Stort fremskritt for pasientbiblioteket ved Ullevål sykehus. [Great progress for patients' library in Ullevål hospital.] *Bok og Bibliotek*, 26 July 1959, 188.

1143 Library services. [Woolwich and Croydon.] *Hospital*, London, 55 (12) Dec. 1959, 1035 – 1036.

1144 MERI, Sirkka-Liisa. Sairaalakirjastoista. [Hospital libraries in Finland.] *Sairaala*, 22 (11) 1959, 525 – 527.

1145 MOODY, M. Recent books for older readers. *ALA Hospital and Institution Book Guide*, 2 Oct. 1959, 31 – 33.

1146 NESS, Charles H. New resources for blind readers. *Libr. J.*, 84 (17) Oct. 1 1959, 2882 – 2884.
LSA 1959/9749

1147 NIEMAN, D. E. Reading aids for the handicapped. *Rehabilitation Literature*, 20 Nov. 1959, 330 – 334.

1148 NIKOLUSSI, Rudolf. Centralbibliothek für Blinde–Blindenhörbücherei. [Central library for the blind–audio library.] *Bücherei und Bildung*, 11 (5) May 1959, 238 – 240.

1149 Organizing and maintaining hospital library services: panel discussion presented at the upper Midwest hospital library conference: summaries of papers. *ALA Hospital and Institution Book Guide*, 2 Oct. 1959, 27 – 29.

1150 ØRVIG, Axela. Hospitalsbiblioteksarbejde. [Hospital library work.] *In*: Jensen, E. A., *editor. Lærebog i biblioteksteknik.* København, Dansk Bibliografisk Kontor, 1959, vol. 3, 527 – 540. English transl. by Brian Selby, Oct. 1962 in MS in Library Association Library, London.

1151 PHINNEY, Eleanor. Trends in library service to the aging. *ALA Bull.*, 53 June 1959, 534 – 535, 539.

1152 PRILLER, R. A reading list for maternity patients. *Hospital Progress*, 40 Oct. 1959, 96 – 100.

1153 PROTOČKOVÁ, Věra. Poznámky ke zlepšení práce knihovny pro nemocné. [How to improve library work in hospitals.] *Knihovnik*, 4 (9) 1959, 273 – 277. LSA 1959/9651

1154 RANTASALO, V. [Hospital libraries.] *Suomen Lääkärilehti*, 14 Nov. 20 1959, 1441 – 1444. (In Finnish.)

1155 RUCKS, P. Libraries for psychiatric patients, North Little Rock division, Consolidated VA hospital, Little Rock. *Arkansas Libraries*, 16 Oct. 1959, 17 – 18.

1156 Savetovanie bibliotekara pokretnih bolničkih biblioteka Narodne Republike Srbije. [Consultation of travelling hospital libraries in Serbia.] *Bibliotekar* (Belgrade) 11 Jan. 1959, 109 – 110.

1157 SCHMID-SCHÄDELIN, I. [Hospital libraries.] *Veska Zeitschrift*, 23 Aug. 1959, 666 – 668.

1158 SPÅNGBERG. M. Göteborgs sjukhusbibliotek. [Gothenburg's hospital libraries.] *Biblioteksbladet,* 44 (10) 1959, 749 – 751. LSA 1959/9665

1159 TEWS, Ruth M. Organizing and maintaining hospital library patient services. *Hospital Progress*, 40 Dec. 1959, 79 – 80, 107.

1160 THIEKÖTTER, Hans. Die Blindenhörbücherei des Landes Nordrhein – Westfalen. [The talking book library for the blind in North Rhine Westphalia.] *Milteilungsblatt* (Nordrhein – Westfalen), 9 (4) Dec. 15 1959, 118 – 119. LSA 1960/9934

1161 TICKNOR, William E. Program for troubled people. *Libr. J.*, 84 (18) Oct. 15 1959, 3078 – 3080. LSA 1959/9669

1162 UNKILA, Enni. Kirjaston merkitys mielisairaalassa. [Significance of the library in the mental hospital.] *Kirjastolehti*, 52 (9) Nov. 1959, 233 – 235; English summary (10) Dec. 1959, 286.

1163 UPTON, M. E. Library service in a VA hospital, Little Rock division, Consolidated VA hospital, Little Rock. *Arkansas Libraries*, 16 Oct. 1959, 13 – 17.

1164 VOGULYS, B. R. de. Las bibliotecas de hospitales. [Hospital libraries.] *Asociación Colombiana de Bibliotecarios. Boletin*, 3 Oct. 1959, 109 – 112.

1165 WILLIAMS, M. J. Library work in a children's hospital. *ALA Hospital and Institution Book Guide*, 1 (5) Jan. 1959, 79 – 85.

1960

1166 ALLUM, Nancy. Books for hospitals. *British Books*, 174 April 1960, 18 – 19, 24.

1167 ANASTASIA, M., *sister*. Bibliotherapy. *Catholic Nurse*, 9 Dec. 1960, 34 – 36.

1168 BASSET, R. S. Bibliothèques des malades dans les hôpitaux de l'Assistance Publique à Paris. [Patients' libraries in Assistance Publique hospitals in Paris.] *L'Hôpital et l'Aide Sociale à Paris*, (1) Jan./Feb. 1960, 49 – 53.
Hosp. Abstr. 1961/125

1169 BEATTY, W. K. Professional reading for library staff and volunteers in hospital and institution libraries. *ALA Hospital and Institution Book Guide*, 2 April 1960, 172 – 176.

1170 BEERENS, Anne-Marie. *Rôle de la bibliothécaire assistante sociale à l'hôpital psychiatrique*. [Role of the librarian, social assistant in the psychiatric hospital.] Bruxelles, Rapport de fin d'études de l'Institut d'Etudes sociale de l'Etat, 1960. 116 pp.

1171 BERRY, J. *Annotated bibliography and buying list of books for use with the mentally ill*. Thesis (M.S. in L.S.) Western Reserve University, 1960. 159 pp.

1172 BLACKSHEAR, Orrilla T. Public libraries serve the aging. *Geriatrics*, 15 May 1960, 390 – 397.

1173 *Boek en bejaarde; gids bij de lectuurvoorziening van de bejaarde: 2e geheel herz. dv.* [List of titles suitable for the aged; 2nd edition.] 's Gravenhage, Prot. Stichting tot bevordering van het bibliotheekwezen en de lectuurvoorlichting in Nederland, [1960]. 20 pp.

1174 Books for hospitals. *British Books*, 174 April 1960, 18 – 19+.

1175 COHOE, Edith. Bibliotherapy for handicapped children. *National Educational Association Journal*, 49 May 1960, 34 – 36.

1176 CORNEY, R. Library service to shut-ins in Poughkeepsie. *Bookmark*, 19 March 1960, 153 – 155.

1177 CORY, Patricia B. *School library services for deaf children*. Washington DC, Alex. Graham Bell Assoc. for the Deaf, 1960. 142 pp.

1178 CRACKNELL, E. G. 'Talking' stories for ophthalmic patients. *Hospital*, London, 56 May 1960, 374 – 375.

1179 CROIX ROUGE DE BELGIQUE. Conseil National des Bibliothèques d'Hôpitaux. Activités pendant l'exercice 1958. *In*: *Actes du Conseil de la Fiab XXIV, 25e session Varsovie, 1959*, La Haye, Martinus Nijhoff, 1960, Annexe XIV, 119.

1180 DARR, F. Die Krankenbücherei. [The hospital library.] *Krankenhaus-Umschau*, 29 (7) July 1960, 367 – 368.

1181 DOCKHORN, Berthold. Die Patientenbücherei im Krankenhaus. [The patients' library in a hospital.] *Krankenhaus-Umschau*, 29 (3) March 1960, 118 – 120.

1182 DOCKHORN, Berthold *and* GÖTTSCHE, E. Büchereiarbeit in einem Hamburger Krankenhaus. [Library work in a Hamburg hospital.] *Bücherei und Bildung*, 12 (7) July 1960, 280 – 283.
Hosp. Abstr. 1961/447

1183 EASON, Helga H. Workshop on aging. *ALA Bull.*, 54 (6) June 1960, 475 – 477.

1184 EULER, Karl Friedrich. Krankenlektüre. [Reading for patients] [intro. to a quarterly suppl. of this journal]. *Münchener Medizinische Wochenschrift*, 102 Jan. 1 1960, 56 – 57.

1185 EULER, Karl Friedrich. Das Problem der Krankenlektüre. [The problem of patients' reading.] *Bücherei und Bildung*, 12 (7) July 1960, 274 – 277. Hosp. Abstr. 1961/445

1186 FÉDÉRATION INTERNATIONALE DES ASSOCIATIONS DE BIBLIOTHÉCAIRES. Commission Bibliothèques d'Hôpitaux. [Rapport par Mme. Schmid-Schädelin.] *In*: *Actes du Conseil de la Fiab XXIV 25e session Varsovie, 1959*. La Haye, Martinus Nijhoff, 1960, 26 – 27.

1187 FONDERIE-TIERIE, E. Bibliotheekwerk met bejaarden. [Library work with the aged.] *De Openbare Bibliotheek*, 3 (6) June 1960, 162 – 167.

1188 GARDNER, F [rank] M. More books for hospitals. [Implications of King Edward's Hospital Fund for London survey of hospital library services.] *British Books*, 174 July 1960, 28 – 29.

1189 GÖTTSCHE, Elfriede. Die Krankenbücherei. [The hospital library.] *Krankenhaus-Umschau*, 29 (3) March 1960, 121 – 123.

1190 GRAVES, J. A. Librarian: a part of the health team in the rehabilitation of the narcotic addict. *Kentucky Library Association Bulletin*, 24 Jan. 1960, 21 – 22+.

1191 GROVE, Louise, *compiler*. Professional reading for the library staff and volunteers in hospital and institution libraries. *ALA Hospital and Institution Book Guide*, 2 May 1960, 192 – 201; June 1960, 216 – 223.

1192 HEINZE, H. Krankenlektüre in psychiatrischen Abteilungen. [Patient literature in the psychiatric unit.] *Münchener Medizinische Wochenschrift*, 102 Nov. 25 1960, 2420 – 2422.

1193 Hospital libraries (editorial). *Hospital*, London, 56 (1) Jan. 1960, 3 – 6.

1194 HUNTER, Judith. The hospital library service of the New South Wales Department of Public Health. *Aust. Libr. J.*, 9 (1) Jan. 1960, 43 – 47.

1195 INTERNATIONAL FEDERATION OF LIBRARY ASSOCIATIONS. Mémoire indicateur sur les bibliothèques d'hôpitaux. [Memorandum on hospital libraries.] *Libri*, 10 (2) 1960, 141 – 146. Hosp. Abstr. 1961/1063

1196 JAMES, *sister* Mary. Why a library? *Canadian Hospital*, 37 March 1960, 44 – 46, 86.

1197 JOHNSON, Barbara Coe. The integrated hospital library. *Spec. Libr.*, 51 (8) Oct. 1960, 440 – 443.

1198 KENT COUNTY COUNCIL. Education Committee. *Books and publications recommended for use with dull and backward children; 2nd edition*. Maidstone, Kent Education Committee, 1960. 24 pp.

1199 KŘIVINKOVÁ, Julie. Problémy výstavby knihoven ve zdravotnických zǎ\-řízeních. [The problems of library construction in health care institutions.] *Československé Zdravotnictví*, 8 (7) 1960, 380 – 391.

1200 KŘIVINKOVÁ, Julie. Some problems of patients' libraries in Czechoslovakia. *AHIL Quarterly*, 1 (1) Fall 1960, 16 – 19.

1201 KŘIVINKOVÁ, Julie. Spolupráce knohovníka a architekta při výstavbe knihoven, tentokrát v restortu ministerstva zdravotnictví. [Co-operation of librarians and architects in the building of hospital libraries.] *Knihovník*, 5 (3) 1960, 81 – 89.
LSA 1960/10246

1202 LANGFELDT, Johannes, *and others*. Krankenhausbüchereiarbeit: Leitsätze Probleme und Erfahrungen. [Hospital library work: principles, problems and practical experience.] *Bücherei und Bildung*, 12 (7) July 1960, 273 – 285.
LSA 1960/10432

1203 MARY GERMAINE, *sister*. Hospital librarian: duties and responsibilities. *The Hospitaller*, 8 Sept. 1960, 1 – 3.

1204 MILES, N. M. Professional reading for library staff and volunteers in hospital and institution libraries. *ALA Hospital and Institution Book Guide*, 2 March 1960, 146 – 149.

1205 MÜLLER, Christa. Wer nicht zu uns kommen kan, zu dem gehen wir. (Kooperationsbeziehungen zwischen der Stadtbibliothek Wittenberg u.d. Kreiskrankenhaus.) [We go to those who cannot come to us: cooperation between Wittenberg City Library and the district hospital] *Bibliothekar*, 14 (9) 1960, 963 – 965.

1206 MUNRO, Jean. Hospital library service in Dunedin. *New Zealand Libraries*, 23 (1) Jan./Feb. 1960, 16 – 18.

1207 NATIONAL INSTITUTES OF HEALTH. Furious children and the library. *Top of the News*, 16 March 1960, 12 – 15; May 1960, 24 – 30; 17 Oct. 1960, 48 – 49.

1208 *Romanliteratur für Patientenbüchereien: eine Empfehlungsliste*. [A list of novels recommended for hospital libraries.] Hrsg. von d. Arbeitsstelle f.d. Büchereiwesen in Zusammenarbeit mit dem Arbeitskreis Krankenhausbüchereien, zusammengestellt von der Krankenhausbüchereien München, 1960. 35 pp.

1209 SCHMIDT, Hannelore. Bücherwagen für Krankenhausbüchereien. [Book trolleys for hospital libraries.] *Bücherei und Bildung*, 12 (7) July 1960, 293 – 294.

1210 SCHMIDT, Hannelore. Die Krankenhausbüchereien der Stadt München. [The hospital libraries of Munich.] *Bücherei und Bildung*, 12 (7) July 1960, 277 – 280.
Hosp. Abstr. 1961/446

1211 SPÅNGBERG, M. Från sjukhusbibliotekssektionen. [From the hospital library department.] *Biblioteksbladet*, 45 Nov. 1960, 741.

1212 STURT, Ronald. Hospital library service. *Libr. Ass. Rec.*, 62 (12) Dec. 1960, 410.

1213 WINGBORG, Olle. Läsning for handikappade barn. [Reading for handicapped children.] *Biblioteksbladet*, 45 Sept. 1960, 584 – 588; English transl. in *Illinois Libraries*, 43 April 1961, 235 – 241.

1961

1214 ALDRICH, Lorna. Saxondale: a mental hospital library. *Libr. Ass. Rec.*, 63 (7) July 1961, 248 – 253.
LSA 1961/11430

1215 ARBORELIUS, B. Lund: i ortopediskt grannskap. [Lund: hospital library located near the orthopaedic clinic.] *Biblioteksbladet*, 46 (5) 1961, 333 – 334.

1216 BAATZ, W. H. Patients' library services and bibliotherapy. *Wilson Libr. Bull.*, 35 Jan. 1961, 378 – 379.

1217 BOŽOVIĆ, Z. Povodom petogodišnjice od osnivanja stalnih pokretnih bolničkih biblioteka Crvenog Križa. [On the fifth anniversary of the establishment of Red Cross travelling libraries.] *Bibliotekar* (Belgrade), 13 Nov. 1961, 626 – 629.

1218 BRENDAN, M., *sister*. Public relations – the heart of library service. *The Hospitaller*, 8 June 1961, 25 – 26+.

1219 BROEKMAN, L. Welfarewerk in de R.K. O.L.B. te Utrecht. [Welfare work in the R.C. P.L. Utrecht.] *De Openbare Bibliotheek*, 4 (6) Aug. 1961, 218 – 219.

1220 DE SELLIERS DE MORANVILLE, N. Les bibliothèques d'hôpitaux de la Croix-Rouge de Belgique. *Libri*, 11 (1) 1961, 83 – 86.

1221 DOLCH, Elaine T. Books for the hospitalized child. *American Journal of Nursing*, 61 Dec. 1961, 66 – 68.

1222 EBERT, Eloise. Library service to state institutions. *ALA Bull.*, 55 (4) April 1961, 332 – 335.

1223 ETHELREDA, *sister*. Library meets a challenge. *Cath. Libr. Wld.*, 32 March 1961, 369 – 372.

1224 FÉDÉRATION INTERNATIONALE DES ASSOCIATIONS DE BIBLIOTHÉCAIRES. Commission Bibliothèques d'Hôpitaux. [Rapport par Mme. Schmid-Schädelin.] *In: Actes du Conseil de la Fiab XXV, 26e session Lund – Malmö, 1960.* La Haye, Martinus Nijhoff, 1961, 35 – 36.

1225 FORSSELL, Kerstin. Några sjukhusbibliotek i Baltimore. [Some hospital libraries in Baltimore.] *Biblioteksbladet*, 46 (6) 1961, 416 – 420.
LSA 1961/11431

1226 GARTLAND, Henry J. Notes on education for hospital librarianship. *ALA Bull.*, 55 (4) April 1961, 345 – 346.
LSA 1961/11123

1227 GEERDTS, Hans Jürgen. Der kranke Mensch und das Buch. [The sick person and the book.] *In: Greifenalmanach 1961.* Rudolstadt, Greifenverl., 1961, 256 – 264.

1228 GREAT BRITAIN. MINISTRY OF HEALTH. *Hospital library service.* London, The Ministry, 1961. (H.M. (61) 62.)

1229 GREENAWAY, Emerson. Library services to the blind and other handicapped groups. *ALA Bull.*, 55 (4) April 1961, 320 – 323.
LSA 1961/11173

1230 GUZIK, K. Biblioteka zdrojowa. [Health resort library.] *Bibliotekarz*, 28 (5) 1961, 141 – 144.

1231 HANSEN, O. R. B. Mer om de glemte lånere. [More about the forgotten borrowers.] *Bogens Verden*, 43 (6) Oct. 1961, 340 – 343.

1232 HARRISON, K. C. *Libraries in Scandinavia*. London, Deutsch, 1961, 147 – 149.

1233 HARVEY, B. C. Hospital administrator's view of hospital libraries to-day. *Kentucky Library Association Bulletin*, 25 April 1961, 25 – 27.

1234 HUNT, E. Hospital library serves veterans. *Oklahoma Librarian*, 11 April 1961, 34 – 35+.

1235 INTERNATIONAL FEDERATION OF LIBRARY ASSOCIATIONS. Hospital Libraries Committee [Conference, 1960, Malmö]. *Bogens Verden*, 43 May 1961, 145 – 149.

1236 JANSSEN, C. E. Les bibliothèques d'hôpitaux de la Croix Rouge de Belgique. [Hospital libraries run by the Belgian Red Cross.] *Hôpital Belge*, 5 (33) Sept./Oct. 1961, 19 – 21.
Hosp. Abstr. 1962/1186

1237 JONES, L. E. Hospital library service in the Veterans Administration neuropsychiatric hospital, Jefferson barracks, St. Louis, Missouri. *Missouri Library Association Quarterly*, 22 Dec. 1961, 104 – 107.

1238 KEARNS, M. M. Observations on bibliotherapy in a VA hospital library. *Kentucky Library Association Bulletin*, 25 April 1961, 22 – 24.

1239 *Krankenhausbüchereiarbeit der öffentlichen Büchereien in der Bundesrepublik und West-Berlin. Stand November 1960*. [Hospital library work of the public libraries in West Germany and West Berlin.] Büchereidienst/Dt. Büchereiverband, 1 (1) 1961. Ziffer 70.

1240 LAFAY, F. [Magnetic-tape libraries for the blind.] *Presse Médicale*, 69 April 1 1961, 748.

1241 LARSEN, J. Lydbogen og dens muligheder i hospitalsbiblioteksarbejdet. [Talking books and their possibilities in hospital library work.] *Bibliotekaren*, 23 (5) 1961, 133 – 138.

1242 Lectuurvoorziening voor bejaarden per boekenbus. [Reading provision for the aged by mobile library.] *De Openbare Bibliotheek*, 4 (4) May 1961, 143.

1243 Librarians are concerned about service to an aging population. *ALA Bull.*, 55 (2) Feb. 1961, 198 – 200.

1244 The library and librarians as resources in rehabilitation (Symposium). *AHIL Quarterly*, 1 Spring 1961, 9 – 14.

1245 LIMPER, Hilda K. The public library at work with children in hospitals and institutions. *ALA Bull.*, 55 (4) April 1961, 329 – 331.
LSA 1961/11239

1246 LUCIOLI, Clara E. Full partnership on the educational and therapeutic team – the goal of hospital and institution libraries. *ALA Bull.*, 55 (4) April 1961, 313 – 315.

1247 LUNDEEN, Alma. General reference books for hospital and institution libraries. *AHIL Quarterly*, 1 Winter 1961, 9 – 18.

1248 MCCOLVIN, L. R. *Libraries in Britain*. London, Longmans Green for the British Council, 1961, 27 – 28.

1249 MASTERS, Anthony. Mental hospital library. *Library Review*, (137) Spring 1961, 29 – 31.
LSA 1961/11176

1250 MENNINGER, Karl. Reading as therapy. *ALA Bull.*, 55 (4) April 1961, 316 – 319.
LSA 1961/11340

1251 MOUNTS, Ann. The librarian in the psychiatric hospital. *Hospital Progress*, 42 June 1961, 106 – 108.

1252 NAGÓRSKA, I. *and* SZYMÁNSKA, G. Ksiązka w poradniach przeciwalkoholowych. [Books in anti-alcoholic dispensaries.] *Bibliotekarz*, 28 Nov. 1961, 325 – 328.

1253 NENADOVIĆ, L. Bibliotekar na humanom postu. [The librarian on a humanitarian job.] *Bibliotekar* (Belgrade) 13 Nov. 1961, 630 – 634.

1254 NIELSEN, Ove. De glemte lånere: bogen til de handicappede. [The forgotten borrowers: books for the handicapped.] *Bogens Verden*, 43 (5) Sept. 1961, 264 – 268.

1255 Norges Blindeforbunds biblioteker. [Libraries of the Norwegian Association for the Blind.] *Bok og Bibliotek*, 28 (1) Jan. 1961, 64 – 65.
LSA 1961/11171

1256 PEART, D. R. The hospital library: a privilege and opportunity. *Canadian Hospital*, 38 (4) April 1961, 50 – 51, 86.
Hosp. Abstr. 1961/1064

1257 PELTIER, Marie *and* YAST, Helen T. Hospital library service: a selected bibliography. *ALA Bull.*, 55 (4) April 1961, 347 – 349.
LSA 1961/11328

1258 SCHMID-SCHÄDELIN, Irmgard. Wegleitung für Spitalbibliotheken. [Guiding principles for hospital libraries.] *Bücherei und Bildung*, 13 (4) April 1961, 164 – 167.
LSA 1961/11175

1259 SEXTON, Kathryn. Library service to the blind. *Libr. J.*, 86 Feb. 1 1961, 527 – 530.

1260 SMITH, Anne Marie. *Play for convalescent children in hospitals and at home*. A. S. Barnes, 1961, 116 – 121.

1261 Smittefare ved utlån til tuberkuloseramte patienter. [Infection through loan of books to TB patients.] *Bogens Verden*, 43 Dec. 1961, 506 – 507.

1262 SWIFT, Helen Pruitt. Trends in hospital library service. *ALA Bull.*, 55 (4) April 1961, 338 – 340.
LSA 1961/11177; Hosp. Abstr. 1961/1826

1263 WILES, Juanita Ziegler. The case for a hospital library. *ALA Bull.*, 55 (4) April 1961, 341 – 344.

1962

1264 AMERICAN LIBRARY ASSOCIATION. *New horizons expanded: readable books for and about the physically handicapped.* Chicago, ALA, 1962.

1265 Arbeitstagung 'Krankenhausbüchereien' [Conference on hospital libraries]. *Das Krankenhaus*, 54 (4) April 1962, 158 – 160.
Hosp. Abstr. 1962/1810

1266 BEATTY, W. K. A historical review of bibliotherapy. *Library Trends*, 11 (2) Oct. 1962, 106 – 117.

1267 Bejaarden – bibliotheekdienst Noord – Holland. [Library service for the aged in the county Noord – Holland.] *Mens en Boek*, 14 (6) June 1962, 117 – 127.

1268 BERG-SONNE, V. Nordisk sygehusbibliotekarkursus. [Hospital librarians course in Scandinavia.] *Bibliotekaren*, 24 (2) 1962, 43 – 49.

1269 Bibliotheekwerk voor bejaarden: een geslaagde studiedag van de Prot. Stichting tot bevordering van het bibliotheekwezen en de lectuurvoorlichting in Nederland, te Utrecht. [Library work with the aged: account of a conference.] *Boek en Vorming*, 8 (2) March 1962, 23 – 26.

1270 BLÖSS, Edith. Krankenhausbüchereien. [Hospital libraries.] *Bücherei und Bildung*, 14 (4) April 1962, 200 – 203.
LSA 1962/12413

1271 BOORER, David. Librarian at Moorhaven hospital. *Outpost*, 14 (1) April 1962, 7 – 15.
LSA 1962/12148

1272 BRAY, Robert S. Books for the blind. *Florida Libraries*, 13 (1) March 1962, 13 – 14, 29 – 30.
LSA 1962/12495

1273 BROOKS, E. H. Bibliotherapy seminar. *AHIL Quarterly*, 2 Summer 1962, 7 – 8.

1274 BULLOCK, J. Y. *Résumé of the history, growth and development of library service to hospital patients by the Queens Borough (New York) public library.* Thesis (M.S. in L.S.) Atlanta University, 1962. 37 pp.

1275 CHUDEK, K. Z polskich doświadczeń w zakresie książki mówionej dla niewidomych. [Polish experiences with talking books for the blind.] *Bibliotekarz*, 29 Feb. 1962, 46 – 48.

1276 COWLES, B. Library service to aged out-patients. *AHIL Quarterly*, 2 Winter 1962, 15 – 16.

1277 CROIX ROUGE DE BELGIQUE. Conseil National des Bibliothèques d'Hôpitaux. *Un livre vous a plu, vous l'avez lu, donnez-le nous.* Bruxelles, Croix Rouge de Belgique, [1962?].

1278 CROIX ROUGE DE BELGIQUE. Conseil National des Bibliothèques d'Hôpitaux. Rapport jumelé des années 1960 et 1961. *In: Actes du Conseil de la Fiab XXVI, 27e session Edimbourg, 1961.* La Haye, Martinus Nijhoff, 1962, Annexe XXII, 139.

1279 DANEBIUS-SCHADEE, H. H. Ziekenhuisbibliotheken te Stockholm. [Hospital libraries in Stockholm.] *De Openbare Bibliotheek*, 5 (10) Dec. 1962, 395 – 398.

1280 FÉDÉRATION INTERNATIONALE DES ASSOCIATIONS DE BIBLIOTHÉCAIRES. Commission Bibliothèques d'Hôpitaux. [Résolutions.] *In*: *Actes du Conseil de la Fiab XXVI, 27e session Edimbourg, 1961*. La Haye, Martinus Nijhoff, 1962, 34.

1281 FICKEL, Gerhard. *Die kulturelle Betreuung der Patienten als Heilfaktor*. [The cultural care of the patient as an aid to recovery.] Potsdam, Institut für Fachschullehrerbildung d. Ministeriums f. Gesundheitswesen, 1962. (Studienmaterial zur Weiterbildung des mittleren medizinischen Personals, 1/1962.) Suppl. to *Die Heilberufe*, Berlin, 14 (1) 1962. 14 pp.

1282 GOING, Mona E. The needs of other handicapped readers. *In*: *Book provision for special needs: papers read at the weekend conference of the London and Home Counties Branch of the Library Association . . . April 1962*. London, LA, 1962, 62 – 64.
Hosp. Abstr. 1963/728

1283 GOING, Mona E. The new group. *Kent News Letter*, 13 (4) Aug. 1962.
LSA 1962/12326

1284 GROVE, H. H. Materials selection policy and procedure, report of a study by the Book selection policy committee, AHIL. *AHIL Quarterly*, 3 Fall 1962, 10 – 12.

1285 GUTHRIE, D[uncan]. Book needs of the physically handicapped. *In*: *Book provision for special needs: papers read at the weekend conference of the London and Home Counties Branch of the Library Association . . . April 1962*. London, LA, 1962, 53 – 56.
Hosp. Abstr. 1963/729

1286 HANNIGAN, Margaret C. The librarian in bibliotherapy: pharmacist or bibliotherapist? *Library Trends*, 11 (2) Oct. 1962, 184 – 198.
LSA 1963/13445

1287 HANNIGAN, Margaret C. Using books for mental health in your community. *Bookmark*, 29 June 1962, 251 – 254.

1288 HAYCRAFT, Howard. Books for the blind. *ALA Bull.*, 56 (9) Oct. 1962, 795 – 802. For abbreviated and updated version *see* no. 1405.

1289 HENRY, Robert P. Talking book services in Florida. *Florida Libraries*, 13 (1) March 1962, 12, 35.
LSA 1962/12496

1290 HOFFMAN, Karl Franz. Die Lektüre des Kranken. [Patients' reading.] *Medizinische Welt*, Stuttgart, 9 March 3 1962, 496 – 498.

1291 *The hospital library in Sweden: a symposium originally issued by the Swedish Library Association in 1958* . . . transl. into English by Mr. and Mrs. Frykman. London, LA, 1962. (LA pamphlet, 23.) For original in Swedish *see* no. 1113.

1292 JUNIER, A. J. Bibliotherapy: projects and studies with the mentally ill patient. *Library Trends*, 11 (2) Oct. 1962, 136 – 146.
[Largely based upon her unpublished thesis, *see* no. 1138.]

1293 KINNEY, M. M. The bibliotherapy program: requirements for training. *Library Trends*, 11 (2) Oct. 1962, 127 – 135.

1294 KRAUS, Eileen, *compiler*. Bibliotherapy for beginners in hospital library work. *AHIL Quarterly*, 2 Winter 1962, 10 – 12.

1295 LANGE, K. 3. nordiske kurs for pasientbibliotekarer Helsingfors 12 – 17 Juni 1962. [Third Scandinavian course for patients' librarians, Helsinki, June 12 – 17, 1962.] *Bok og Bibliotek,* 29 July 1962, 204 – 206.

1296 Lectuur voor visuel gehandicapten. [Reading matter for the visually handicapped.] *Mens en boek*, 14 (9) Sept. 1962, 193 – 199.

1297 LEWIS, M. Joy. Book needs of the physically and mentally handicapped. *In: Book provision for special needs: papers read at the weekend conference of the London and Home Counties Branch of the Library Association . . . April 1962*. London, LA, 1962, 57 – 61.
LSA 1962/12486; Hosp. Abstr. 1963/730

1298 LEWIS, M. Joy. From trolley to truck: some impressions of an English hospital librarian in America. *Libr. Ass. Rec.*, 64 (1) Jan. 1962, 1 – 9.
LSA 1962/11998

1299 LUCIOLI, Clara E. Workshop notes . . . library services to the aging. *Kansas Library Bulletin*, 31 Sept. 1962, 8 – 10.

1300 MARKUS, Florence. Library publicity at Wood. *Special Libraries Association. Wisconsin Chapter Bulletin*, 31 Jan. 1962, 7 – 9.

1301 MERI, Sirkka-Liisa. Ihminen ja kirja. [The book and human beings.] *Kirjastolehti*, 55 (6) 1962, 158 – 159.
LSA 1962/12335

1302 MERI, Sirkka-Liisa. Sairaalakirjastojen perustamiseen liittyviä näkökohtia. [Some viewpoints on the founding of hospital libraries.] *Kirjastolehti,* 55 (3) 1962, 58 – 62.
LSA 1962/11898

1303 MILLWARD, R. H. The Westminster delivery service to old people. *Libr. Ass. Rec.,* 64 (11) Nov. 1962, 419 – 420.
LSA 1962/12704

1304 MONTELIN, Y. Den tredje nordiska sjukhusbibliotekariekursen. [The third Scandinavian course for hospital librarians.] *Biblioteksbladet*, 47 (10) Dec. 1962, 760 – 761.

1305 MOODY, M. T. Bibliotherapy: modern concepts in general hospitals and other institutions. *Library Trends*, 11 (2) Oct. 1962, 147 – 158.

1306 MORROW, W. A. Some thoughts on the efficacy of bibliotherapy in the hospital setting. *North Carolina Libraries*, 21 Fall 1962, 22 – 24.

1307 NENADOVIĆ, L. Beogradske pokretne bolničke biblioteke Crevenog Križa. [Hospital libraries of the Red Cross in Belgrade.] *Bibliotekar* (Belgrade), 14 July 1962, 362 – 363.

1308 NYBORG, Karen. Nordisk hospitalsbibliotekarkursus i Finland. [Scandinavian course for hospital librarians in Finland.] *Bogens Verden*, 44 (6) 1962, 388 – 389.

1309 PHILOMENE, *sister*. The librarian's duties: an administrator's view. *Hospital Progress*, 43 (7) July 1962, 122, 124, 126.
Hosp. Abstr. 1962/1811

1310 PHINNEY, Eleanor. *Study of current practices in public library service to an aging population: an evaluative report*. University of Illinois Graduate Library School, 1962. 20 pp. (Occasional paper, 62.)

1311 RIEMSDIJK, G. A. van. Het bejaardenwerk in de Openbare Bibliotheek. [Work with old people in the public library.] *Volksopvoeding*, 11 (4) March 1962, 214 – 220.

1312 *Romanliteratur für Patientenbüchereien: eine Empfehlungsliste: 2 Auflage.* [A list of novels recommended for hospital libraries; 2nd edition.] Hrsg. von d. Arbeitsstelle f.d. Büchereiwesen in Zusammenarbeit mit dem Arbeitskreis 'Krankenhausbüchereien'; zusammengestellt von den Krankenhausbüchereien München. 1962. 19 pp.

1313 ROOS, S. de. Het boek de bejaarden en mijn ervaring. [The book, the aged and my experience.] *Boek en Vorming*, 8 (3) June 1962, 45 – 48.

1314 SPOKES, Ann. Libraries and the elderly. *Libr. Ass. Rec.*, 64 (11) Nov. 1962, 417 – 418.
LSA 1962/12703

1315 STEPHENS, Maureen. Books are everybody's business! (Editorial). *Canadian Hospital*, 39 March 1962, 33 – 34.

1316 TEIRICH, H. R. 'Gezieltes' und 'ungezieltes' Verleihen von Büchern als psychotherapeutische bzw. psychoheygienische Massnahme. ['Directed' and 'non-directed' lending of books as a psycho-therapeutic or mental health measure. *Zeitschrift für Psychotherapie und Medizinische Psychologie*, 12 (1) Jan. 1962, 21 – 30.

1317 TEWS, Ruth M. The questionnaire on bibliotherapy. *Library Trends*, 11 (2) Oct. 1962, 217 – 227.

1318 TEWS, Ruth M., *issue editor*. Bibliotherapy. *Library Trends*, 11 (2) Oct. 1962, 97 – 228.
For contents *see* nos. 1266, 1286, 1292, 1293, 1305, 1317.

1319 UNITED STATES. VETERANS ADMINISTRATION. Department of Medicine and Surgery. Medical and General Reference Library. *Bibliotherapy in hospitals: an annotated bibliography 1900 – 1961*. Washington DC, Veterans Administration, 1962. 59 pp.

1320 URCH, M. E. Libraries in hospitals. (3) The general hospital library. *In*: Library Association. *Proceedings, papers and discussions at the Llandudno conference, 25 – 28 September 1962*. London, LA, 1962, 51 – 54.

1321 VOLIN, L. K. Architectural barriers. *Libr. J.*, 87 Dec. 1 1962, 4396.

1322 WILSON, K. Hospitalsbibliotekarmødet i Odense 21-10-62. [Hospital librarians' annual meeting in Odense, 21-10-62.] *Bibliotekaren*, 24 (4 – 5) 1962, 105 – 106.

1963

1323 BABCOCK, K. B. Library standards, a symposium: The joint commission on accreditation of hospitals. *Bull. Med. Libr. Ass.*, 51 Jan. 1963, 81 – 83.

1324 *Bibliotheekvoorziening, De voor bejaarden in Gelderland: de resultaten van een onderzoek: met een voorw. van A. D. W. Tilanus.* [Library service for the aged in the county Gelderland: results of an investigation.] Arnhem, Stichting Gelderland voor maatschappelijk werk, 1963. 24 pp.

1325 *Bibliotheekwerk voor bejaarden: doel en methoden in kort bestek.* [Library work for the aged: aim and methods in a nutshell.] Voorburg, Prot. stichting tot bevordering van het bibliotheekwezen en de lectuurvoorlichting in Nederland, 1963. 14 pp.

1326 *Boek en bejaarde: gids bij de lectuurvoorziening van bejaarden: ze geheel nieuwe dr. met bijdragen van A. A. Koolhaas en C. van Dijk.* [List of titles suitable for the aged; 3rd edition prefaced by two lectures.] Voorburg, Prot. Stichting tot bevordering van het bibliotheekwezen en de lectuurvoorlichting in Nederland, 1963. 60 pp.

1327 BOW, Amelae. Serving the handicapped child. *Wilson Libr. Bull.*, 38 (2) Oct. 1963, 170 – 172.
LSA 1963/13765

1328 BUTTERWORTH, Margaret *and* STUCKEY, Elizabeth. The mental hospital and its library. *In*: Going, Mona E., *editor. Hospital libraries and work with the disabled.* London, LA, 1963, 78 – 85.

1329 CHAMBERLIN, J. A. The chest hospitals. *In*: Going, Mona E., *editor. Hospital libraries and work with the disabled.* London, Library Association, 1963, 86 – 95.

1330 CHAMBERS, D. C. Disability and bibliotherapy. *Cath. Libr. Wld.,* 35 Oct. 1963, 93 – 94.

1331 COWLES, Barbara. Starting a patients' library from scratch. *Auxiliary Leader,* 4 June 1963, 1 – 5.

1332 CROIX ROUGE DE BELGIQUE. Conseil National des Bibliothèques d'Hôpitaux. Rapport des activités de l'année 1961. *In: Actes du Conseil de la Fiab XXVII, 28e session Berne, 1962.* La Haye, Martinus Nijhoff, 1963, Annexe XIX, D.231; Annexe XX, 232.

1333 CROUCH, Marcus S. Work with disabled children and slow learners. *In*: Going, Mona E., *editor. Hospital libraries and work with the disabled.* London, Library Association, 1963, 155 – 161.

1334 EULER, Karl Friedrich. Bericht über die 2. Arbeitstagung Krankenhausbücherei. [Report on the second conference on the hospital library]. *Die Evangelische Krankenpflege,* 13 (1) May 1963, 22.

1335 EULER, Karl Friedrich. Wenn Kranke lesen . . . [When patients read . . .] *Bücherei und Bildung,* 15 (9) Sept. 1963, 397 – 400.
LSA 1962/13702

1336 FARROW, V. L., *compiler.* Bibliotherapy: an annotated bibliography. *Curriculum Bulletin* (Univ. of Oregon). 19 (234) May 1963. 32 pp.

1337 FÉDÉRATION INTERNATIONALE DES ASSOCIATIONS DE BIBLIOTHÉCAIRES. Commission Bibliothèques d'Hôpitaux. [Rapport et résolutions présenté par Mme. Schmid-Schädelin.] *In*: *Actes du Conseil de la Fiab XXVII, 28e session Berne, 1962*. La Haye, Martinus Nijhoff, 1963, 57 – 58.

1338 GOING, Mona E., *editor. Hospital libraries and work with the disabled*. London, Library Association, 1963. 198 pp.
For contents *see* nos. 1328, 1329, 1333, 1351, 1352, 1353, 1365, 1367, 1372, 1380.
Hosp. Abstr. 1963/1345

1339 GRAY, J. D. Allan. *The Central Middlesex Hospital*. London, Pitman Medical, 1963, 190 – 191 Library services.

1340 GUBALKE, Wolfgang. Probleme der Patientenbibliotheken. [Problems of patients' libraries.] *Krakenhaus – Umschau*, 32 (8) Aug. 1963, 363 – 364.

1341 HANNIGAN, Margaret C. *and* HENDERSON, William, T. Narcotic addicts take up reading. *Bookmark*, 22 July 1963, 281 – 286.

1342 HARRISON, K. C. *Public libraries to-day*. London, Crosby Lockwood, 1963, 95 – 97.

1343 HILL, A. Marjorie. Library service at Lancaster Moor Hospital. *Nursing Mirror*, 116 July 26 1963, 359.
Hosp. Abstr. 1963/1819.

1344 In the patients' good books: St. John and Red Cross hospital library service. *Nursing Mirror*, 116 Sept. 27 1963, 556.

1345 JEKIČ, U. Pokretne bolničke bibliotheke Crvenog Križa i njihov udeo u lečenju bolesnog čoveka. [Ambulatory hospital libraries of the Red Cross and their contribution in curing patients.] *Bibliotekar* (Belgrade), 15 (3) 1963, 163 – 165.

1346 KABELL, Margaret. Old folks library. *Books* (345) Jan./Feb. 1963, 36 – 37.
LSA 1963/13166

1347 KERSTEN, Hans-Hermann. Das Buch soll der Genesung dienen. Tagung des arbeitskreises 'Krankenhausbuchereien'. [Conference of hospital librarians.] *Bücherei und Bildung*, 15 Sept. 1963, 406 – 410.

1348 KING, Mary E. When reading is a handcraft. *Books* (345) Jan./Feb. 1963, 29 – 31.
LSA 1963/13355

1349 KŘIVINKOVÁ, Julie. Několik poznámek o plánovaní zdravotnických knihoven. [The planning of hospital libraries.] *Knihovnik*, 8 (3) 1963, 91 – 96.
LSA 1963/13515

1350 KŘIVINKOVÁ, Julie. Příspěvek k typizaci knihovnické buňky ve zdravotnických zařízeních. [A contribution to the standardisation of library units in Health care institutions.] *Ceskoslovenské Zdravotnictví*, 11 (2) 1963, 80 – 84.

1351 LEWIS, M. Joy. Book trolleys. *In*: Going, Mona E., *editor. Hospital libraries and work with the disabled*. London, LA, 1963, 115 – 121.

1352 LEWIS, M. Joy, Reading aids and equipment for handicapped and partially-sighted readers. *In*: Going, Mona E., *editor. Hospital libraries and work with the disabled.* London, LA, 1963, 122 – 133.

1353 LEYS, Duncan. The place of literature in healing. *In*: Going, Mona E., *editor. Hospital libraries and work with the disabled.* London, LA, 1963, 44 – 50.

1354 LINDBLAD, I. Statistikföring vid sjukhusbibliotek. [Keeping statistics in hospital libraries.] *Biblioteksbladet*, 48 (7) 1963, 488 – 489.

1355 LINDERBERG, Kerstin. Shut-in-verksamhet i Västerås. [House-bound service in Västeras.] *Biblioteksbladet*, 48 (3) 1963, 180 – 181.

1356 LYONS, G. J. Children's library, the Kings Park State Hospital. *Bookmark*, 23 Nov. 1963, 29 – 31.

1357 MCARTHUR, Thelma. Starting (public) library service to hospitals. *ALA Bull.*, 57 Oct. 1963, 859 – 860.

1358 MCINNES, E. M. *St. Thomas' Hospital.* London, Allen & Unwin, 1963, 180 – 181.

1359 MAHLOW, Johanna. Büchereipraxis: Die Mannheimer Krankenhausbücherei. [The hospital library in Mannheim.] *Bücherei und Bildung*, 15 Sept. 1963, 439 – 440.

1360 MAHON, M. W. Bedridden people need library services. *Mississippi Library News*, 27 March 1963, 29 – 30.

1361 MARCHI, Lorraine. NAVH helps the visually handicapped. *Libr. J.*, 88 (22) Dec. 15 1963, 4821 – 4822, 4838.
LSA 1964/14095

1362 MARY CONCORDIA, *sister*. Book selection: bibliography. *Cath. Libr. Wld.*, 34 March 1963, 363 – 364; April 1963, 410 – 412.

1363 MATTHEWS, Ann. Bibliotherapy gives a new lease on life. *Hospital Management*, 95 Jan. 1963, 56 – 58.

1364 MERI, Sirkka-Liisa. *Sairaalakirjastotoiminnan opas: 2nd edition.* [A manual for hospital librarians; 2nd edition.] Helsinki, Suomen Kirjastoseura, 1963. 31 pp.

1365 MILLWARD, R. H. The library service to old people. *In*: Going, Mona E., *editor. Hospital libraries and work with the disabled.* London, LA, 1963, 148 – 154.

1366 MORRIS, Effie Lee. Serving the handicapped child. *Wilson Libr. Bull.*, 38 (2) Oct. 1963, 165 – 169.
LSA 1963/13758

1367 MUNFORD, W. Library service to the blind. *In*: Going, Mona E., *editor. Hospital libraries and work with the disabled.* London, LA, 1963, 162 – 171.

1368 NIELSEN, Helga. Mødet for hospitalsbibliotekarer den 20 Oktober 1963 i Odense. [Meeting for hospital librarians Oct. 20 1963 in Odense.] *Bibliotekaren*, 25 (4) 1963, 167 – 168.

1369 NYBERG, Mirjam (afterwards Mirjam Grundstroem). Biblioteksarbetet på sjukhus och kommunalhem. [Library work in hospitals and old people's homes.] *Kommunaltidningen*, (6) 1963, 139 – 142.

1370 OXENER, R. A. Vitnodiging, bibliotheekwerk voor bejaarden – waarom? – hoe? [Invitation, library work for the elderly – why? how?] *Boek en Vorming*, 9 (3) April 1963, 45 – 48.

1371 Plaatselijke lectuurdiensten ten behoeve van niet mobilen. [Local reading services for the non mobile.] *Mens en Boek*, 15 (6) June 1963, 77 – 83.

1372 Planning of hospital libraries. *In*: Going, Mona E., *editor. Hospital libraries and work with the disabled*. London, Library Association, 1963, 106 – 114.

1373 RAUSSENDORF, Christa *and* STARK, Elisabeth. Stiefkind Patientenbibliotheken. [Patients' libraries – the Cinderella.] *Bibliothekar*, 17 (11) 1963, 1210 – 1211.

1374 RUTHERFORD, *Mrs.* Herbert W. Creating and operating a library cart service. *Auxiliary Leader*, 4 Dec. 1963, 10 – 13.

1375 SCHMID-SCHÄDELIN, Irmgard. Die Krankenhausbücherei als Sondergebiet der Büchereiarbeit. [The hospital library as a special aspect of library work.] *Bücherei und Bildung*, 15 Sept. 1963, 393 – 397.

1376 SIEMEN, U. *and* DUX, W. Der Bibliothekar im Krankenhaus. Gedanken zur bibliothekarischen Wirksamkeit im Gesundheitswesen. [The librarian in hospital. Thoughts on library efficiency in the health service.] *Bibliothekar*, 17 (11) Nov. 1963, 1134 – 1140.

1377 SIMPSON, Virginia. Books for the blind. *News notes of California Libraries*, 58 (4) Fall 1963, 387 – 394.
LSA 1964/14445

1378 SINDIK, N. Jedan osvrt na rad beogradskih pokretnih bolničkih biblioteka. [Review of 'Bookmobiles' in hospital libraries.] *Bibliotekar* (Belgrade), 15 (4) 1963, 328 – 330.

1379 STOVALL, M. W. Play-reading as a library activity in a psychiatric hospital. *AHIL Quarterly*, 3 Winter 1963, 20 – 22.

1380 STURT, Ronald. History of hospital libraries. *In*: Going, Mona E., *editor. Hospital libraries and work with the disabled*. London, Library Association, 1963, 17 – 32.

1381 THORNTON, John L. *Medical librarianship: principles and practice*. London, Crosby Lockwood, 1963, 30 – 49, libraries in hospitals.

1382 URCH, M. E. Hospital library services in Great Britain: the present and the future. *AHIL Quarterly*, 4 Fall 1963, 9 – 14.

1383 WHITE, Ruth W. Light in a dark world: how you can help the visually handicapped child. *Libr. J.*, 88 (22) Dec. 15 1963, 4817 – 4820, 4825.
LSA 1964/13979.

1384 WINNBERG, A. M. *Survey of the literature concerning the work of the public library with the community hospital*. Thesis (M.S. in L.S.) Catholic University of America, 1963. 61 pp.

1385 WINOWICH, Nicholas. Bringing public library service to the hospital. *Auxiliary Leader*, 4 June 1963, 6 – 9.

1386 ZANGERLE, J. Von der Bibliotherapie zur Krankenbücherei. [From bibliotherapy to the hospital library.] *Osterreichische Krankenhauszeitung*, 4 (9) 1963, 259 – 264.

1964

1387 AMERICAN LIBRARY ASSOCIATION. Adult Services Division. Committee on Library Services to an Aging Population. Statement on the library's responsibility to the aging. *ALA Bull.*, 58 April 1964, 321.

1388 BEATTY, W. K., *editor*. A.L.A. bibliotherapy workshop. St. Louis, June 25 – 27, 1964 . . . proceedings. *AHIL Quarterly*, 4 (4) Summer 1964. 60 pp. (special issue).

1389 BOLITHO, H. Writing and reading aids for the paralysed. *Unesco Bull. Libr.*, 18 (1) Jan./Feb. 1964, 45 – 48.

1390 Books – one more aspect of patient care. *Hospital Administration in Canada*, 6 March 1964, 24 – 25.

1391 CANFIELD, A. A. 'Unused channels' in hospitals. *Cath. Libr. Wld.*, 35 March 1964, 458 – 461.

1392 COSGROVE, J. M. *Study of library service to children in selected large general hospitals.* Thesis (M.S. in L.S.) Southern Connecticut State College, 1964. 70 pp.

1393 COWBURN, Lorna M. Books for blind readers. *In*: *The library in the hospital and care in the community: papers given at the Hospital Libraries and Handicapped Readers Group conference . . . Nottingham, 1963.* London, LA, 1964, 27 – 29.

1394 COWLES, Barbara. Library is new tool for rehabilitation. *Nursing Home Administrator*, 18 Nov./Dec. 1964, 53 – 55.

1395 CZECHOSLOVAKIA. MINISTRY OF PUBLIC HEALTH. Regulations for patients libraries in inpatient health institutions. (Decree of the Czechoslovak Ministry of Public Health of the first of June 1953). *In*: *Actes du Conseil . . . XXVIII, 29e session Sofia, 1963.* La Haye, Martinus Nijhoff, 1964, 73 – 76.

1396 DUFFEY, K. I. Deposit libraries and state library extension services. *AHIL Quarterly*, 4 Winter 1964, 12 – 14.

1397 EULER, Karl Friedrich. *Krankenlektüre: erfahrungen – folgerungen – ratschläge.* [Patients' reading; experience, conclusions, recommendations.] Stuttgart, Hippokrates – Verl., 1964. 103 pp. (Schriftenreihe zur Theorie und Praxis der Psychotherapie.)

1398 FÉDÉRATION INTERNATIONALE DES ASSOCIATIONS DE BIBLIOTHÉCAIRES. Sous – Section des Bibliothèques d'Hôpitaux Pour Les Malades. Report and resolutions of meeting of September 3. *In*: *Actes du Conseil . . . XXVIII, 29e session Sofia, 1963.* La Haye, Martinus Nijhoff, 1964, 71 – 72.

1399 FINGERET, Rose W. Aids for the reader with changing vision. *ALA Bull.*, 58 (9) Oct. 1964, 792 – 794.

1400 GALE, Selma R. The hand extended. *ALA Bull.*, 58 (9) Oct. 1964, 777 – 780.

1401 GOING, Mona E. Care in the Community. *In*: *The library in the hospital and care in the community: papers given at the Hospital Libraries and Handicapped Readers Group conference, Nottingham, 1963.* London, LA, 1964, 17 – 18.

1402 GUBALKE, Wolfgang. Sollen Bücher Kranke heilen helfen? [Should books help patients to recover?] *Bayerisches Ärzteblatt* (2) 1964, 158 – 162.

1403 GÜNNEL, P. Bibliotheksarbeit in Krankenhäusern: Krankenhausbibliotheken in anderen ländern. [Library work in hospitals: hospital libraries in foreign countries.] *Bibliothekar*, 18 Jan. 1964, 100 – 102.

1404 HANNIGAN, Margaret C. The reader with mental and emotional problems. *ALA Bull.*, 58 (9) Oct. 1964, 798 – 803.

1405 HAYCRAFT, Howard. Books for the blind. *New Outlook for the Blind*, 58 April 1964, 106 – 110. Abbreviated and updated version of no. 1288.

1406 Hospital libraries abroad. *AHIL Quarterly*, 4 Winter 1964, 16 – 17.

1407 INTERASSOCIATION HOSPITAL LIBRARIES COMMITTEE, CHICAGO. *Basic list of guides and information sources for setting up hospital, medical and nursing libraries.* Chicago, The Committee, 1964. 13 pp.

1408 IRISH REPUBLIC. HOSPITAL LIBRARY COUNCIL. *Report on meeting held Tuesday, April 28 1964.* Dublin, The Council, 1964. 7 pp.

1409 JOHRDEN, J. A. *Bibliotherapy for children: a selective annotated bibliography, 1950 – 1962.* Thesis (M.S. in L.S.) Catholic University of America, 1964. 34 pp.

1410 *Katalog över talböcker, 1955 – 1964.* [Catalogue of talking books, 1955 – 1964.] Stockholm, De Blindas Förening, 1964.

1411 KENT COUNTY COUNCIL. Education Committee. *Books and publications recommended for use with dull and backward children: 3rd edition.* Maidstone, Kent County Council, 1964. 22 pp.

1412 KLAGES, W. Zur Bibliotherapie bei psychiatrisch Kranken. [Bibliotherapy for the mentally ill.] *Psychiatria et Neurologia*, Basel 148 (3) 1964, 178 – 190.

1413 *Krankenhausbücher.* [Books in hospital.] *Artikel 103 im Nachrichtendienst des Deutschen Städtebundes*, May 1964, 86.

1414 KROESE-BELTMAN, F. L. Het boek als belangrijkste facer van de tijdsbesteding van bejaarden. [The book as important part of spare time occupation for the aged.] *Volksontwikkeling*, 39 (1) Jan. 1964, 14 – 15.

1415 LARSSON, Estrid. *Sjukhusbibliotek i de nordiska länderna: organisation och administration.* [Hospital libraries in Scandinavia: organisation and administration.] Lund, Bibliotekstjänst, 1964. (Sveriges allmänna biblioteksforenings småskrifter, 63.)

1416 LAURIE, Gini. Aids for quads and respos. *ALA Bull.*, 58 (9) Oct. 1964, 785 – 759.

1417 LEEUWENBURGH, P. B. Het bejaardenhuis krijgt zijn bibliotheek. [The old people's home gets its library.] *De Bejaarden*, 10 (10) Oct. 1964, 225.

1418 LEWIS, M. Joy. A hospital library. [Gowers Library, National Hospital, Queen Square, London.] *British Hospital & Social Service Journal*, 74 Feb. 21 1964, 237.
Hosp. Abstr. 1964/877

1419 LEWIS, M. Joy. The hospital library. *Nursing Times*, 60 Oct. 9 1964, 1343 – 1344.

1420 LEYS, Duncan. Literature in healing. *Libr. Ass. Rec.*, 66 (4) April 1964, 161 –
166.
LSA 1964/14442

1421 Lezen houdt geest actief: geen aparte bejaarden lectuur. [Reading makes the
mind active: no separate old age reading matter.] *Op Leeftijd*, 1 (3) Jan./Feb.
1964, 48 – 49.

1422 LIBRARY ASSOCIATION. Hospital Libraries and Handicapped Readers Group.
*The library in the hospital and care in the community: papers given at the Hospital
Libraries and Handicapped Readers Group conference ... Nottingham 1963.*
London, LA, 1964. 32 pp. For papers presented *see* nos. 1393, 1401, 1434,
1440, 1443, 1445, 1451.

1423 LUCIOLI, Clara E. *and* FLEAK, Dorothy H. The shut-in – waiting for what?
ALA Bull., 58 (9) Oct. 1964, 781 – 784.

1424 Mensen en boeken: een gesprek. [People and books.] *De Bejaarden*, 10 (7)
July 1964, 161 – 163.

1425 MEYLING, A. Per boekenbus naar bejaarden centra. [With a book bus to old
people's centre.] *De Bejaarden*, 10 (11) Nov. 1964, 255; (12) Dec. 1964, 267;
also in *De Openbare Bibliotheek*, 10 (7/8) Sept./Oct. 1967, 272 – 273.

1426 MITCHELL, Dorothy. Dorothy Mitchell reminisces about library service to
the blind. *Canadian Library*, 21 (3) Nov. 1964, 131.

1427 The modern hospital library: functions considered at Scottish meeting.
British Hospital and Social Service Journal, 74 Feb. 7 1964, 178.

1428 MOODY, Mildred T. Bibliotherapy for chronic illness. *Hospital Progress*, 45
Jan. 1964, 62.

1429 MOODY, Mildred T. The reader who needs remotivation. *ALA Bull.*, 58 (9)
Oct. 1964, 795 – 797.

1430 MUNFORD, W. A. Library services for the blind, sighted and partially sighted.
In: Library Association. *Proceedings, papers and summaries of discussions held at
the public libraries conference held at Rothesay, 30 Sept. – 2 Oct. 1964.* London,
LA, 1964, 16 – 23.

1431 New specialty is born; clinical librarian (Editorial). *New York State Journal
of Medicine*, 64 Dec. 15 1964, 2977 – 2978.

1432 NYE, P. W. Reading aids for blind people: a survey of progress with tech-
nological and human problems. *Medical Electronics & Biological Engineering*, 2
(3) July 1964, 247 – 264.
LSA 1964/14443

1433 *Oudere mens, De en zijn lectuur*; bijdragen K. J. M. van de Loo, A. P. F. M.
Kemme en D. Reumer. [The old person and his reading matter: 3 papers.]
Utrecht, Katholiek bibliotheekcentrum in samenw. met de Katholieke
nationale federatie voor bejaardenzorg, 1964. 94 pp.

1434 PAGET, S. J. A book service for housebound readers. *In*: *The library in the
hospital and care in the community: papers given at the Hospital Libraries and Handicapped Readers Group conference ... Nottingham, 1963.* London, LA, 1964
23 – 26.

Bibliography

1435 PANSE, Friedrich *and others. Das psychiatrische Krankenhauswesen* . . . [Psychiatric hospitals. . . .] Stuttgart, Thieme, 1964, 202 – 208 Die Bücherei [The library]. Hosp. Abstr. 1965/1071

1436 PODGÓRECZNY, J. Refleksje bibliotekarza na wczasach. [Reflections of a librarian on vacation.] *Bibliotekarz*, 31 (1) 1964, 15 – 17.

1437 *Romanliteratur für Patientenbüchereien: eine Empfehlungsliste: 3 Auflage.* [A list of novels recommended for hospital libraries; 3rd edition.] Hrsg. von d. Arbeitsstelle f.d. Büchereiwesen in Zusammenarbeit mit dem Arbeitskreis 'Krankenhausbüchereien', zusammengestellt von der Krankenhausbüchereien München. 1964. 40 pp.

1438 RUSSELL, W. R. *and* SCHUSTER, E. Page-turner for patients with paralysed hands. *Lancet*, ii Oct. 24 1964, 893 – 894.

1439 SAINTE-LEONIE, *sister*. Bibliothèque des malades. [A l'hôtel-dieu de Quebec.] [Patients' library in Quebec hospital.] *Association Canadienne des Bibliothécaires de Langue Française. Bulletin*, 10 June 1964, 56 – 58.

1440 SANDERS, Brenda. The library and its work. *In: The library in the hospital and care in the community: papers given at the Hospital Libraries and Handicapped Readers Group conference, Nottingham, 1963.* London, LA, 1964, 8 – 12.

1441 SCHROERS, Herbert. *Die Arbeit mit dem Buch in der Nervenklinik der Medizinischen Fakultät (Charité) der Humboldt – Universität, Berlin, als wichtiger Erziehungs – Bildungs – und Heilfaktor bei der kulturellen Betreeung der Patienten.* [Work with books in the Nervenklinik. . . .] Meissen/Siebeneichen, Fachschul für Klubleiter, 1964. 20 pp. (Abschlussarbeit.)

1442 SCHROERS, Herbert. Patientenbibliotheken: kein unlösbares Problem. [Patients' libraries: not an unsolvable problem.] *Bibliothekar*, 18 (6) June 1964, 657 – 659.

1443 SCRIVENS, Barbara. In the wards. *In: The library in the hospital and care in the community: papers given at the Hospital Libraries and Handicapped Readers Group conference . . . Nottingham, 1963.* London, LA, 1964, 13 – 16.

1444 STURT, Ronald. Libraries in hospitals. *Libr. Ass. Rec.*, 66 (4) April 1964, 158 – 160.
LSA 1964/14199

1445 STURT, Ronald. The library in the hospital. *In: The library in the hospital and care in the community: papers given at the Hospital Libraries and Handicapped Readers Group conference . . . Nottingham, 1963.* London, LA, 1964, 5 – 7.

1446 TEIRICH, H. R. Ein Beitrag zur sogenannten 'Bibliotherapie'. [A contribution to so-called 'bibliotherapy'.] *Österreichische Arztezeitung*, 19 1964, 1 – 6.

1447 UNITED STATES. VETERANS ADMINISTRATION. Office of the Chief Medical Director. *Planning criteria for medical facilities.* Washington, DC, VA, 1964, chapter 17 Library service [3] pp. (Manual M – 7.)

1448 VEDSTED, Ingrid. Bør vi ikke tænke lidt mere på særopgaverne? [Shouldn't we pay a little more attention to extension work.] *Bogens Verden*, 46 (8) 1964, 536.

1449 VEGGELAND, U. Pasientbiblioteker ved Ullevål sykehus i nye lokaler. [Patients' library at Ullevål hospital in new premises.] *Bok og Bibliotek*, 31 Nov. 1964, 317–318.

1450 WILSON, Karen. Kursus i hospitalsarbejde. [Course in hospital library work.] *Bogens Verden*, 46 (6) Oct. 1964, 391–393.

1451 WYATT, A. Shirley. The hospital and ancillary services provided by Lewisham Borough Council. *In: The library in the hospital and care in the community: papers given at the Hospital Libraries and Handicapped Readers Group conference . . . Nottingham, 1963.* London, LA, 1964, 19–22.

1965

1452 AMERICAN LIBRARY ASSOCIATION. Adult Services Division. Committee on Reading Improvement for Adults. *Books for adults beginning to read.* Chicago, Ala, 1965.

1453 AMERICAN LIBRARY ASSOCIATION. Association of Hospital and Institution Libraries. Volunteers in hospital and institution libraries [panel discussion]. *AHIL Quarterly*, 5 Winter 1965, 3–9.

1454 BARTELS, Hanna. Das Buch am Krankenbett. [The book by the hospital bed.] *In: Werkheft für die katholische Volksbüchereien des Sankt Michaelsbundes*, Dec. 1965, 3–14.

1455 BELL, Donald. Some aspects of the work of the Royal Institute for the Blind. *In: Hospital library services surveyed: papers given at Hospital Libraries and Handicapped Readers Group conference . . . Sheffield, 1964.* London, LA, 1965, 17–32.

1456 BERRY, Philip. Librarians in mental hospitals. *British Hospital Journal & Social Service Review*, 75 June 18 1965, 1151.

1457 Bibliotherapie? Kulturelle Betreuung als medizinische Aufgabe. [Bibliotherapy? Cultural care as a medical problem.] *Humanitas*, Berlin 5 (24) 1965, 11.

1458 BOGARD, H. M. Bibliotherapy – for whom and by whom. *AHIL Quarterly*, 6 Fall 1965, 11–17.

1459 Books for partially-sighted people. [News and information.] *Unesco Bull. Libr.*, 19 (2) March/April 1965, 111–112.

1460 BOORER, David. Librarian at large – mental hospital library services. *In: Hospital library services surveyed: papers given at Hospital Libraries and Handicapped Readers Group conference . . . Sheffield, 1964.* London, LA, 1965, 33–54.

1461 BRANDT, Eleanor. Effective use of volunteers in hospital and institution libraries. *AHIL Quarterly*, 5 Winter 1965, 4–6.

1462 *Buchauswahl für Krankenhaus-Büchereien.* [Book selection for hospital libraries.] Deutscher Verband Evangelischer Büchereien, 1965. 38 pp.

1463 CHANDLER, G. *Libraries in the modern world.* Oxford, Pergamon, 1965, 70–72.

1464 COLLIS, D. Reading problems of the partially sighted. *In: Hospital library services surveyed: papers given at Hospital Libraries and Handicapped Readers Group conference . . . Sheffield, 1964.* London, LA, 1965, 55–57.

1465 COUNCIL OF NATIONAL LIBRARY ASSOCIATIONS. Joint Committee on Hospital Libraries. *Basic list of guides and information sources for professional and patients' libraries in hospitals.* Chicago, ALA, 1965. 13 pp.

1466 CZECHOSLOVAKIA. MINISTRY OF HEALTH. *Regulations for library and science information services in institutions for curative and preventive care.* [Prague, The Ministry, 1965.] 6 pp. typescript.

1467 DAY, Anne. Library services – 1. Hill End hospital. *Book Trolley*, 1 (3) Sept. 1965, 5 – 7.

1468 DELVALLE, J. *and others.* Reading patterns of the aged in a nursing home environment. *Professional Nursing Home*, 7 June 1965, 46 – 53; also in *AHIL Quarterly*, 6 Winter 1966, 8 – 11.

1469 Disinfecting library books. (Any questions?) *British Medical Journal*, ii Dec. 4 1965, 1354. Reprinted in *Book Trolley*, 1 (5) March 1966, 11.

1470 EPPINGER, Lilli. Therapie mit dem Buch. Auf die zusammenarbeit kommt es an. [Therapy with the book. It depends on co-operation.] *Humanitas*, Berlin, 5 (20) 1965, 13.

1471 ESBECH, Svend. IFLA – møde i Helsingfors 1965. [IFLA – meeting in Helsingfors 1965.] *Bogens Verden*, 47 (8) 1965, 608 – 611.

1472 EULER, Karl Friedrich. Das Buch als Therapie-Helfer im Krankenhaus. [The book as a therapeutic aid in hospital.] *Das Krankenhaus*, 57 (1) Jan. 1965, 25 – 27.

1473 EULER, Karl Friedrich. Bucharbeit am Krankenbett. [Books at the hospital bed.] *Deutsche Schwesternzeitung*, 18 (8) Aug. 1965, 300 – 303.

1474 FLANDORF, Vera S. *Films for hospitalized and institutionalized children.* Chicago, Children's Memorial Hospital, 1965.

1475 FLANDORF, Vera S. Preparing a child for hospitalization. *General Practitioner*, 31 March 1965, 107 – 110.

1476 FLANDORF, Vera S. Up-dating the children's library. *Hospital Management*, Chicago, 100 Oct. 1965, 82 – 84.

1477 GALE, Selma R. Effective use of volunteers in hospital libraries. *AHIL Quarterly*, 5 Winter 1965, 6 – 9.

1478 GARDNER, Frank M. Hospital libraries – the international scene. *In: Hospital library services surveyed: papers given at the Hospital Libraries and Handicapped Readers Group conference . . . Sheffield, 1964.* London, LA, 1965, 58 – 63.

1479 GARTLAND, Henry J. Libraries in hospitals. *World Hospitals,* 1 (4) April 1965, 329 – 332; in French, 332 – 335; summaries in Spanish and German, 335 – 336.

1480 GEISELER, W. Bibliotherapie. *Berliner Medizinische Rundschau*, (3) 1965, 24.

1481 GELDERBLOM, Gertrud. Die Krankenhausbücherei. [The hospital library.] *In:* Langfeldt, J. *editor. Handbuch des Büchereiwesens.* Wiesbaden, Harrassowitz, 1965, vol. 2, 589 – 627.

1482 GÖTTSCHE, Elfriede. Die Patientenbücherei: Aufgabe und Ergebnis. [The patients' library: purpose and effect.] *Krankenhaus-Umschau*, 34 (4) April 1965, 144 – 148.
Hosp. Abstr. 1965/1344

1483 GUTHRIE, Duncan. Reading needs of the physically handicapped. *In: Hospital library services surveyed: papers given at the Hospital Libraries and Handicapped Readers Group conference . . . Sheffield, 1964.* London, LA, 1965, 14 – 16.

1484 HALLQVIST, M. Biblioteksterapi för långliggande barn. [Bibliotherapy for children in long-stay hospitals.] *Biblioteksbladet*, 50 (9) 1965, 666 – 668.

1485 HJELMQVIST, Bengt. Vision och vilja. [Includes information on hospital libraries and the handicapped reader.] *Biblioteksbladet*, 50 (8) 1965, 546 – 556.
LSA 1966/462

1486 HUSBY, Jacob. Lydboger til lammede. [Talking books for the paralysed.] *Bogens Verden*, 47 Nov. 1965, 522 – 523.

1487 JANNASCH, Christine. Die Bucharbeit im St. Markus Krankenhaus Frankfurt/Main. [Library work in St. Markus hospital Frankfurt am Main.] *Deutsche Schwestern – Zeitung*, 18 (8) Aug. 1965, 303 – 304.

1488 JOHNSTON, Nancy. Group reading as a treatment tool with geriatrics. *American Journal of Occupational Therapy*, 19 July/Aug. 1965, 192 – 195.

1489 JUNGE, Richard. Bibliotherapie? Über die Zusammenarbeit des Arztes und der Schwester mit der Bibliothekarin zum Wohle des Patienten. [Bibliotherapy: co-operation of doctors and nurses with the librarian for the good of the patient.] *Humanitas*, Berlin, 5 (23) 1965, 13.

1490 Katholische Krankenhausbüchereien. [Catholic hospital libraries.] *Krankendienst*, 12 1965, 385 – 387.

1491 KELLNER, B. Hospital libraries in Sweden. *Unesco Bull. Libr.*, 19 (4) July/Aug. 1965, 207 – 209.
Hosp. Abstr. 1966/454

1492 LEICH, Helmut. Die Leistungsfähige Patientenbücherei. [The efficient patients' library.] *Krankenhaus-Umschau*, 34 (1) Jan. 1965, 26.

1493 LENTZ, R. T. Hospital librarian: the professional person. *Cath. Libr. Wld.*, 37 Sept. 1965, 79 – 80.

1494 LEWIS, M. Joy. Hospital and medical libraries. *In*: Burkett, J. *editor. Special library and information services in the United Kingdom; 2nd rev. edition.* London, LA, 1965, 270 – 286.

1495 LEWIS, M. Joy. The reading needs of children in hospital: paper presented at IFLA conference, Helsinki, 1965. *De Openbare Bibliotheek*, 8 Nov. 1965, 356 – 359.

1496 LIBRARY ASSOCIATION. *Hospital libraries: recommended standards for libraries in hospitals.* London, LA, 1965. 16 pp.

1497 LIBRARY ASSOCIATION. Hospital Libraries and Handicapped Readers Group. *Hospital libraries surveyed: papers given at the Hospital Libraries and Handicapped Readers Group conference . . . Sheffield, 1964.* London, LA, 1965. 63 pp. For papers presented *see* nos. 1455, 1460, 1464, 1478, 1483.

1498 MARY CHRISTINE, *sister*. Library committee and the patients' library. *Cath. Libr. Wld.*, 36 April 1965, 562 – 564+.

1499 Materials selection for hospital and institution libraries. *AHIL Quarterly*, 6 Fall 1965, 18 – 22.

1500 Moderne sygehusdrift. [Modern hospital operation.] *Bibliotekaren*, 27 (4) 1965, 121 – 123.

1501 MULLEN, Frances A. *and* PETERSON, Miriam. Special education and the school librarian: a co-operative service in the Chicago public schools. *Illinois Libraries*, 47 (5) May 1965, 407 – 416.
LSA 1965/15645

1502 NANNESTAD, Anna (afterwards Anna Nannestad Nicolaysen) *and* HVARDAL, Maren. Bibliotektjenesten ved våre sykehus: pasientbibliotek og medisinsk bibliotek. [Library services for patients and medical staff in our hospitals.] *Sykehuset*, 28 (6) 1965, 121 – 124.
Hosp. Abstr. 1967/676

1503 NEW YORK STATE. INTERDEPARTMENTAL HEALTH AND HOSPITAL COUNCIL. Committee on Library Services in State Institutions. *A plan to provide library service to people in New York State Institutions.* Albany, NY, The Council, 1965. 124 pp.

1504 NIELSEN, Helga. De danske hospitalsbiblioteker og deres organisation. (Foredrag.) [Danish hospital libraries and their organisation. (Lecture to hospital library course, 1964, abbreviated version.)] *Bogens Verden*, 47 1965, 517 – 522.

1505 OLSEN, D. *and* O'TOOLE, M. Picture and easy reading books for adults: a selected list. *AHIL Quarterly*, 5 Winter 1965, 10 – 11.

1506 PAULIN, L. V. Recommended standards for libraries in hospitals. *Book Trolley*, 1 (4) Dec. 1965, 2 – 4.
LSA 1966/88

1507 PETERS, Marianne. Büchereiarbeit mit alten menschen. [Library service for the elderly.] *Bücherei und Bildung*, 17 1965, 608 – 609.

1508 RAYMOND, E. A branch library in a psychiatric hospital. *Nursing Mirror*, 121 Nov. 26, 1965, IX.
Hosp. Abstr. 1966/968

1509 Reading as a restorative. *Canadian Hospital*, 22 Nov. 1965, 56 – 58.

1510 RIEFF, Donald. The librarian and the mentally ill. *Cath. Libr. Wld.*, 36 (5) Jan. 1965, 313 – 317, 334.
LSA 1965/15289

1511 ŠAPOŠNIKOV, A. E. Library services for the blind in the Soviet Union. *Unesco Bull. Libr.*, 19 (5) Sept./Oct. 1965, 246 – 250.
LSA 1965/15843

1512 SCHMIDT, Hannelore. Nochmals: die leistungsfähige Patientenbücherei. [Once again the efficient patients' library.] *Krankenhaus-Umschau*, 34 (7) July 1965, 288.

1513 SCHMITZ, T. Der Kranke und das Buch, wer sind unsere Kranken und welche Bücher brauchen sie. [The patient and the book, who are our patients and what sort of books do they need?] *Die Diakonieschwester*, 61 (6) June 1965, 114.

1514 STEGMANN, [   ] von *and* STEIN, B. Erfahrungen aus der praktischen Arbeit mit der Krankenbücherei. [Experiences from practical work in the hospital library.] *Die Diakonieschwester*, 61 (6) June 1965, 114 – 115.

1515 SVENSSON, Marianne. Boken kommer: kontaktdagar kring bibliotekens sociala sector. [Books are coming: conference on social services of libraries.] *Biblioteksbladet*, 50 (5) 1965, 299 – 301.
LSA 1965/15912

1516 TAIT, Lilias. Library services – 2. The Edinburgh hospitals. *Book Trolley*, 1 (4) Dec. 1965, 6 – 7.

1517 THIEKÖTTER, Hans. Die Blindenbücherei. [Library for the blind.] *In*: Langfeldt, J. editor. *Handbuch des Büchereiwesens*. Wiesbaden, Harrasowitz, 1965, vol. 2, 577 – 588.

1518 THOMPSON, Godfrey. Library services – 2. Not by these standards alone. *Book Trolley*, 1 (4) Dec. 1965, 4 – 6.

1519 TOULSON, S. Reading in bed: the hospital library service. *British Books*, Feb. 1965, 17 – 19.

1520 WALMER, John D. Psychology of illness and the use of reading in the treatment plan. *AHIL Quarterly*, 5 (3) Spring 1965, 4 – 9.
LSA 1966/98

1521 WEIMERSKIRCH, Philip J. Benjamin Rush and John Minson Galt II: pioneers of bibliotherapy in America. *Bull. Med. Libr. Ass.*, 53 Oct. 1965, 510 – 526.

1522 WIGHT, B. L. Library service to hospitals. *California Librarian*, 16 July 1965, 253 – 254.

1523 YELLAND, M. editor. *Large and clear: a list of large-type books*. London, LA, 1965. 31 pp.

1966

1524 AVERY, Chester *and* LYMAN, Helen H. Libraries and the visually handicapped [report of a meeting]. *Wilson Libr. Bull.*, 40 (9) May 1966, 854 – 856.

1525 BERGMANN, Bärbelies. Bücher in unserer Psychotherapie. [Books in our psychotherapy.] *Humanitas*, Berlin, 6 (10) 1966, 11.

1526 Blind like all others. *Kansas Library Bulletin*, 35 (1) Spring 1966, 16 – 17.
LSA 1966/682

1527 BÖTHIG, Siegfried. Das richtige Buch: ein Teil der psychologischen Krankenführung. [The right book: part of the psychological management of ill health.] *Humanitas*, Berlin, 6 (8) 1966, 16.

1528 BOURDIN, Geneviève. Les bibliothèques d'hôpitaux: resultats d'une enquête. [Hospital libraries: results of a survey.] *Association des Bibliothécaires Français Bulletin d'Informations*, (50) March 1966, 25 – 29. LSA 1966/668

1529 BOUTON, E. N. *Library service to hospitalized children in the city of Baltimore.* Thesis (M.S. in L.S.) Catholic University of America. 1966. 57 pp.

1530 BROOKE, G. A. G. Is your library accessible to all? *Libr. Ass. Rec.*, 68 (3) March 1966, 86 – 87.

1531 BURGESS, David G. The hospital library service in Lincoln. *Library World*, 67 (790) April 1966, 290 – 294. LSA 1966/416

1532 A card catalog for the blind. *Wilson Libr. Bull.*, 40 (9) May 1966, 830 – 831.

1533 CARNER, C. Reaching troubled minds through reading. *To-day's Health*, 44 Dec. 1966, 32+.

1534 CLARKE, Jean M. The Hospital Libraries and Handicapped Readers Group of the Library Association. *Library World*, 67 (790) April 1966, 288 – 290.

1535 COUNCIL OF NATIONAL LIBRARY ASSOCIATIONS. Joint Committee on Hospital Libraries. *Basic list of guides and sources for setting up hospital, medical and nursing libraries.* Chicago, 1966.

1536 DAVIS, Ellen L. This library open 24 hours a day, serves staff, students, patients: Harper Hospital, Detroit. *Hospital Topics*, 44 (7) July 1966, 48 – 50.

1537 DEWE, Michael, *and others, compilers.* Library service to children in hospital: a list of related references; compiled by Michael Dewe, M. Joy Lewis, Lisa-Christina Persson. *In*: IFLA Sub-Section on Library Work With Children. *Library service to children.* Lund, Bibliotekstjänst, 1966, vol. 2, 86 – 92.

1538 DONALIES, Christian. Über den Einfluss von Büchern und andere Gedanken zur 'Bibliotherapie'. [The influence of books and other thoughts on bibliotherapy.] *Humanitas*, Berlin, 6 (11) 1966, 13.

1539 EPSTEIN, R. Hospital libraries; Cape Province. *Cape Librarian*, April 1966, 14 – 16.

1540 FAVAZZA, A. R. Bibliotherapy: a critique of the literature. *Bull. Med. Libr. Ass.*, 54 April 1966, 138 – 141.

1541 FÉDÉRATION INTERNATIONALE DES ASSOCIATIONS DE BIBLIOTHÉCAIRES. Sous – Section des Bibliothèques d'Hôpitaux pour les Malades. Committee report. *In*: *Actes du Conseil General . . . XXI, 31e session Helsinki, 1965.* La Haye, Martinus Nijhoff, 1966, 106 – 107.

1542 FINZEL, Siegfried. Bibliotherapie und Berufsausbildung. [Bibliotherapy and professional training.] *Humanitas*, Berlin, 6 (13) 1966, 11.

1543 FITCH, William C. The new look in aging. *Wilson Libr. Bull.*, 40 (9) May 1966, 833 – 835.

1544 FLANDORF, Vera S. Use of audio-visual materials with children in hospitals and institutions. *Cath. Libr. Wld.*, 37 Feb. 1966, 398 – 399+.

1545 FREIBERGER, H. *and* MURPHY, E. F. Reading machines for the blind. *Science*, 152 April 29 1966, 679 – 680.

1546 GOING, Mona E. Library services – 3, Kent. *Book Trolley*, 1 March 1966, 9 – 10.

1547 GOSTYŃSKA, Danuta. Czytelnictwo chorych i biblioterapia w szpitalach. [Reading interests of patients and bibliotherapy in hospitals.] *Bibliotekarz*, 33 (11) 1966, 322 – 327.

1548 GREAT BRITAIN. MINISTRY OF HEALTH. *Hospital library service*. London, The Ministry, 1966. (H.M. (66) 77.)

1549 GREENAWAY, E. Report on my work in the school at High Wick Hospital, 1961 – 65. *New Era in Home and School*, 47 Jan. 1966, 1 – 16.

1550 HAAS, Dorothy B. That the blind may read. *Wisconsin Library Bulletin*, 62 (3) May/June 1966, 152 – 154.

1551 HAVENS, Shirley. A library for the blind. *Libr. J.*, 91 (13) July 1966, 3333 – 3338.
LSA 1966/681

1552 Hospital libraries (editorial). *British Medical Journal*, i Feb. 19 1966, 437 – 438.

1553 Hospital libraries: report of a conference at the Hospital Centre, London, 1966. *British Hospital Journal & Social Service Review*, 76 Feb. 25 1966, 362 – 363.

1554 ILLINOIS DEPARTMENT OF MENTAL HEALTH *and* ILLINOIS STATE LIBRARY. *Summary: first joint workshop for community public librarians and librarians serving patients at Illinois Mental Health Institutions: 'Improving library services for those with mental health problems'* . . . Springfield, Ill., 1966, 28 pp.

1555 JANSEN, Mogens. De sidste procenter analfabeter. Let læselige bøger for voksne. [The last percentage illiterates. Easy-readers for adults.] *Bogens Verden*, 48 (4) 1966, 281 – 282.

1556 JONES, John W. The visually handicapped child. *Wilson Libr. Bull.*, 40 (9) May 1966, 824 – 828.

1557 JUNG, H. D. Bibliotherapie im modernen Geburtskrankenhaus auf dem Lande. [Bibliotherapy in a modern maternity hospital.] *Humanitas*, Berlin, 6 (7) 1966, 13.

1558 KAUPPI, Hilkka. *Några principer vid sjukhusbibliotekets bokval*. [Hospital library book selection.] Den Nordiske Fortsættelsesskole for Bibliotekarer, 1966. (Duplicated.)

1559 KINNEY, M. M. Patients' library in a psychiatric setting. *AHIL Quarterly*, 6 Winter 1966, 12 – 17.

1560 KUHLMANN, F. Der kranke Mensch und das Buch. [The sick person and the book.] *Die Evangelische Krankenpflege*, 16 (6) Nov. 1966, 149 – 155.

1561 KÜNZEL, D. Bibliotherapie und medizinische Publizistik. [Bibliotherapy and medical publications.] *Humanitas*, 6 (14) 1966, 13.

1562 LEUSCHNER, Lucille K. Bibliotherapy and patient libraries: the growth of hospital library services. *In*: O'Morrow, G. S., *compiler. Administration of activity therapy service.* Springfield, Ill., Thomas, 1966, 137 – 172.

1563 LEWIS, M. Joy. Hospital librarian and the child. *In*: *IFLA*. Sub-section on Library Work With Children. *Library service to children.* Lund, Bibliotekstjänst, 1966, vol. 2, 82 – 85.

1564 LEWIS, M. Joy. Hospital libraries the world over. [Report of IFLA conference, Helsinki.] *British Hospital Journal & Social Service Review*, 77 (3973) June 10 1966, 1069.
Hosp. Abstr. 1966/2055

1565 LEWIS, M. Joy. Służba biblioteczna w szpitalach angielskich. [Hospital libraries in England; transl. into Polish by M. Minkiewicz.] *Bibliotekarz*, 33 (7 – 8) 1966, 217 – 222.

1566 Libraries in hospitals: Scottish Hospital Centre conference. *SLA News*, (76) Oct. 1966, 14 – 15.

1567 Libraries: report on a conference at the Hospital Centre, London, Feb. 1966. *Nursing Times*, 62 Feb. 18 1966, 230 – 231; also in *Hospital*, London, 62 (3) March 1966, 103 – 104.

1568 LIMPER, Hilda K. Library services to deaf children. *AHIL Quarterly*, 7 (1) Fall 1966, 7 – 10.
LSA 1967/180

1569 LINNOVAARA, Leena. *Synpunkter på sanatoriernas biblioteksverksamhet: en principiell diskussion på grundval av finska förhallanden.* [Aspects of libraries in TB sanatoria in Finland.] Den Nordiske Fortsættelsesskole for Bibliotekarer, 1966. (Duplicated.)

1570 LUCIOLI, Clara E. *Patients' libraries, an extended role.* New York, United Hospital Fund of New York, 1966. 9 pp.

1571 LUCIOLI, Clara E. Step up – keep up – move up. *AHIL Quarterly*, 6 Winter 1966, 6 – 8.

1572 MAHONEY, Sally M. *and* STOKES, Liselotte Z. A school library program for the blind. *Wilson Libr. Bull.*, 40 (9) May 1966, 829, 857.

1573 MUNFORD, W. A. Services old and new (National Library for the Blind.) *Book Trolley*, 1 (6) June 1966, 1 – 3.

1574 NATIONAL ASSOCIATION OF GROUP SECRETARIES. South Western Regional Branch. *Notes on a study of hospital libraries in the South Western Region.* Northampton, The Association, 1966. 7 pp.

1575 NIELSEN, Hanne Grove. Ordblindebøger for voksne. [Books for dyslexic adults.] *Bogens Verden*, 48 (3) 1966, 209 – 210.

1576 NOAKES, Edward H. Making libraries useable. *Wilson Libr. Bull.*, 40 (9) May 1966, 851 – 853.

1577 NORTHERN IRELAND. MINISTRY OF EDUCATION. *The public library service in Northern Ireland: report of the committee . . . [chairman: Dr. J. S. Hawnt]*. Belfast, HMSO, 1966. (Cmd. 494) paras. 29; 70 – 77, Services to hospitals, institutions, the elderly and the handicapped.

1578 NYBERG, Mirjam [afterwards Mirjam Grundstroem]. Hospital libraries in Finland. *Book Trolley*, 1 (7) Sept. 1966, 3 – 5.

1579 OLIVER, Beryl. *The British Red Cross in action*. London, Faber & Faber, 1966, 305, Red Cross war library; 485 – 486, Hospital library service.

1580 ORR, J. M., compiler. *Books for the bed: a selective and annotated reading list of fiction for those confined to bed*. Manchester, Manchester College of Commerce, Dept. of Librarianship, 1966. 15 pp.

1581 [PARLAND, Oscar.] Kirjallisuus, psykiatrinen hoito ja mentaalihygienia. [An analysis of the relation between literature and mental health.] *Mielenterveys*, 6 (2) 1966, 15 – 20.

1582 PARTINGTON, W[ylva] W. Library services – 4. Queen Elizabeth II hospital. *Book Trolley*, 1 June 1966, 4 – 6.

1583 PARTINGTON, Wylva W. The Queen Elizabeth II hospital library. *Postgraduate Medical Journal*, 42 (491) Sept. 1966, 537 – 542.

1584 PRICE, P. P. Library services and Construction Act amendments of 1966 (P.L. 89 – 511). *Health Education and Welfare Indicators*, (9) Sept. 1966, 1 – 12.

1585 *Rapport van de commissie ad hoc bibliotheekwerk bejaarden uitgebracht aan het Studiecentrum voor Openbare Bibliotheken*. [The committee on library work for the aged reports to the Dutch L.A. on standards.] 's Gravenhage, C.V., 1966. 68 pp.

1586 Reading for older persons. *Wilson Libr. Bull.*, 40 May 1966, 836 – 837.

1587 RIGDEN, M. S. Recommended standards for libraries in hospitals. *Book Trolley*, 1 (4) March 1966, 3 – 4.

1588 RONNIE, M. Library service to hospitals in Dunedin. *New Zealand Libraries*, 29 (7 – 8) Aug. – Sept. 1966, 133 – 139.
LSA 1966/723

1589 SANDERS, Brenda M. *Library services in hospitals: a survey of their present provision and possible future development in the South East Metropolitan Region*. London, LA, 1966. 45 pp (LA pamphlet, 27.)

1590 SCHMIDT, Hannelore. Die Krankenhausbücherei. [The hospital library.] *Die Neue Bücherei*, (3) 1966, 249 – 251.

1591 SCHYRA, B. Krankenhausbibliothek, eine therapeutische Notwendigkeit. [Hospital library, a therapeutic necessity.] *Das Deutsche Gesundheit*, 21 (23) June 1966, 1096 – 1099.

1592 SMITH, Frederick W. Library services to housebound readers. *Libr. Ass. Rec.*, 68 (12) Dec. 1966, 433 – 434.

1593 STRESNO, [   ]. Library service to old age homes. *Cape Librarian*, May 1966, 24 – 25.
LSA 1967/181

1594 STURT, Ronald. Hospital libraries: the state of the art. *Library Review*, 20 (7) Autumn 1966, 473 – 481; also shortened version in *British Hospital Journal & Social Service Review*, 77 Aug. 18 1967, 1539 – 1541.
LSA 1966/937

1595 UNITED HOSPITAL FUND OF NEW YORK. *Bibliography on patients' libraries*. New York, The Fund, 1966. 10 pp.

1596 UNITED HOSPITAL FUND OF NEW YORK. *Essentials for patients' libraries: a guide*. New York, The Fund, 1966. 103 pp.

1597 VELLEMAN, Ruth A. A library for the handicapped. *Libr. J.*, 91 (16) Sept. 15 1966, 4200 – 4204.
LSA 1966/988

1598 VRHOVAC, N. Društveni značaj bolničke biblioteke. [Social importance of hospital libraries.] *Bibliotekar* (Belgrade) 18 Jan. 1966, 78 – 80.

1599 WALLIS, Jean. The library comes to you. *Camden Journal*, 1 (6) April 1966, 140 – 143.

1600 WOLFF, Hildegard. Büchereipraxis: Büchereiarbeit im Krankenhaus. [Library work in hospital.] *Bücherei und Bildung*, 18 (3) March 1966, 159 – 160.

1967

1601 ALEXANDER, R. H. *and* BUGGIE, S. E. Bibliotherapy with chronic schizophrenics. *Journal of Rehabilitation*, 33 Nov. – Dec. 1967, 26+.

1602 AMERICAN LIBRARY ASSOCIATION. Library Administration Division. *Standards for library services for the blind and visually handicapped*. Chicago, ALA, 1967. 54 pp.

1603 American standard specifications for making buildings and facilities accessible to, and usable by, the physically handicapped. *Library News Bulletin*, 34 (1) Jan. – March 1967, 60 – 65.

1604 ANDREWES, J. Bibliotherapy. *In*: *Reading and health: papers given at the Hospital Libraries and Handicapped Readers Group conference . . . Southampton, 1965*. London, The Group, 1967, 42 – 51.

1605 ARBEITSKREIS 'KRANKENHAUSBÜCHEREIEN'. *Büchereiarbeit im Krankenhaus. 3. öffentliche Arbeitstagung für Krankenhausbüchereien, Düsseldorf 1967*. [Library work in hospitals, 3rd public conference on hospital libraries, Düsseldorf 1967.] Berlin, D.B.V. Arbeitsstelle für das Büchereiwesen, 1967, 115 pp. (Bibliotheksdienst Beiheft 29/30.)
For papers presented *see* nos. 1653, 1665, 1666, 1681, 1684
LSA 1968/393; Hosp. Abstr. 1968/409

1606 ARBEITSKREIS 'KRANKENHAUSBÜCHEREIEN'. Richtlinien für Krankenhausbüchereien. [Guidelines for patients' libraries in hospitals.] *Krankenhaus-Umschau*, 36 (11) Nov. 1967, 1016, 1025 – 1027.
Hosp. Abstr. 1968/1854

1607 BARE, Nancy J. Pierce County will serve nursing homes. *Library News Bulletin* (Washington State Library), 34 (3) July/Sept. 1967, 241 – 243. LSA 1968/210

1608 BERRY, J. Bibliotherapy. *Cath. Libr. Wld.*, 39 Oct. 1967, 123 – 127.

1609 BOORER, David. *The mental hospital library.* London, LA, 1967. 43 pp. (LA pamphlet, 31.)
Hosp. Abstr. 1968/738

1610 BOURDIN, Geneviève *and* GARIEL, Elisabeth. Bibliothèques d'hôpitaux: une enquête. [Hospital libraries: an enquiry.] *Lecture et Bibliothèques*, (2) July 1967, 25 – 29.
LSA 1967/673

1611 BUNCH, Antonia J. Hospital libraries. *In: Proceedings of the annual conference of the Scottish library association, 1967.* Glasgow, University of Strathclyde, 1967, 27 – 33.
LSA 1968/122

1612 CALIFORNIA LIBRARY ASSOCIATION. Hospitals and Institutions Round Table. Patients' libraries in California county hospitals: a report. *California Librarian*, 28 Jan. 1967, 33 – 37; excerpts in *AHIL Quarterly*, 7 Spring 1967, 74 – 76.

1613 CLARKE, J[ean] M. The Library Association: a policy statement. *Book Trolley*, 1 (10) Summer 1967, 3 – 4.

1614 COUNCIL OF NATIONAL LIBRARY ASSOCIATIONS. Joint Committee for Hospital Libraries. *Basic list of guides and information sources for professional and patients' libraries in hospitals.* Chicago, American Hospital Association, 1967. 15 pp.

1615 CRITCHLEY, W. E. G. Library service to the handicapped. *In: Proceedings of the annual conference of the Scottish library association, 1967.* Glasgow, University of Strathclyde, 1967, 35 – 39.
LSA 1968/203

1616 DEUTSCHER BÜCHEREIVERBAND. *Richtlinien für Krankenhausbüchereien.* [Guidelines for hospital libraries.] Berlin, DBV, 1967. 17 pp. (Bibliotheksdienst Beiheft 20.)
LSA 1968/394

1617 ELLSWORTH, R. H. Library service in Danish mental hospitals. *AHIL Quarterly*, 7 Winter 1967, 46 – 47.

1618 Evangelischen Krankenhausbüchereien. Die evangelischen Krankenhausbüchereien in dem Deutschen Evangelischen Krankenhausverband angeschlossenen Krankenanstalten in der Bundesrepublik und Berlin (West). Eine Bestandsaufnahme. Stand August 1966. [Protestant hospital libraries in West Germany and West Berlin.] *Die Evangelische Krankenpflege*, 17 (6) Nov. 1967, 139 – 144.

1619 FÉDÉRATION INTERNATIONALE DES ASSOCIATIONS DE BIBLIOTHÉCAIRES. Sous-Section des Bibliothèques d'Hôpitaux. Report and resolutions. *In: Actes du Conseil General ... XXXII, 32e session La Haye, 1966.* La Haye, Martinus Nijhoff, 1967, 74 – 75.

1620 FLANDORF, Vera S., *compiler. Books to help children adjust to a hospital situation.* Chicago, AHIL, 1967. 56 pp.

1621 FROMMER, E. A. The needs of children in hospital. *In: Reading and health: papers given at the Hospital Libraries and Handicapped Readers Group Conference... Southampton, 1965.* London, The Group, 1967, 30 – 39.

1622 GALLOZZI, Charles. New hope for the handicapped. *Libr. J.*, 92 (7) April 1 1967, 1417 – 1420.
LSA 1967/458

1623 GOTTHARDSEN, Marthe Overgaard. Centralbiblioteket for Tuberkulose-patienter: 25 ars jubilæm. [The central library for TB patients 25th anniversary.] *Bogens Verden*, 49 (4) July 1967, 293 – 294.

1624 GRAHAM, Earl C. Public library services to the handicapped. *ALA Bull.*, 61 (2) Feb. 1967, 170 – 179.
LSA 1967/457

1625 GRANGER, E. M. Düsseldorf: hospital library conference. *Book Trolley*, 1 (11) Sept. 1967, 13 – 15.

1626 GRAY, P. G. *and* TODD, Jean E. *Mobility and reading habits of the blind: an enquiry made for the Ministry of Health covering the registered blind of England and Wales in 1965.* London, HMSO, 1967. 119 pp. (Government social survey.)

1627 HAGLE, A. D. Large print revolution. *Libr. J.*, 92 Sept. 15 1967, 3008 – 3010.

1628 HEATHFIELD, Shirley. Library services: Lewisham. *Book Trolley*, 1 (12) Dec. 1967, 9 – 11.
LSA 1968/454

1629 HEWITT, Marion. Working with handicapped children. *L.A. Youth Libraries Group News*, 11 (1) March 1967, 3 – 5.

1630 IFLA and hospital libraries. *Book Trolley*, 1 (9) March 1967, 1.

1631 IRISH REPUBLIC. HOSPITAL LIBRARY COUNCIL. *Summary of thirty years' service, 1937 – 1967.* Dublin, The Council, 1967. 1 p.

1632 JACK, Alexandra *and* KEWLEY, Peter D. Libraries and the housebound: a report on Stockport. *Book Trolley*, 1 (12) Dec. 1967, 19 – 24.

1633 KAUPPI, Hilkka. Biblioterapia. *In: Psykiatrinen kuntoutus.* [Psychiatric rehabilitation.] Porvoo – Helsinki, Werner Söderström, 1967, 168 – 172.

1634 KŘIVINKOVÁ, Julie. Biblioteki dla pacjentów w szpitalach czechosławackich. [Patients' libraries in Czechoslovak hospitals.] *Bibliotekarz*, 34 (9) 1967, 270 – 272.

1635 Large print: trends in a new field. *Libr. J.*, 92 (16) Sept. 15 1967, 3011 – 3013.
LSA 1968/221

1636 LATTANZI, Angela Daneu. Le biblioteche ospedaliere. [Hospital libraries. *AIB Boll.*, 6 (6) Nov. – Dec. 1967, 153 – 162.
LSA 1968/125; Hosp. Abstr. 168/1521

1637 LEICH, Helmut G. R. Bibliotherapie im Krankenhaus. [Bibliotherapy in the hospital.] *Das Krankenhaus*, 59 (11) Nov. 1967.

1638 LEICH, Helmut, G. R. Die Patientenbücherei im Krankenhaus. [The patients' library in the hospital.] *Krankenhausforschung/Krankenhauspraxis* (1) 1967, 1 – 12 issued with *Krankenhaus*, Koln, 59 (3) March 1967.
Hosp. Abstr. 1967/1371

1639 LEITH, Marian *and* VON OESEN, Elaine. Library services for the blind and handicapped. *Southeastern Librarian*, 17 (1) Spring 1967, 17 – 21.
LSA 1967/678

1640 LIBRARY ASSOCIATION. Hospital Libraries and Handicapped Readers Group. *Reading and health: papers given at the Hospital Libraries and Handicapped Readers Group conference . . . Southampton, 1965*. London, The Group, 1967. 51 pp.
For papers presented *see* nos. 1604, 1621, 1648, 1675.

1641 LIBRARY ASSOCIATION. Hospital Libraries and Handicapped Readers Group. Survey of public library service to hospitals, the housebound and prisons. *Libr. Inf. Bull.*, 1 (4) 1967, 113 – 118; also shortened version in *Book Trolley*, 1 (11) Sept. 1967, 3 – 9.
LSA 1968/453

1642 The London declaration [on hospital patients' library service]. *Book Trolley*, 1 (12) Dec. 1967, 3 – 5.
LSA 1968/395

1643 LUCIOLI, Clara E. Out of isolation. *Libr. J.*, 92 (7) April 1 1967, 1421 – 1423.
LSA 1967/396

1644 LUCIOLI, Clara E. *and* DORR, M. M. Begin with one child. [To expose people to the meaning of reading.] *Top of the News*, 23 Jan. 1967, 150 – 153.

1645 LYONS, G. J. Psychiatric librarianship at Kings Park State Hospital. *Odds & Bookends*, (54) Summer 1967, 4 – 5.

1646 MATTHEWS, D. A. Library services for the blind. *In*: Collison, Robert L., editor. *Progress in library science 1967*. London, Butterworths, 1967, 134 – 150.

1647 MATTHEWS, D. A. Reading habits of the blind. ii. It stops where it begins to get interesting. *Book Trolley*, 2 (2) June 1968, 31 – 34.

1648 MICHELL, R. A. The hospital and the child. *In*: *Reading and health: papers given at the Hospital Libraries and Handicapped Readers Group conference . . . Southampton, 1965*. London, The Group, 1967, 21 – 29.

1649 National Library of the Blind in Jordan. [News and information.] *Unesco Bull. Libr.*, 21 (4) July – Aug. 1967, 222.

1650 NYBERG, Mirjam (afterwards Mirjam Grundstroem). Englannin sairaalakirjastomaailmassa tapahtuu. [Observations on hospital library work in England.] *Kirjastolehti*, 60 (10) 1967, 354 – 356.
LSA 1967/949

1651 NYBERG, Mirjam (afterwards Mirjam Grundstroem). Service to groups cut off from the public library. *Book Trolley*, 1 (10) Summer 1967, 11 – 17.
LSA 1967/951

1652 ODESCALCHI, E. K. Fun for the housebound through Uncle Sam's generosity. *Bookmark*, 26 May 1967, 255 – 257.

1653 PANSE, Friedrich. Lektüre als Heilfaktor. [Reading as a therapy.] *In*: *Büchereiarbeit im Krankenhaus 3 öffentliche Arbeitstagung für Krankenhausbüchereien, Dusseldorf 1967*. Berlin, D.B.V. Arbeitsstelle für das Büchereiwesen, 1967, 11 – 21. (Bibliotheksdienst Beiheft, 29/30); also in *Krankenhaus-Umschau*, 37 (1) Jan. 1968. 40 – 44.

1654 Patients' libraries in California county hospitals. *AHIL Quarterly*, 7 Spring 1967, 74 – 76.

1655 PÖYSÄLÄ, Pirkko. Kirjastotyötä vanhusten ja sokeitten hyväksi. [Library work for old people and for the blind.] *Kirjastolehti*, 60 (8) 1967, 261 – 265. LSA 1967/949

1656 PÖYSÄLÄ, Pirkko. Laistoskirjastotoimintamme laadusta ja laajuudesta. [Hospital library work in Finland.] *Kirjastolehti*, 60 (3) 1967, 66 – 69; English summary, 96 LSA 1967/455

1657 Printed texts for the partially sighted. *British Printer*, 80 (2) Feb. 1967, 55 – 59.

1658 RADFORD, David. Reading habits of the blind. iii. The implications for the future. *Book Trolley*, 2 (2) June 1968, 34 – 37.

1659 REES, Leslie M. Read well before shaking. *Book Trolley*, 1 (10) Summer 1967, 6 – 11. LSA 1967/950

1660 Relationship and responsibilities of the state library agency to state institutions. *AHIL Quarterly*, 7 Spring 1967, 67 – 71.

1661 ROGERS, J. A. The library and the ESN child. *L.A. Youth Libraries Group News*, 11 (1) March 1967, 7 – 10.

1662 ROSSINI, G. Il servizio di biblioteca in ospedale per il benessere morale de malato. [The effect of library service in hospital in improving the patients' morale.] *Ospedale*, 20 (1) Jan. 1967, 21 – 26. Hosp. Abstr. 1967/1859

1663 RYNELL, A. Symposium för sjukhusbibliotekarier. [Symposium for hospital librarians.] *Biblioteksbladet*, 52 (9) 1967, 872 – 874.

1664 *Sachliteratur für Patientenbüchereien: eine Empfehlungsliste: 2 Auflage*. [Non fiction for hospital libraries: a recommended list; 2nd edition.] Berlin, D.B.V. Arbeitsstelle für das Büchereiwesen, 1967. 71 pp.

1665 SCHMIDT, Hannelore. Krankenhausbüchereien in der Bundesrepublik und Berlin (West). Ergebnisse einer Umfrage. [Hospital libraries in West Germany and West Berlin: results of a survey.] *In*: *Büchereiarbeit im Krankenhaus. 3. öffentliche Arbeitstagung für Krankenhausbüchereien. Dusseldorf 1967*. Berlin, D.B.V. Arbeitsstelle für das Buchereiwesen, 1967, 33 – 39. (Bibliotheksdienst Beiheft 29/30.)

1666 SCHÖNE, Heinz. Krankenhausverwaltung und Krankenhausbücherei. [The hospital administration and the patients' library.] *In: Büchereiarbeit im Krankenhaus 3. öffentliche Arbeitstagung für Krankenhausbüchereien, Düsseldorf 1967.* Berlin, D.B.V. Arbeitsstelle für das Büchereiwesen, 1967, 65 – 73. (Bibliotheksdienst Beiheft 29/30), also in *Krankenhaus-Umschau,* 36 (11) Nov. 1967, 1013 – 1016.
Hosp. Abstr. 1968/1856

1667 SCOTTISH HOSPITAL CENTRE. Libraries in hospitals. *In: Collected conference reports, 1966.* Edinburgh, The Centre, [1967], 41 – 44.

1668 SHAW, Alison. The design of reading material for the partially-sighted. *Book Trolley,* 1 (11) Sept. 1967, 10 – 12.
LSA 1968/479

1669 SHAW, Alison. Reading habits of the blind. i. The first of its kind. *Book Trolley,* 2 (2) June 1968, 28 – 31.

1670 SHORE, H. Books on wheels. *Professional Nursing Home,* 9 July 1967, 12 – 13.

1671 SWENSON, R. P. Activity therapist's library. *AHIL Quarterly,* 7 Winter 1967, 37 – 40; Summer 1967, 93 – 96.

1672 SYDENHAM, J. H. St. John and Red Cross hospital library county organisation. *Book Trolley,* 1 (10) Summer 1967, 18 – 19.

1673 SYDENHAM, J. H. St. John and Red Cross hospital library service. *Book Trolley,* 1 (9) March 1967, 3 – 5.
LSA 1967/395

1674 TEWS, Ruth M. Bibliotherapy: a link with the community. *Hospital Progress,* 48 Jan. 1967, 88 – 94.

1675 THOMAS, Barbara. Planning libraries in hospitals. *In: Reading and health: papers given at the Hospital Libraries and Handicapped Readers Group conference . . . Southampton, July 1965.* London, The Group, 1967, 5 – 13.

1676 TOFAN, Antoaneta. Organizarea si functionarea bibliotecilor de spitale. [Organization and function of hospital libraries.] *Revista Bibliotecilor,* Bucharest, 20 (4) 1967, 208 – 213.

1677 UNITED STATES. VETERANS ADMINISTRATION. Department of Medicine and Surgery. *Planning criteria for medical facilities.* Washington, DC, VA, 1967, chapter 17 Library service [5] pp. (Department of Medicine and Surgery manual M – 7.)

1678 UNITED STATES. VETERANS ADMINISTRATION. Department of Medicine and Surgery. Medical and General Reference Library. *We call it bibliotherapy: an annotated bibliography . . . 1900 – 1966* [compiled by Rosemary Dolan]. Washington, DC, VA, 1967, 50 pp.

1679 VIG-NIELSEN, Ingeborg. Udvalget for hospitalsbiblioteksarbejde. [The committee for hospital work.] *Bogens Verden,* 49 (4) 1967, 295 – 296.

1680 WALLIS, Jean. Experiments and developments in social work. I. Books meet people. *Social Service Quarterly,* Winter 1966 – 1967, 106 – 107.

1681 WECHSELBERG, K. *and* PUYN, Ulrike. Lektüre im Kinderkrankenhaus. [Reading in children's hospitals.] *In: Büchereiarbeit im Krankenhaus. 3. öffentliche Arbeitstagung für Krankenhausbüchereien, Dusseldorf 1967.* Berlin, D.B.V. Arbeitsstelle für das Büchereiwesen, 1967, 23 – 32. (Biblioteksdienst Beiheft 29/30.)

1682 WINNICK, P. *and* HUGUENOR, H. H. Library services to the disadvantaged and handicapped. *ALA Bull.*, 61 (9) Oct. 1967, 1064 – 1074.

1683 WISCONSIN UNIVERSITY. School of Library and Information Science. *Library service to the unserved: papers presented at a library conference held at the University of Wisconsin – Milwaukee, School of Library and Information Science, Nov. 16 – 18 1967.* New York and London, R. R. Bowker, 1970. (Library and information science studies, 2.)

1684 WOLFF, Hildegard. Selbstkritische Betrachtungen über die Krankenhausbüchereiarbeit in Dusseldorf. [Consideration of hospital library work in Dusseldorf.] *In: Büchereiarbeit im Krankenhaus. 3. öffentliche Arbeitstagung für Krankenhausbüchereien, Dusseldorf, 1967.* Berlin, D.B.V. Arbeitsstelle für das Büchereiwesen, 1967, 75 – 87.

1968

1685 ALEXANDER, Rose Horn. Bibliotherapy with chronic schizophrenics. *AHIL Quarterly*, 8 (2) Winter 1968, 39 – 44.
LSA 1968/397

1686 AMERICAN LIBRARY ASSOCIATION. Hospital Libraries Division. *Hospital libraries: objectives and standards:* Chicago, ALA, 1953. 19 pp. Reprinted with prefatory note on proposed revision and updating, Association of Hospital and Institution Libraries, 1968.

1687 BERGGREN, Gösta. *Handikapp och rehabilitering.* [Handicap and rehabilitation: a bibliography.] Lund, 1968. 105 pp.

1688 BIRKHOLZ, Ulrich. Gegenwartsprobleme der Krankenhausbüchereiarbeit. [Actual problems of the work in hospital libraries.] *Der Krankenhausarzt*, (3) 1968, 64 – 67.

1689 BLOM, Marianne. Tekniska hjälpmedel. [Reading aids.] Biblioteksbladet, 53 (3) 1968, 233 – 238.

1690 BLUME, Alfred. Was ist Bibliotherapie und was sollte der Leiter der Patientenbücherei davon wissen? [What is bibliotherapy?] *Krankendienst*, 41 (5) May 1968, 139 – 146.

1691 BRIGGS, Allan H. Through a glass darkly. *Book Trolley*, 2 Dec. 1968, 69 – 71.

1692 BRITISH LIBRARY OF TAPE RECORDINGS FOR HOSPITAL LIBRARIES. [*Brochure*]. London, The Library, 1968, various paging.

1693 BROWN, Roy. Westminster City Libraries: hospital libraries and the housebound reader service. *Book Trolley*, 2 (1) March 1968, 8 – 12.

1694 BUNGENBERG, de JONG, C. J. Ontstaan en werkzaamheden van het Lectuurdepot Rode Kruis. [Establishment and activities of the Red Cross Library depot.] *De Openbare Bibliotheek*, 11 (7) Aug. 1968, 235 – 243.
LSA 1968/720

1695 CAMDEN PUBLIC LIBRARY. *Smoothing the path: a booklist for children entering hospital.* London, Camden P.L., 1968. 4 pp.

1696 CLARKE, Jean M. Library services: St. Thomas' hospital, London. *Book Trolley,* 2 (1) March 1968, 3 - 8.

1697 CLEVELAND PUBLIC LIBRARY. *Second sight through books in large print.* Cleveland, Public Library, 1968 (typescript).

1698 COUNCIL OF NATIONAL LIBRARY ASSOCIATIONS. Joint Committee on Hospital Libraries. *Basic list of guides and sources for setting up hospital medical and nursing libraries.* Chicago, 1968.

1699 COX, E. H. Patients library at the Arkansas tuberculosis sanatorium. *Arkansas Libraries,* 24 Spring 1968, 18 - 19.

1700 CRITCHLEY, W. E. G. Library services for housebound readers in Scotland. *Book Trolley,* 2 (3) Sept. 1968, 54 - 58.
Lisa 1969/765

1701 CROIX-ROUGE DE BELGIQUE. Conseil National des Bibliothèques d'Hôpitaux. *Bibliothèques d'hôpitaux de Belgique: standards.* [Hospital libraries of Belgium.] [Bruxelles, Croix-Rouge de Belgique, 1968.] 12 pp. Text in French, Flemish, English.

1702 DU MONCEAU DE BERGENDAL, I. G., *comtesse.* Book selection methods as used by the Belgian Red Cross. *In: Librarianship and therapy: papers given at the Hospital Libraries and Handicapped Readers Group conference . . . Cambridge, 1967.* London, The Group, 1968, 39 - 46.

1703 ERIKSSON, S. Bibliotek på sjukhus. [Libraries in hospitals.] *Biblioteksbladet,* 53 (6) 1968, 714 - 716.

1704 EULER, Karl Friedrich. Krankenhausbücherei und Krankenlektüre. [The hospital library and literature for patients.] *Deutsches Zentralblatt f. Krankenpflege,* 12 (3) 1968, 129 - 130.

1705 FÉDÉRATION INTERNATIONALE DES ASSOCIATIONS DE BIBLIOTHÉCAIRES. Sous - Section des Bibliothèques d'Hôpitaux. Report. *In: Actes du Conseil General . . . XXXIII, 33e session Toronto, 1967.* La Haye, Martinus Nijhoff, 1968, 71.

1706 GASKING, A. F. J. *and* ROCKALL, F. W. Page turner built by model makers. *Occupational Therapy,* 31 (3) March 1968, 38 - 39.

1707 GOING, Mona E. Hospital libraries and libraries for readers with special needs. *In:* Sewell, P. H., *editor. Five years' work in librarianship, 1961 - 1965.* London, LA, 1968, 190 - 212.

1708 GRANNIS, Florence. Philosophical implications of book selection for the blind. *Wilson Libr. Bull.,* 43 (4) Dec. 1968, 330 - 339.
Lisa 1969/318

1709 GROGAN, J. Libraries serve the handicapped. *Wisconsin Library Bulletin,* 64 (5) Sept. - Oct. 1968, 350 - 351.

1710 GÜNTHER, Jutta, *compiler.* Bibliotherapie: eine literaturauswahl. [Bibliotherapy: a select bibliography.] *Bibliothekar,* Berlin, 22 (12) 1968, 1286 - 1287.

1711 HAHN, Hanne. Kursus i hospitalsbiblioteksarbejde. [Course in hospital librarianship.] *Bogens Verden*, 50 Sept. 1968, 411 – 414.

1712 HAMILTON, Aileen. Books for the retarded child. *Libr. J.*, 93 (4) Feb. 15 1968, 838 – 839.
LSA 1968/450

1713 HANNIGAN, M. C. Has Public Law 89 – 522 affected your library? 'Books for the blind and other physically handicapped.' *AHIL Quarterly*, 9 (1) Fall 1968, 4 – 5.

1714 HARDING, Gösta. Biblioterapi-mentalhygienisk effekt av skönlitteratur. [Bibliotherapy – effect of literature on mental health.] *Psykisk Hälsa*, 1968, 199 – 213.

1715 HAYCRAFT, Howard. *Books for the blind and physically handicapped: a postscript and an appreciation; 3rd edition revised*. New York, H. W. Wilson, 1968. 16 pp.

1716 HÖÖK, Lisbet. Läge, förhoppningar. [Present situation – hopes for the future.] *Biblioteksbladet*, 53 (3) 1968, 209 – 211.

1717 HÖÖK, Lisbet. Omsorger om psykiskt utvecklingsstörda. [Care of the mentally handicapped.] *Biblioteksbladet*, 53 (3) 1968, 239 – 243.

1718 HUETTENBUEGEL, Johannes. Rund um die Krankenhausbücherei. [Around the hospital library.] *Krankendienst*, 41 (5) May 1968, 152 – 154.

1719 KELLNER, B. Einige gedanken über die Bibliotherapie und über Krankenhausbibliotheken. [Thoughts on bibliotherapy and hospital libraries.] *Bibliothekar*, 22 May 1968, 463 – 468.

1720 KJERRSTRÖM, Ulla. Det kombinerade sjukhusbiblioteket. [The combined hospital library.] *Biblioteksbladet*, 53 (3) 1968, 216 – 225; discussion, 226 – 232.

1721 KJERRSTRÖM, Ulla, *compiler*. Yrkeslitteratur för sjukhusbibliotekarier. [Professional literature for hospital librarians.] *Biblioteksbladet*, 53 (3) 1968, 244 – 245.

1722 KNIGHT, N. H. Powered hospital book trucks. *AHIL Quarterly*, 8 Summer 1968, 96 – 98.

1723 Ett kombinerat sjukhusbibliotek? [A combined hospital library.] (Editorial.) *Biblioteksbladet*, 53 (3) 1968, 203 – 204.

1724 KOZAKIEWICZ, Wanda. *Czytelnictwo chorych*. [Patients' reading.] Warszawa, Stowaryszenie Bibliotekarzy Polskich, 1968, 76 pp.

1725 Książka w służbie chorych. *Biblioteki szpitalne za granicą*. [The book in the service of the sick. Hospital libraries in other countries.] Warszawa, Biblioteka Norŏdowa, 1968. 96 pp. (Zeszyty przekładow, 122.)

1726 LEDGARD, Doreen. Escape from the public library to a psychiatric hospital library. *Library Review*, 21 (5) Spring 1968, 247 – 249.
LSA 1968/716

1727 LEWIS, M. Joy. Library service to handicapped readers. *Libr. Ass. Rec.*, 70 (5) May 1968, 120 – 123.
LSA 1968/758

1728 LEWIS, M. Joy. 60 – talets sjukhusbibliotek i England. [Hospital libraries in England; transl. into Swedish by Sonja Pleijel.] *Biblioteksbladet*, 53 (9) 1968, 1096 – 1101.

1729 LIBRARY ASSOCIATION. Hospital Libraries and Handicapped Readers Group. *Librarianship and therapy: papers given at the Hospital Libraries and Handicapped Readers Group conference . . . Cambridge, 1967*. London, The Group, 1968. 61 pp. For papers presented *see* nos. 1702, 1740, 1749. Hosp. Abstr. 1968/1855

1730 LUCIOLI, Clara E. Strengthening existing programs. *AHIL Quarterly*, 8 Summer 1968, 98 – 102.

1731 MCCROSSAN, John *and others*. *Library services for the handicapped in Ohio*. Ohio, Kent State University, Center for Library Studies, 1968.

1732 MOODY, M. T. Bibliotherapy clearinghouse. *AHIL Quarterly*, 8 Winter 1968, 39 – 44.

1733 MOODY, M. T. Librarian as a communication analyst. *AHIL Quarterly*, 9 Fall 1968, 14 – 17.

1734 MULLEN, Marjorie M., *editor*. *Reading aids for the handicapped; 5th revision A.H.I.L. special committee on reading aids for the handicapped*. Chicago, ALA, 1968, 21 pp.

1735 MULLER, R. J. Large print books. *ALA Bull.*, 62 June 1968, 735 – 738.

1736 NATIONAL BOOK LEAGUE. *Help in reading: books for the teacher of backward children and for pupils backward in reading*. London, N.B.L., 1968. 33 pp.

1737 National program for blind and physically handicapped children. *AHIL Quarterly*, 8 Spring 1968, 72 – 74.

1738 NIEMEIJER, J. Bejaardenbibliotheekwerk, waarom? [Library work with the old, why?] *De Openbare Bibliotheek*, 11 (1) Jan. 1968, 3 – 5.

1739 NUIVER, J. Bejaardenbibliotheekwerk, hoe? [Library work with the old, how?] *De Openbare Bibliotheek*, 11 (1) Jan. 1968, 6 – 10.

1740 NYBERG, Mirjam (afterwards Mirjam Grundstroem). Hospital library book selection in Finland: *In*: *Librarianship and therapy: papers given at the Hospital Libraries and Handicapped Readers Group conference . . . Cambridge, 1967*. London The Group, 1968, 28 – 33.

1741 NYE, P. W. Research on reading aids for the blind: a dilemma. *Medical & Biological Engineering*, 6 Jan. 1968, 43 – 50.

1742 ODESCALCHI, E. K. The library can brighten the lives of the homebound. *New York Library Association Bulletin*, 16 July 1968, 102 – 103.

1743 OLSSON, K. Ny organisation i Västernorrland. [New organisation in West Norrland.] *Biblioteksbladet*, 53 (3) 1968, 248 – 250.

1744 PATON, W. B. The public library and the hospital. *Book Trolley*, 2 (3) Sept. 1968, 49 – 50. Lisa 1969/757

1745 PEIFER, David B. Meeting the needs of the physically handicapped. *Library Occurrent*, 22 (11) Aug. 1968, 289 – 290.

1746 PERS, Mats. Bibliotekets plats i långtidsvården. [The role of the library in the treatment of the chronic sick.] *Biblioteksbladet*, 53 (10) 1968, 1225 – 1233; also in *Tidskrift for Sveriges Sjuksköterskor*, 36 (1) Jan. 1969, 50 – 60.
Lisa 1969/317; Hosp. Abstr. 1969/915

1747 PÉTURSDÓTTIR, Kristín H. *and* THORSTEINSDÓTTIR, Kristín. Sjúkrahúsabóka-söfn. [Hospital libraries.] *Samvinnan*, 62 (2) March – April 1968, 25 – 26.

1748 *Romanliteratur für Patientenbüchereien: eine Empfehlungsliste; 4. Auflage.* [A list of novels recommended for hospital libraries; 4th edition.] Berlin, D. B. V. Arbeitsstelle für das Büchereiwesen, 1968. 56 pp.

1749 RYNELL, Aina. Policy governing book selection at Swedish hospital libraries. *In*: *Librarianship and therapy: papers given at the Hospital Libraries and Handicapped Readers Group conference . . . Cambridge, 1967.* London, The Group, 1968, 34 – 38.

1750 Sjukhusbiblioteken och Bibliotekstjänst. [Hospital libraries and Bibliotekstjänst.] *Biblioteksbladet*, 53 (3) 1968, 277 – 279.

1751 SMOKOSKI, Fred J. The school librarian and the mentally retarded student. *AHIL Quarterly*, 8 (2) Winter 1968, 33 – 35.
LSA 1968/449.

1752 STURT, Ronald. Access for the disabled. *Book Trolley*, 2 (4) Dec. 1968, 71 – 73.

1753 TAIT, Lilias. Recordings in hospital through volunteer help: an experiment at the patient's library Western general hospital, Edinburgh. *Book Trolley*, 2 (3) Sept. 1968, 50 – 53.
Lisa 1969/756

1754 TEBBEL, J. Large-type books an expanding horizon. *Saturday Review*, 51 July 13 1968, 55 – 56.

1755 THULIN, Kjerstin. Den sociala verksamheten vid Malmö stadsbibliotek. [Social activity at Malmö public library.] *Biblioteksbladet*, 53 (5) 1968, 529 – 533.

1756 Two new book trolleys. *British Hospital Journal & Social Service Review*, 78 Jan. 19 1968, 120.

1757 UNITED HOSPITAL FUND OF NEW YORK. *Library service for hospitalized children: principles, patterns, goals. Proceedings of the annual meeting committee on patients' libraries.* New York, The Fund, 1968. 19 pp.

1758 UNITED STATES. LIBRARY OF CONGRESS. Division for the Blind and Physically Handicapped. *That all may read.* Washington DC, Library of Congress, 1968. 2 pp.

1759 UPTON, M. E. Multi-faceted service from Little Rock VA hospital strives towards reading as therapy. *Arkansas Libraries*, 24 Spring 1968, 20 – 22.

1760 WEGENER, Sigrid. *Auswahlanalyse einiger Literatur zur Bibliotherapie im Hinblick auf die Patientenbibliothek.* [Book selection for bibliotherapy with regard to the patients' library.] Leipzig, Fachschule für Bibliothekare 'Erich Weinert', 1968. 20 pp. (Abschluss-Hausarbeit.)

1761 WILSON, Bertha. History of AHIL. *AHIL Quarterly*, 8 (2) Winter 1968, 48 – 54.
LSA 1968/611

1762 ZACCARIA, Joseph S. *and* MOSES, Harold A. *The use of bibliotherapy in teaching and counseling.* Champaign, Ill., Stipe's Pub. Co., 1968. 270 pp.

1969

1763 AALTO, Rauni. Mitä kirjoja mielisairaalaan? [Which books for mental hospitals?] *Kirjastolehti*, 62 (4) 1969, 122 – 124; English summary, 157.

1764 Advisory Council librarians discuss service to handicapped people and institutions. *Mississippi Library News*, 33 (3) Sept. 1969, 125 – 126.

1765 AHLNÄS, Benita. Johannesbergin kirjastokerho Porvoossa. [Library club activities at an old people's home in Poorvoo.] *Kirjastolehti*, 62 (4) 1969, 124 – 125; English summary, 157.

1766 AMERICAN LIBRARY ASSOCIATION. Association of Hospital and Institution Libraries. Annual report of the division, 1968 – 1969. *AHIL Quarterly*, 9 (4) Summer 1969, 83 – 90.

1767 ANDREE, O. Die Wirkung von Literatur und Dichtung auf Patienten in einer rationalen Psychotherapie. [The effect of literature and poetry on patients with efficient psychotherapy.] *Psychiatrie, Neurologie und Medizinische Psychologie, Leipzig*, 21 (4) 1969, 152 – 156.

1768 ANDERSEN, Liv. Finnmarks lydavis for blinde. [Finnmark's talking newspaper for the blind.] *Bok og Bibliotek*, 36 (1) Jan. 1969, 25 – 26.
Lisa 1969/767

1769 Arkansas state hospital patients' library work-shop. *Arkansas Libraries*, 25 Spring 1969, 25 – 26.

1770 BEKKER, Johan. Leesstof vir Swaksiendes: die Verskyning van grootdruk-boeke in Afrikaans. [Reading matter for the partially-sighted: the publication of large-print books in Afrikaans.] *S. Afr. Libr.*, 37 (1) July 1969, 2 – 11, 41.
Lisa 1969/2075

1771 BEST, D. de. Bibliotheekwerk: bij uitstek sociaal-cultureel vormend. [Library work: pre-eminently social-cultural education.] *Op Leeftijd*, V (5) Sept./Oct. 1969, 262 – 263.

1772 Bibliotekslokaler inom sjukhus. [Library accommodation in hospitals.] *Spri Informerar*, (5) 1969, 7.

1773 BJERRE, Aase. Hospital library services in Denmark and library service in special areas of social care. *Libri*, 19 (4) 1969, 246 – 248.
Lisa 1970/1421

1774 BOELKE, Joanne, *compiler. Library service to the visually and physically handi-capped: a bibliography.* Minneapolis, Minn., University of Minnesota and ERIC clearing House for Library and Information Sciences, 1969. 20[1] pp. (Bibliography ser., no. 4 ERIC Acc no. ED 031615.)

1775 Buch und Büchereiarbeit im Krankenhaus. [The book and library work in the hospital.] *Die Evangelische Krankenpflege*, 19 (1) Jan. 1969, 28.

1776 BUNCH, Antonia J. *and* CUMMING, Eileen E. Libraries in hospitals: a review of services in Scotland. Edinburgh, Scottish Hospital Centre, 1969, 76 pp. Hosp. Abstr. 1969/1229

1777 BURGESS, David. Libraries in hospitals: a review of the Scottish Hospital Centre report. *SLA News*, (91) 1969, 302 – 305.

1778 BURNS, L. Toward the free world: a library program for the hospital patient. *AHIL Quarterly*, 10 Fall 1969, 18 – 20.

1779 CAMPBELL, H. C. *and* LUDLOW, Virginia F. IFLA, Libraries in Hospitals Sub-section: hospital library surveys, pt. 3: the Canadian library scene. *Int. Libr. Rev.*, 1 (2) April 1969, 213 – 223. Lisa 1969/1656

1780 CASEY, Genevieve. Libraries in the therapeutic society. *ALA Bull.*, 63 (8) Sept. 1969, 1085 – 1086.

1781 COUNCIL OF NATIONAL LIBRARY ASSOCIATIONS. Joint Committee on Library Service in Hospitals. *Basic list of guides and information sources for professional and patients' libraries in hospitals; 6th edition.* [Chicago, American Hospital Association], 1969. 15 pp.

1782 DUDLEY, E. *and* MOUNCE, M. W. Visiting librarian and thereafter. *ALA Adult Services Division Newsletter*, 6 (4) Summer 1969, 53 – 55.

1783 DU MONCEAU DE BERGENDAL, I. G., *comtesse.* IFLA, Libraries in Hospitals Sub-section: hospital library surveys, pt. 2: Education and training for hospital libraries in Belgium. *Int. Libr. Rev.*, 1 (2) April 1969, 209 – 212. Lisa 1969/1657

1784 The education of the visually handicapped: the Library Association's memorandum of evidence to the Department of Education and Science ... *Book Trolley*, 2 (5) March 1969, 83 – 92.

1785 FÉDÉRATION INTERNATIONALE DES ASSOCIATIONS DE BIBLIOTHÉCAIRES. Sous-Section des Bibliothèques d'Hôpitaux. The joint business meeting. Resolutions. Area of responsibility of Sub-Section (draft/project). Rules of the Sub-Section (draft/project). *In: Actes du Conseil Général ... XXXIV, 34e session Frankfurt-Am-Main, 1968.* La Haye, Martinus Nijhoff, 1969, 77 – 82. For papers read *see* nos. 1783, 1789, 2126.

1786 *75 Jahre Deutsche Zentral bücherei für Blinde zu Leipzig, 1894 – 1969.* [75 years of the German Central Library for the Blind, Leipzig.] Leipzig, Deutsche Zentralbücherei für Blinde zu Leipzig, 1969. 159 pp.

1787 GARDNER, F[rank] M. IFLA, Libraries in Hospitals Sub-section: the integrated hospital library, pt. 2: England. *Int. Libr. Rev.*, 1 (1) Jan. 1969, 61 – 65. Lisa 1969/1654

1788 GARDNER, Frank M. *and* LEWIS, M. Joy, *editors. Reading round the world: a set of international reading lists compiled by members of the International Federation of Library Associations.* London, Clive Bingley for IFLA, 1969. 260 pp.

1789 GARTLAND, Henry J. IFLA, Libraries in HospitalsSu b-section: hospital library surveys, pt. 1: the training of hospital librarians in the USA. *Int. Libr. Rev.,* 1 (2) April 1969, 201 – 208.
Lisa 1969/1655

1790 GELDERBLOM, Gertrud. Krankenhausbüchereiarbeit. Immer noch Neuland für uns. [Hospital library work. Still a new ground for us.] *Bücherei und Bildung,* 21 (1/2) Jan./Feb. 1969, 31 – 35.

1791 GOING, Mona E. A day in my library. *Book Trolley,* 2 (8) Dec. 1969, 14 – 16.

1792 GOING, Mona E. Hospital libraries: looking forward. *In: Proceedings, papers and summaries of discussions at the public libraries conference held at Southport, 22nd – 25th September, 1969.* London, LA, 1969, 34 – 38.
Lisa 1969/2532

1793 GOSTYŃSKA, Danuta. Bibliotekarstwo i biblioterapia w szpitalu. [Librarianship and bibliotherapy in the hospital.] *Bibliotekarz,* 36 (5) 1969, 147 – 151.
Lisa 1970/1409

1794 GRANNIS, Florence. Book selection for the blind. *Cath. Libr. Wld.,* 40 April 1969, 491 – 495.

1795 GREAT BRITAIN. SCOTTISH EDUCATION DEPARTMENT. *Standards for the public library service in Scotland: report of a working party appointed by the Secretary of State for Scotland [chairman: I. M. Robertson].* Edinburgh, HMSO, 1969, 27 – 29.

1796 *Grossdruckbücher: eine Zusammenstellung von Büchern in grosser Schrift; 2 Auflage.* [Large print: a collection of books in large print; 2nd edition.] Berlin, D.B.V. Arbeitsstelle für das Büchereiwesen, 1969. 34 pp.

1797 HANNIGAN, Margaret C. Institutional libraries, U.S.A. *Book Trolley,* 2 (6) June 1969, 103 – 108.
Lisa 1970/445

1798 HANNIGAN, Margaret C. Library services to the physically handicapped. *AHIL Quarterly,* 10 Fall 1969, 16 – 17.

1799 HAPP, F. William. Multi-media services for retardates in institutions. *Top of the News,* 25 (3) April 1969, 268 – 272.
Lisa 1969/1667

1800 HARRISON, K. C. *Libraries in Scandinavia; 2nd rev. edition,* London, Grafton Books, 1969, 77 – 79, 142, 153 – 155, 175, 237, 257 – 258, 262.

1801 HIRN, Sven. Kirjastolaitos ja laitoskirjasto. [The library institution and institutional libraries.] *Kirjastolehti,* 62 (4) 1969, 113; English summary, 157.

1802 HOLMSTRÖM, Bengt. IFLA. Libraries in Hospitals Sub-section: the [integrated] hospital library, pt. 3. Scandinavia. *Int. Libr. Rev.,* 1 (1) Jan. 1969, 67 – 70.
Lisa 1969/1658

1803 INTERNATIONAL FEDERATION OF LIBRARY ASSOCIATIONS. Libraries in Hospitals Sub-section. IFLA standards for libraries in hospitals (general service). *Unesco Bull. Libr.*, 23 (2) March/April 1969, 70 – 76.
Lisa 1969/1098

1804 IFLA Libraries in Hospitals Sub-section; hospital library surveys, pt. 4: hospital libraries in the Federal Republic of Germany 1960 to 1968. *Int. Libr. Rev.*, 1 (2) April 1969, 225 – 227.
Lisa 1969/1653

1805 JAKOB, Herbert. 75 Jahre Deutsche Zentralbücherie für Blinde zu Leipzig. [75 years of the German Central Library for the Blind at Leipzig.] *Zentralblatt für Bibliothekswesen*, 83 (12) Dec. 1969, 720 – 725.
Lisa 1970/992

1806 JANKOWSKA, E. Biblioteki szpitalne dla chorych na terenie Łodzi. [Hospital libraries in Lodz.] *Bibliotekarz*, 36 (2) 1969, 47 – 51.

1807 KARJALAINEN, Vappu. Maalaiskuntien sivukirjastojen ja laitoskirjastojen huoneistot. [Rural branch library and hospital library buildings.] *Kirjastolehti*, 62 (11) 1969, 376 – 377.
Lisa 1970/426

1808 *Kinderbücher für die Patientenbüchereien: eine Empfehlungsliste.* [Children's books for hospital libraries: a recommended list.] Berlin, Deutscher Büchereiverband. Arbeitsstelle für das Büchereiwesen, 1969. 60 pp.

1809 Konferens om sjukhusbibliotek. [Conference on hospital libraries.] *Tidskrift for Sveriges Sjuksköterskor*, 36 (1) Jan. 1969, 61 – 62.

1810 LA BAUVE, Lois F. Helping them to help themselves: a report on the Division for the blind and physically handicapped of the Texas state library. *Tex. Libr.*, 31 (2) Summer 1969, 60 – 74.
Lisa 1969/2542

1811 LEEUWENBURGH, P. B. Normen voor ziekenhuisbibliotheken van de IFLA. [IFLA's standards for hospital libraries.] *De Openbare Bibliotheek*, 12 (7/8) Sept./Oct. 1969, 292 – 297.

1812 LEWIS, M. Joy. Equipment for hospital libraries and allied service points. *Unesco Bull. Libr.*, 23 (2) March/April 1969, 84 – 87.
Lisa 1969/1168

1813 LEWIS, M. J. Hospital librarianship courses and education for librarianship in the United Kingdom with special reference to the School of Librarianship, North-Western Polytechnic. *In*: Krol, J. L. P. M. *and* Nachbar, V. H., *eds. International librarianship: Liber Amicorum in honour of G. A. van Riemsdijk.* Amsterdam, School of Librarianship, 1969, vol. 2, pt. 2, 308 – 316.

1814 LEWIS, M. Joy. *Libraries for the handicapped: 1967 Sevensma prize essay.* London, LA, 1969. 48 pp. (LA pamphlet, 33.)

1815 LEWIS, M. Joy. Library services to hospital patients and housebound readers: minimum requirements and future provision. *In*: *Our essential services: report of annual weekend conference and school, 18th to 20th April 1969.* London, LA, London & Home Counties' Branch, 1969, 30 – 45.
Hosp. Abstr. 1970/721

1816 LOHMANN, Victor L. How to identify the special reading needs of library users. *Minnesota Libraries*, 22 (6) Summer 1968, 165 – 169; also in *AHIL Quarterly*, 9 (2) Winter 1969, 40 – 46.

1817 LUDLOW, Felicy. Library services to hospitals and the handicapped. *Ontario Library Review*, 53, (2) June 1969, 60 – 65.
Lisa 1969/2074

1818 MCCLASKEY, Harris C. Education of librarians for work with exceptional children. *Top of the News*, 25 (3) April 1969, 273 – 278.
Lisa 1969/1666

1819 MONROE, Margaret E. Services in hospital and institution libraries: libraries in the therapeutic society. *ALA Bull.*, 63 (9) Oct. 1969, 1280 – 1283; also in Casey, Genevieve, *comp. Libraries in the therapeutic society.* Chicago, ALA, AHIL, 1971, 11 – 13.
Lisa 1969/2541

1820 NANNESTAD, Anna (afterwards Anna Nannestad Nicolaysen) *and* STANGE, Ragnhild Holme. Bibliotekene ved Ullevål sykehus. [The libraries at Ullevål hospital.] *Ullevål Nytt*, 2 (2) Dec. 1969, 16 – 20. For English translation *see* no. 2019.

1821 NIELSEN, Helga. Hospital libraries in Denmark. *Scandinavian Publ. Libr. Q.*, 2 (3) 1969, 165 – 174.
Lisa 1969/2533

1822 NYBERG, Mirjam (afterwards Mirjam Grundstroem). Favoured by law: an outline of hospital library activity in Finland. *Scandinavian Publ. Libr. Q.*, 2 (4) 1969, 201 – 210.
Lisa 1970/1410

1823 NYBERG, Mirjam (afterwards Mirjam Grundstroem). Katsaus kansainvälisiin sairaalakirjastonormeihin. [Survey of international hospital norms.] *Kirjastolehti*, 62 (4) 1969, 117 – 119; English summary, 157.

1824 NYBERG, Mirjam (afterwards Mirjam Grundstroem). Library service for old people's homes in Finland. *Libri*, 19 (4) 1969, 260 – 264.
Lisa 1970/1418

1825 ØPDAHL, Synnøve. Library service for the blind in Norway. *Scandinavian Publ. Libr. Q.*, 2 (3) 1969, 149 – 158.
Lisa 1969/2544

1826 ØRJASÆTER, T. *and* FEYDT, A. *Handicappede barn og bøkene.* [Handicapped children and books.] Oslo, Statens Bibliotekstilsyn, 1969. 55 pp.

1827 PERHEENTUPA, Liisa. Äänikirjatoimintaa Suomessa. [Talking books in Finland.] *Kirjastolehti*, 62 (4) 1969, 119 – 122; English summary, 157.

1828 PERHEENTUPA, Liisa. The Finnish Library for the Blind. *Scandinavian Publ. Libr. Q.*, 2 (3) 1969, 159 – 164.
Lisa 1969/2543

1829 PERSSON, Eva. Kulturprogram för döva. [Cultural programme for the deaf.] *Biblioteksbladet*, 54 (10) 1969, 1002 – 1003.

1830 PÖYSÄLÄ, Pirkko, Laitoskirjastonhoitajien koulutuksesta. [Training of institutional librarians.] *Kirjastolehti*, 62 (4) 1969, 114 – 116; English summary, 157

1831 REIXACH, K. Talking books bridge the communication gap for blind and handicapped patients. *Modern Nursing Home*, 23 July/Aug. 1969, 77 – 80.

1832 RESEARCH INSTITUTE FOR CONSUMER AFFAIRS. *Reading aids: page turners.* London, National Fund for Research into Crippling Diseases, 1969. 15 pp. (Rica comparative test report, 2.)

1833 ROSSEM, J. van. De Blindenbibliotheek in een zich snel ontwikkelende samenleving. [The library for the blind in a quickly developing society.] *De Openbare Bibliotheek*, 12 (2) Feb. 1969, 37 – 40.
Lisa 1969/766

1834 SCHARIOTH, Joachim. *Das Lesen alter Menschen. Eine empirische Untersuchung über das Bücherlesen in Hamburg.* [The reading of old people. An analysis about the reading of books in Hamburg.] Hamburg, Verl. f. Buchmarkt-Forschung, 1969.

1835 SCHAUDER, D. E. The South African Library for the Blind: its future as a national library. *S. Afr. Libr.*, 37 (2) Oct. 1969, 80 – 87, 89.
Lisa 1969/2545

1836 SHAW, Alison. *Print for partial sight: a report to the Library Association subcommittee on books for readers with defective sight.* London, LA, 1969, 92 pp.

1837 SHAW, Alison. The visually handicapped reader: print for partial sight. *Libri*, 19 (4) 1969, 249 – 253.
Lisa 1970/1441

1838 SMITH, D. Co-operative efforts [among hospital libraries]. *AHIL Quarterly*, 9 Summer 1969, 93 – 99.

1839 STURT, Ronald. Hospital libraries in Wales: readings in history. *Book Trolley*, 2 (6) June 1969, 108 – 118.
Lisa 1970/431

1840 SUTINEN, Kyllikki, Biblioterapiasta. [On bibliotherapy.] *Suomen Lääkärilehti-Finlands Läkartidning*, (6) 1969, 495 – 500.

1841 TAFFEL, Roslyn. The Royal palm school library. *Top of the News*, 25 (3) April 1969, 279 – 281.
Lisa 1969/1665

1842 THORPE, Frederick. Books for the partially-sighted. *Cape Librarian*, Oct. 1969, 3 – 4.

1843 THULIN, Kjerstin. Library service for housebound readers. *Libri*, 19 (4) 1969, 254 – 259.
Lisa 1970(1423

1844 TOMA, I. Egyesitett szakszervezeti és betegkönyvtár a tatai Városi Kórházban. [Unified trade union and hospital library in the City hospital of Tata.] *Könyvtáros* 19 (1) 1969, 32.

1845 TOMA, I. A kórházi betegkönyvtárak néhány kérdése. [Some problems of hospital libraries.] A magyar orvosi könyvtárügy és dokumentáció 20 éve, 1969, 105 – 112.

1846 TOMA, I. *A magyarországi kórházi betegek könyvtárainak megszervése.* [The organisation of Hungarian hospital libraries.] Draft, 1969. 18 pp.

1847 VARGA, A. M. A kórházi könyvtárak helyzetérol. [The situation of hospital libraries.] *Kortárs,* 13 (6) 1969, 942 – 947.

1848 WALSH, Mary A. Organisation of library services for hospital patients. *Unesco Bull. Libr.,* 23 (2) March/April 1969, 77 – 83.
Lisa 1969/1167

1849 WOLFF, Hildegard. Die Aufgabe der Bücherei im Krankenhaus. [The function of the hospital library.] *Krankenhaus Umschau,* 38 (12) Dec. 1969, 1376, 1379.
Hosp. Abstr. 1970/719

1970

1850 AALTO, Rauni. The book selection problem in a mental hospital. *Scandinavian Publ. Libr. Q.,* 3 (3/4) 1970, 168 – 175.
Lisa 1971/2287

1851 AMERICAN LIBRARY ASSOCIATION. Association of Hospital and Institution Libraries. Hospital Library Standards Committee. *Standards for library services in health care institutions.* Chicago, ALA, 1970. 25 pp.

1852 ANDERSSON, Gunder. Böcker för blinda. [Books for the blind.] *Biblioteksbladet,* 55 (9) 1970, 285 – 288.
Lisa 1971/451

1853 AREVAD, Bodil. Biblioteksarbejde på Ebberødgaard. [Library work at Ebberødgaard.] *Ungdom og Bøger,* (4) 1970, 1 – 3.

1854 BABER, A. Patient's library, Logansport state hospital. *Library Occurrent,* 23 Nov. 1970, 292+.

1855 BASKIN, Barbara Holland. Library response to the challenge of mental retardation: libraries in the therapeutic society. *Am. Libr.,* 1 (1) Jan. 1970, 65 – 68; also in Casey, Genevieve M., *comp. Libraries in the therapeutic society.* Chicago, ALA, AHIL, 1971, 43 – 48.
Lisa 1970/1427

1856 BEATTY, W. K., *compiler.* Professional reading for library staff members in hospital libraries: an annotated list. *AHIL Quarterly,* 11 Fall 1970, 3 – 5.

1857 BECKER, Mary Justa. Book power: libraries for the mentally retarded. *AHIL Quarterly,* 10 (3) Spring 1970, 73 – 74.
Lisa 1970/1913

1858 BELLINGER, Robert C. Workshop on library service to the visually and physically handicapped, Milwaukee, Wisconsin, April 23 – 25 1969. *AHIL Quarterly,* 10 (2) Winter 1970, 35 – 36.

1859 BERECZKY, L. *Javaslat a betegek könyvtári ellátására.* [Proposal for providing the patients with a library]. Budapest, Centre for Library Science and Methodology, 1970. 15 pp.

1860 Bijeenkomst van de leden van het Studiecentrum voor O.b. en; gewijd aan lectuurvoorziening voor bejaarden en zieken. [Session of the Dutch LA about hospital library work.] *De Openbare Bibliotheek*, 13 (2) Feb. 1970, 39 – 45.

1861 BJERRE, Aase. IFLA normer for hospitalsbiblioteker. [IFLA standards for hospital libraries.] *Bogens Verden*, 52 (3/4) 1970, 258 – 260.

1862 Bookrests for handicapped readers. *Round and About* (Lincoln City Libraries), 6 Jan. 1970, 16 – 20.

1863 BOORER, David. The challenge of the psychiatric hospital. *Assistant Librn.*, 63 (10) Oct. 1970, 150 – 152, 154, 156.
Lisa 1970/2337

1864 BOURDIN, Geneviève. *L'association des Bibliothèques d'Hôpitaux.* [Association of Hospital Libraries.] Lyon, 1970. 3 pp. typescript.

1865 BUNCH, Antonia J. *Hospital and health sciences libraries in the United States. (Sir Evelyn Wrench travelling fellowship for librarians, 1969.)* Edinburgh, Scottish Hospital Centre, 1970, typescript.

1866 BYLUND, Rolf. Likvärdig och utökad bibiloteksservice för patienter och personal vid sjukhusen. [Expanded library service for hospital patients and staff.] *Landstingens Tidskrift*, 57 (1) Jan. 15 1970, 53 – 57.
Hosp. Abstr. 1970/1190

1867 CAHLING, Ulla. The supply of books to the blind and partially sighted in Sweden. *Scandinavian Publ. Libr. Q.*, 3 (2) 1970, 84 – 95.
Lisa 1971/452

1868 CASEY, Genevieve M. If we are serious . . . a response to the library education and manpower policy proposal. *Am. Libr.*, 1 (7) July/Aug. 1970, 706 – 709; also in Casey, Genevieve M., comp. *Libraries in the therapeutic society*. Chicago, ALA, AHIL, 1971, 53 – 59.
Lisa 1970/2826

1869 CHAPMAN, K. Tulsa library has shut-in service. *Oklahoma Librarian*, 20 (4) Oct. 1970, 17 – 18.

1870 DESCHAMPS, Marie-Claire. La bibliothèque universitaire centrale des étudiants malades. [The central university library for invalid students.] *Bull. Bib. Fr.*, 15 (2) Feb. 1970, 75 – 78.
Lisa 1970/1417

1871 DUNNE, Michael. The optimum values and range needed for the angle and height of book-rests. *Book Trolley*, 2 (10) June 1970, 12 – 14.
Lisa 1970/2334

1872 EGAS, C. Sociaal cultureel werk voor bejaarden. [Social cultural work for the aged.] *De Openbare Bibliotheek*, 13 (2) Feb. 1970, 34 – 38.

1873 FIDDER, H. Het werk van de blindenbibliotheken in Nederland. [Activities of the libraries for the blind in the Netherlands.] *De Openbare Bibliotheek*, 13 (1) Jan. 1970, 1 – 7.
Lisa 1970/1426

1874 GEERTS, W. Lezen op leeftijd. [Reading in old age.] *De Openbare Bibliotheek*, 13 (2) Feb. 1970, 22 – 25.

1875 GOING, Mona E. Therapeutic value of reading. *Assistant Librn.*, 63 (7) July 1970, 108, 110.
Lisa 1970/1903

1876 GREAT BRITAIN. DEPARTMENT OF HEALTH AND SOCIAL SECURITY. *Hospital Library service*. London, DHSS, 1970. 1 p. (HM (70) 41.)

1877 GREAT BRITAIN. DEPARTMENT OF HEALTH AND SOCIAL SECURITY. *Library services in hospitals*. London, DHSS, 1970. (HM (70) 23.)
Lisa 1970/2322

1878 GRECO, Constance M. Barred from the library. *Am. Libr.*, 1 (9) Oct. 1970, 908 – 910.
Lisa 70/2830

1879 HEDEMANN, Anne-Grete. Et skritt på rett veg. [A step in the right direction.] *Bok og Bibliotek*, 37 (1) Jan. 1970, 34 – 38.
Lisa 1970/990

1880 INTERNATIONAL FEDERATION OF LIBRARY ASSOCIATIONS. Libraries in Hospitals Sub-section. [Annual reports, business meeting, abstracts of papers read, Copenhagen 1969.] *In: IFLA annual 1969. Proceedings of the General Council . . .* Copenhagen, Scandinavian Library Center, 1970, 63 – 72. For papers in full *see* nos. 1773, 1824, 1837, 1843.

1881 JACKSON, W. S. Beatty resident library. *Library Occurrent*, 23 Nov. 1970, 295 – 296.

1882 JANICKI, Andrzej. O biblioterapii w szpitalach psychiatrycznych. [Bibliotherapy in psychiatric hospitals.] *Szpitalnictwo Polskie*, 14 (3) 1970, 116 – 120.

1883 JAVELIN, Muriel C. Services to the senior citizen: libraries in the therapeutic society. *Am. Libr.*, 1 (2) Feb. 1970, 133 – 137; also in Casey, Genevieve M., *comp. Libraries in the therapeutic society*. Chicago, ALA, AHIL, 1971, 14 – 20.
Lisa 70/1420

1884 JOHANSEN, Anna. Biblioteksarbejde blandt syge og handicappede børn. [Library work among sick and handicapped children.] *Bogens Verden*, 52 (3 – 4) 1970, 262 – 263.

1885 KELLNER, B. A kórházi könyvtárügy is meggyógyul egyszer? [Will the matter of hospital libraries be cured once?] *Könyvtáros*, 20 (8) 1970, 476 – 478.

1886 KIRSTEIN, Kirsten. Eventyrtimer for børn på Ebberødgaard. [Story hours for children from Ebberødgaard.] *Ungdom og Bøger* (4) 1970, 3 – 4.

1887 KJERRSTRÖM, Ulla. Sjukhusbiblioteket flyttar in i nya lokaler. [The hospital library moves into new accommodation.] *Mixturen*, (3) 1970, 12 – 16.

1888 KOVÁCS, P. A kórházi könyvtárakról. [On hospital libraries.] *Könyvtáros*, 20 (8) 1970, 475 – 476.

1889 KOZAKIEWICZ, Wanda. Biblioteki szpitalne wobec realizacji Ustawy. [Hospital libraries in Poland on the eve of implementation of the new libra ries act.] *Bibliotekarz*, 37 (3) 1970, 72 – 76.
Lisa 1970/1904

1890 KOZAKIEWICZ, Wanda. Stan bibliotek szpitalnych w Polsce w przededniu realizacji nowej Ustawy Bibliotecznej. [Rank of hospital libraries in Poland on the eve of realisation of new Library Law.] *Szpitalnictwo Polskie*, 14 (4) 1970, 181 – 183; summaries in Russian and English, 184.

1891 LANDAU, Robert A. *and* NYREN, Judith S., *editors*. *Large type books in print*. New York and London, R. R. Bowker, 1970. 193 pp.

1892 LATTANZI, Angela Daneu. Il servizio di lettura ai minorati. [Reading services for the disabled.] *Accademie e Biblioteche d'Italia*, 38 May 1970, 230 – 234.

1893 LEEUWENBURGH, P. B. Bibliotheekvoorziening zieken en bejaarden: kant-tekeningen n.a.v. een bezoek aan Engeland. (1969.) [Library work with the old and ill in England.] *De Openbare Bibliotheek*, 13 (2) Feb. 1970, 53 – 60.

1894 LEEUWENBURGH, P. B. Bibliotheekwerk in ziekenhuizen en bejaardentehuizen. [Library work in hospitals and old people's homes.] *Instelling en Management*, 2 (5) May 1970, 269 – 272.

1895 LEEUWENBURGH, P. B. IFLA Congres. Kopenhagen 24 – 30 Aug. 1969. *De Openbare Bibliotheek*, 13 (2) Feb. 1970, 67 – 69.

1896 LIBRARY ASSOCIATION. West Midland Branch. *Library services to hospitals and handicapped people: a report*. [Birmingham, The Branch, 1970.] 17 pp.

1897 LONDON, W. A. Samenwerking en coördinatie (van bejaardenwerk). [Co-ordination with other bodies in library work with the aged.] *De Openbare Bibliotheek*, 13 (2) Feb. 1970, 46 – 47.

1898 LUCIOLI, C. Minority of minorities: library service for the handicapped. *AHIL Quarterly*, 10 Summer 1970, 42 – 45.

1899 MCCROSSAN, John A. Extending public library services to the homebound: libraries in the therapeutic society. *Am. Libr.*, 1 (5) May 1970, 485 – 490; also in Casey, Genevieve M., *compiler*. *Libraries in the therapeutic society*. Chicago, ALA, AHIL, 1971, 27 – 34.
Lisa 1970/1911

1900 MCCULLOUGH, F. Patients' library. *Cath. Libr. Wld.*, 41 April 1970, 531 – 533.

1901 MADSEN, Charlotte. Hospitalsbibliotekarer: en slags supermennesker? [Hospital librarians: a kind of supermen?] *Bogens Verden* (7) 1970, 604.

1902 MADSEN, Charlotte *and* HØGH, Hanne. Patientbiblioteket på Statshospitalet i Glostrup. [The patients' library at the Mental Hospital in Glostrup.] *Ungdom og Bøger* (4) 1970, 4 – 7.

1903 MATTHEWS, David. Indecent exposure? Observations on a tour of hospitals. *Book Trolley*, 2 (9) March 1970, 3 – 6.
Lisa 1970/1905

1904 MOLENAAR, Th. K. Leeshulpmiddelen voor zieken en gehandicapten. [Reading aids for the ill and handicapped.] *De Openbare Bibliotheek* 13 (2) Feb. 1970, 61 – 66.

1905 MOLIN, Brita *and* MOLIN, Lars. Läsvanor och bibliotekskontakter hos sjukhusvårdade patienter: en enkätstudie. [An enquiry into the reading habits and library contacts of hospitalised patients.] *Sjukhuset*, 47 (12) Dec. 1970, 646 – 648.

1906 MORAN, Audrey. The Red Cross picture library in Scotland. *Book Trolley*, 2 (9) March 1970, 8 – 9.

1907 MÜLLER-HARNEY, Hildegard. Mit dem Bücherwagen unterwegs auf Krankenstation. [With the trolley on the ward.] *In*: *Öffentliche Büchereien in Baden-Württemberg, 1970*, 82 – 86.

1908 NEFEDČENKO, M. Hospital libraries in the Union of Soviet Socialist Republics. *Unesco Bull. Libr.*, 24 (5) Sept./Oct. 1970, 248 – 250, 283.
Lisa 1970/2814

1909 NIELSEN, Nina Thuesen. Hospitalsbibliotekarkursus 1969. [Hospital librarianship course 1969.] *Bogens Verden*, 52 (1) 1970, 29 – 30.

1910 NIEMAN, D. E., *compiler. Reading aids for the handicapped.* Chicago, ALA Audio-Visual Committee, [1970].

1911 NIEMINEN, Raija. Kuulovamaisten kirjastopalvelusta. [Library service to persons with defective hearing.] *Kirjastolehti*, 63 (9) 1970, 259 – 260.
Lisa 1971/97

1912 PARTINGTON, Wylva W. The Southern hospital library: reminiscences of an assistant. *Book Trolley*, 2 (11) Sept. 1970, 7 – 10.
Lisa 1970/2812

1913 PAYNE, Joan. Dunstable and 'Topsy'. *Book Trolley*, 2 (11) Sept. 1970, 10 – 12.
Lisa 1970/2828

1914 PERSSON, Eva. Konferens om biblioteksverksamhet bland sjuka och handikappade barn samt bland psykiskt utvecklingsstörda. [Conference on library activity with ill and handicapped children.] *Biblioteksbladet*, 55 (1) 1970, 2.

1915 Producing books for the visually handicapped reader. *Bookseller*, (3384) Oct. 31 1970, 2230 – 2232.
Lisa 1970/2842

1916 RESEARCH INSTITUTE FOR CONSUMER AFFAIRS. *Reading aids: microfilm projectors, reading aids: prismatic spectacles.* London, National Fund for Research into Crippling Diseases, 1970. 9 pp. (Rica comparative test report, 3 and 4.)

1917 RETIEF, H. J. M. Die Openbare Biblioteek en sy Gebruikers: Bejaardes. [The public library and its users: the aged.] *S. Afr. Libr.*, 38 (3) Dec. 1970, 184 – 191.
Lisa 1971/98

1918 ROMANI, Dorothy. Guidelines for library service to the institutionalized aging: libraries in the therapeutic society. *Am. Libr.*, 1 (3) March 1970, 286 – 289; also in Casey, Genevieve M., *compiler. Libraries in the therapeutic society*. Chicago, ALA, AHIL, 1971, 21 – 26.
Lisa 1970/1419

1919 RYÖMÄ, Seija. Vammaisten kirjastopalvelu. [Libraries and the handicapped reader.] *Kirjastolehti*, 63 (3) 1970, 66 – 68.
Lisa 1970/1425

1920 SCHAUDER, D. E. *Library services for the visually handicapped in the 1970's*. South African Library for the Blind, 1970. [1], 10, [1] p.

1921 SCHICK, Frank L. [IFLA, Copenhagen 1969: a report.] *Bull. Med. Libr. Ass.*, 58 (3) July 1970, 419 – 422.

1922 SCHONEBAUM, A. *and* POORT, E. M. van der. Bijeenkomst van de leden van het Studiecentrum voor openbare bibliotheken: gewijd aan de lectuurvoorziening voor bejaarden en zieken. [Book provision for the aged and sick people.] *De Openbare Bibliotheek*, 13 (2) Feb. 1970, 39 – 45.
Lisa 1970/1424

1923 SCOTTISH HOSPITAL CENTRE. Library services in hospitals. *In: Collected conference reports, 1969*. Edinburgh, The Centre, [1970], 3, 1 – 16; also in *Leabharlann*, 28 (2) June 1970, 40 – 56.

1924 SCOUGALL, J. Place of the library in the hospital family, outline of the paper presented at the Library training institute . . . Sept. 1969. *AHIL Quarterly*, 10 Spring 1970, 67 – 72.

1925 SECCHI, Margaret. 'Zelo zelatus sum . . .': reminiscences of a hospital librarian. *Book Trolley*, 2 (11) Sept. 1970, 3 – 7.
Lisa 1970/2813

1926 SEEGERS, W. Th. De O.B. en de oudere mens en zijn creativiteit. [The public library, the older person and his creativity.] *De Openbare Bibliotheek*, 13 (2) Feb. 1970, 48 – 50.

1927 SÖDERBLOM, Harriette. För rörelsehindrade barn. [For physically handicapped children.] *Biblioteksbladet*, 55 (1) 1970, 22 – 24.
Lisa 1970/991

1928 STEELE, U. M. Services available to the hospitalized from the Regional libraries for the blind and handicapped: an untapped resource? *AHIL Quarterly*, 10 (2) Winter 1970, 36 – 38.
Lisa 1970/1422

1929 STURT, Ronald. The talking newspaper. *Book Trolley*, 2 (10) June 1970, 3 – 12; also in *Library World*, 72 Aug. 1970, 44 – 45.
Lisa 1970/2335

1930 Talking newspaper for blind in Wales. *British Hospital Journal & Social Service Review*, LXXX Aug. 28 1970, 1680.

1931 TEWS, R. M. Progress in bibliotherapy. *In*: Voigt, M. J., *editor. Advances in librarianship vol. 1*. London, Academic Press, 1970, 171 – 188.

1932 THULIN, Kjerstin. Sjuka barn och barn med handikapp. [Sick and handicapped children.] *Biblioteksbladet*, 55 (5) 1970, 173 – 175.

1933 Training for library service to the institutionalized and handicapped. Short-term institution, the handicapped, the aging and exceptional children. *AHIL Quarterly*, 11 (4) Fall 1970, 7 – 8.

1934 VAN DER RIET, F. G. Public library service to blind readers. *S. Afr. Libr.*, 38 (3) Dec. 1970, 192 – 197.
Lisa 71/96

1935 VEDSTED, Ingrid. Hospitalsbiblioteksarbejdets organisation. [The organisation of hospital library work.] *Bogens Verden*, 52 (3/4) 1970, 260 – 262.
Lisa 1970/2324

1936 VOLLANS, R. F. Print for the visually handicapped reader: a one-day conference. *Library World*, 72 (846) Dec. 1970, 180 – 183.
Lisa 1971/344

1937 WASHINGTON STATE LIBRARY. *Guide lines for introducing mentally retarded persons to the public library*. Olympia, Washington State Library, 1970. [3] pp.

1938 WENDT, Harro *Psychotherapie – Anwendung und Methoden. Lehrmaterialen für Aus-und Weiterbildung von mittleren medizinischen personal*; 2 Aufl. [Psychotherapy: application and technique . . .] Potsdam, Institut für Weiterbildung mittlerer medizinischer Fachkräfte, 1970, 32 pp.

1971

1939 AITKEN, W. R. *A history of the public library movement in Scotland to 1965*. [*Submitted to University of Edinburgh as Ph.D. thesis, 1955*.] Glasgow, Scottish Library Association, 1971, 204 – 205, Provision for the blind; 205 – 207, Hospital libraries.

1940 AMERICAN LIBRARY ASSOCIATION. Association of Hospital and Institution Libraries. *Bibliotherapy: methods and materials*. Chicago, ALA, 1971. 161 pp.

1941 AMERICAN LIBRARY ASSOCIATION. Library Administrative Division. Guidelines for using volunteers in libraries. *Am. Libr.*, 2 (4) April 1971, 407 – 408.

1942 ARAGO, I. Bibliotecas para hospitales y sanatorios. [Libraries in hospitals and sanatoria.] *Policlinica*, Barcelona, (11) July/Sept. 1971, 57, 59, 61, 63.

1943 BATIE, Martha. Biblioteket viktig länk i social kontaktverksamhet. [The library an important link in social contact.] *Socialnytt*, (3) 1971, 48 – 52.

1944 BEASLEY, J. F. Service to state institutions and the physically handicapped. *Illinois Libraries*, 53 (4 – 5) April – May 1971, 340 – 345.

1945 BERRINGTON, J. *and* HARTZENBERG, M. Library service to hospitals. *Cape Librarian*, April 1971, 13 – 16.

1946 BIALAC, V. Public library and the retarded patron. *AHIL Quarterly*, 11 Spring 1971, 31 – 32.

1947 Biblioteksbetjening of åndssvage. Forslag til biblioteksmæssigt samarbejde i Storstrømsamtet mellem Statens åndssvageforsorg og folkebibliotekerne. [Library service to the mentally deficient. Proposal for co-operation in Storstrømsamtet between the public library and the State Welfare for the Mentally Deficient.] *Bogens Verden,* 53 (10) 1971, 640 – 641.

1948 Biblioteksservicen på sjukhus. [Library service in hospitals.] *Moderna Sjukhus,* (3) 1971, 17 – 21.

1949 BRADY, D. Creedence Clearwater helps stir a library revival. *Louisiana Library Association. Bulletin,* 34 Spring 1971, 16+.

1950 BROWN, E. G. Library service for the blind in Canada. *Ontario Library Review,* 55 (4) Dec. 1971, 230 – 233.
Lisa 1972/158

1951 BUNCH, Antonia J. *and* CUMMING, Eileen E. Scotland '69: a review of library services in Scottish hospitals. *In: Libraries for health and welfare: papers given to the Hospital Libraries and Handicapped Readers Group conferences in 1968 and 1969.* London, LA, 1971, 24 – 28.

1952 BUSWELL, Christa H. Our other customers: reading and the aged. *Wilson Libr. Bull.,* 45 (5) Jan. 1971, 467 – 476.
Lisa 1971/453

1953 CAHLING, Ulla. Frågor och svar om talböcker. [Questions and answers on talking books.] *Biblioteksbladet,* 56 (2 – 3) 1971, 51 – 55.
Lisa 1971/1373

1954 CARLSSON, Folke. Planera bibliotek för alla. [Design of libraries for all.] Folke Carlsson, Alf Nilsson, Sten Soderström. *Biblioteksbladet,* 56 (2 – 3) 1971, 44 – 47.
Lisa 1971/1499

1955 CASEY, Genevieve M. Library services to the handicapped and institutionalised. *Library Trends,* 20 (2) Oct. 1971, 350 – 366.

1956 CASEY, Genevieve M. Public library service to the aging: ASD special report. *Am. Libr.,* 2 (9) Oct. 1971, 999 – 1004.
Lisa 1972/159

1957 CASEY, Genevieve M., *compiler. Libraries in the therapeutic society.* Chicago, ALA, Association of Hospital and Institution Libraries, 1971. 67 pp. For contents *see* nos. 1819, 1855, 1868, 1883, 1899, 1918.

1958 CLARKE, Jean M. Hospital libraries – the future. *In: Libraries for health and welfare: papers given to the Hospital Libraries and Handicapped Readers Group conferences in 1968 and 1969.* London, LA, 1971, 18 – 23.

1959 CLARKE, Jean M. IFLA General Council, Liverpool 1971. *Book Trolley,* 3 (4) Dec. 1971, 13 – 16.

1960 CORNWALL COUNTY LIBRARY. *Investigation of requirements for service to the housebound.* Truro, Cornwall County Library, 1971. 25 pp. (Report, 1.)

1961 CRITCHLEY, W. E. G. Is welfare a library's business? *In: Libraries for health and welfare: papers given to the Hospital Libraries and Handicapped Readers Group conferences in 1968 and 1969.* London, LA, 1971, 29 – 33.

1962 CROOKS, S. A 'first' at Rainier School. *Library News Bulletin (Washington State Library)* 38 Oct. 1971, 317 – 319.

1963 CUMMING, Eileen E. Children in hospital: do they need a library service? *Book Trolley*, 3 (3) Sept. 1971, 3 – 9.
Lisa 1971/2302

1964 CUXART, C. La biblioteca de la Clinica mental de Santa Coloma de Gramenet. [Library of the Santa Coloma de Gramenet mental clinic.] *Biblioteconomia*, 28 Jan. 1971, 221 – 226.

1965 DEUTSCHER BÜCHEREIVERBAND. *Richtlinien für Krankenhausbüchereien; 2 auflage.* [Guidelines for hospital libraries; 2nd edition.] Berlin, D.B.V. Arbeitsstelle für das Büchereiwesen und DKl, 1971. 25 pp. (Bibliotheksdienst Beiheft 20.)

1966 DOMNEY, J. M. *and* TOOKER, G. C. Metropolitan state hospital's 'in-depth book collection' project. *News Notes of California Libraries*, 66 Summer 1971, 420 – 422.

1967 FRYKSÉN, Birgitta. Biblioteksverksamhet för barn på sjukhus. [Library work with children in hospital.] *In:* Sewall, Lena. *Att arbeta i sjukhusbibliotek.* Lund, Bibliotekstjänst, 1971, 119 – 126.

1968 GOING, Mona E. On the receiving end. *Book Trolley*, 3 (2) June 1971, 9 – 11.
Lisa 1971/1369

1969 GOSTYŃSKA, Danuta. Zagadnienia biblioterapii w szpitalach. [Problems of bibliotherapy in hospitals.] *Szpitalnictwo Polskie*, 15 (2) 1971, 71 – 73; summaries in Russian and English, 74.

1970 GRAHAM, Earl C. Response to a restive world: health, social and rehabilitation services. *AHIL Quarterly*, 11 Summer 1971, 45 – 47.

1971 Guidelines for using volunteers in libraries: ALA report. *Am. Libr.*, 2 (4) April 1971, 407 – 408.
Lisa 1971/975

1972 HANNIGAN, Margaret C. Counseling and bibliotherapy for the general reader. *In:* Monroe, Margaret E., *editor. Reading guidance and bibliotherapy* . . . Madison, Univ. of Wisconsin, Library School, 1971, 45 – 50.

1973 HANNIGAN, Margaret C. On the plus side: landmark achievements – standards for library services in residential facilities for the mentally retarded. *AHIL Quarterly*, 11 Spring 1971, 35 – 38.

1974 HANSEN, Mogens Bjerring. Skønlitteratur på Statshospitalet. [Fiction at the mental hospital.] *Bogens Verden*, 53 (3) 1971, 201 – 203.

1975 HARRIS, N. G. Audiovisual resources: resident library services for the mentally retarded. *AHIL Quarterly*, 11 Spring 1971, 38 – 40.

1976 HART, Joan A. *and* RICHARDSON, J. A. *Books for the retarded reader; United Kingdom edition prepared by J. A. Hart.* London, Ernest Benn, 1971. 111 pp.

1977 HILLIARD, J. Patient's library, Central state hospital. *Focus on Indiana Libraries*, 25 Sept. 1971, 124 – 125.

1978 HODOCK, I. Services to the deaf. *Focus on Indiana Libraries*, 25 Dec. 1971, 160 – 163.

1979 HØGH, Hanne. Biblioteksbetjening på en børnepsykiatrisk afdeling. [Library service to a children's psychiatric department.] *Bogens Verden*, 53 (10) 1971, 638 – 640.

1980 Internationales seminar über krankenhausbüchereien. [International seminar on hospital libraries.] *Buch und Bibliothek*, 23 Feb. 1971, 169.

1981 INTERNATIONAL FEDERATION OF LIBRARY ASSOCIATIONS. Libraries in Hospitals Sub-section. [Annual reports, abstracts of papers read, Moscow, 1970.] *In*: *IFLA annual 1970. Proceedings of the General Council* . . . Copenhagen, Scandinavian Library Center, 1971, 165 – 169. For papers in full *see* nos. 2121, 2138, 2158.

1982 INTERNATIONAL FEDERATION OF LIBRARY ASSOCIATIONS. Libraries in Hospitals Sub-section. [Annual reports, business meeting, abstracts of papers read, Liverpool 1971.] *In*: *IFLA annual 1971. Proceedings of the General Council* . . . Copenhagen, Scandinavian Library Center, 1971, 68 – 72. For papers in full *see* nos. 2063, 2129, 2131, 2133, 2141.

1983 KENCHINGTON, Susan. The National hospital for nervous diseases and the Gowers library. *Book Trolley*, 3 (2) June 1971, 11 – 13.
Lisa 1971/1368

1984 KLUMB, *Mrs*. David *and others*. Public library works with the retarded. *AHIL Quarterly*, 11 Spring 1971, 32 – 34.

1985 KOEFOED, Ingerlise. Handicappede skal også kunne bruge bibliotekerne. [The handicapped should also have the advantage of using libraries.] *Bogens Verden*, 53 (10) 1971, 651 – 653.

1986 KŘIVINKOVÁ, Julie. *Die Entwicklung der Patientenbibliotheken in der CSSR. Referat, gehalten auf der 7. Mitgliederversammlung der Untersektion Patienten-bibliotheken des DBV in Dresden, 23 – 24, 9, 1971*. [Development of patients' libraries in CSSR: paper . . . Dresden 1971.] Berlin, Humboldt-Universität, Bereich Medizin, Charité, Patienten-u. Gewerkschaftsbibliothek, 1971. 11 pp. typescript.

1987 KUEHN, Melody. Library services casebook: Minot serves aged. *Am. Libr.*, 2 (11) Dec. 1971, 1198.
Lisa 1972/745

1988 KULCZYCKI, Marian. *Psychologiczne problemy człowieka chorego*. [Psychological problems of the sick] Wrocław, 1971, 178 pp.

1989 Large print books for the aged and partially sighted. *Concord*, Winter 1970/71, 113, 115.

1990 LEEUWENBURGH, P. B. IFLA, 1971: Sub-section Libraries in Hospitals. *De Openbare Bibliotheek*, 14 (10) Dec. 1971, 473 – 474.

1991 LEWIS, M. Joy. Large print book publishing (review article). *Libr. Ass. Rec.*, 73 (5) May 1971, 93 – 94.
Lisa 1971/1218

1992 LEWIS, M. Joy. The Libraries in Hospitals Sub-section of the International Federation of Library Associations. *In: Libraries for health and welfare: papers given to the Hospital Libraries and Handicapped Readers Group conferences in 1968 and 1969.* London, LA, 1971, 49 – 54.

1993 LIBRARY ASSOCIATION *and* NATIONAL ASSOCIATION FOR THE EDUCATION OF THE PARTIALLY SIGHTED. *Print for the visually handicapped reader: papers and proceedings of a conference sponsored by the Library Association and the National Association for the Education of the Partially Sighted and held on 28 October, 1970* ... London, LA, 1971. 64 pp. (LA research publication, 6.)

1994 LIBRARY ASSOCIATION. County Libraries Group, Wales. The library and the handicapped child. *In: Proceedings of ... Weekend school, Bangor, 1970.* Dolgellan, Merioneth County Library, 1971, 31 – 33.

1995 LIBRARY ASSOCIATION. Hospital Libraries and Handicapped Readers Group. *Libraries for health and welfare: papers given to the Hospital Libraries and Handicapped Readers Group conferences in 1968 and 1969.* London, LA, 1971. [iii], 67 pp. For individual papers *see* nos. 1951, 1958, 1961, 1992, 2006, 2009, 2037, 2046.
Lisa 1972/153; Hosp. Abstr. 1972/975

1996 Library resources for patient education (symposium). *AHIL Quarterly*, 11 Winter 1971, 11 – 15.

1997 LIEBIG, M. Direct service to mentally retarded residents in an institution. *AHIL Quarterly*, 11 Spring 1971, 34 – 35.

1998 LINDERBERG, Kerstin. *Böcker med stor stil.* [Books with large print.] Lund, Bibliotekstjänst, 1971. (Btj. serien 33.)

1999 LOGAN, M. With a little help among friends: the Atascadero state hospital library program. *News Notes of California Libraries*, 66 Summer 1971, 404 – 408.

2000 LUCIOLI, Clara E. Bibliotherapeutic aspects of public library services to patients in hospitals and institutions. *In*: Monroe, Margaret E., *editor. Reading guidance and bibliotherapy* ... Madison, University of Wisconsin, Library School, 1971, 51 – 56.

2001 LUCIOLI, Clara E. Role of public and institution librarians in helping the patient transfer from institution to the community. *In*: Monroe, Margaret E., *editor. Reading guidance and bibliotherapy* ... Madison, University of Wisconsin, Library School, 1971, 63 – 70.

2002 LUNDSTRÖM, Beata. Samarbeta med handikapprörelse. [Co-operation with aid to the handicapped.] *Biblioteksbladet*, 56 (2 – 3) 1971, 40 – 43.
Lisa 1971/1372

2003 LYMAN, Helen Huguenor. The art of reading guidance. *In*: Monroe, Margaret E., *editor. Reading guidance and bibliotherapy* ... Madison, University of Wisconsin, Library School, 1971, 16 – 32.

2004 LYON, E. Ugly duckling: Fort Wayne State Hospital & training center library. *Focus on Indiana Libraries*, 25 Dec. 1971, 158 – 159.

2005 MCDOWELL, David, J. Bibliotherapy in a patients' library. *Bull. Med. Libr. Ass.*, 59 (3) July 1971, 450 – 457.

2006 MACLEAN, Fiona. Patients as library assistants. *In: Libraries for health and welfare: papers given to the Hospital Libraries and Handicapped Readers Group conferences in 1968 and 1969.* London, LA, 1971, 39 – 41.

2007 MARSHALL, Margaret R. *Story books for retarded readers.* [Leeds] LA, Yorkshire branch, 1971. 16 pp.

2008 MATTHEWS, Geraldine M., compiler. *Library information service programs in residential facilities for the mentally retarded.* Madison, Wisconsin, Wisconsin Dept. of Public Instruction, Divison for Library Services, 1971. 221 pp.

2009 MAY, Margaret. The training of volunteers in hospital libraries. *In: Libraries for health and welfare: papers given to the Hospital Libraries and Handicapped Readers Group conference in 1968 and 1969.* London, LA, 1971, 34 – 38.

2010 MEYER, J. R., compiler. Selected bibliography library services in mental retardation. *AHIL Quarterly*, 11 Spring 1971, 30 – 31.

2011 MEYERS, Arthur S. The unseen and unheard elderly. *Am. Libr.*, 2 (8) Sept. 1971, 793 – 796.
Lisa 1972/160

2012 MINIĆ, V. Sadašnji položaj centralne biblioteke saverza slepih Jugoslavije. [Present state of the central library of the Yugoslav Association for the Blind.] *Bibliotekar* (Belgrade), 23 (2) March – April 1971, 199 – 202.
Lisa 1972/2829

2013 MONROE, Margaret E., editor. *Reading guidance and bibliotherapy in public, hospital and institution libraries: a selection of papers presented at a series of adult services institutes, 1965 – 1968.* Madison, University of Wisconsin, Library School, 1971. 76 pp. For contents *see* nos. 1972, 2000, 2001, 2003, 2014, 2015, 2016, 2043.

2014 MONROE, Margaret E. Reading guidance as a basic library service. *In*: Monroe, Margaret E., editor. *Reading guidance and bibliotherapy* ... Madison, University of Wisconsin, Library School, 1971, 1 – 11.

2015 MONROE, Margaret E. Reader services and bibliotherapy. *In*: Monroe, Margaret E., editor. *Reading guidance and bibliotherapy* ... Madison, University of Wisconsin, Library School, 1971, 40 – 44.

2016 MOODY, Mildred T. Bold new approach. *In*: Monroe, Margaret E., editor. *Reading guidance and bibliotherapy* ... Madison, University of Wisconsin, Library School, 1971, 33 – 39.

2017 MÜLLER-FAHLBUSCH, Hans. Was ist Bibliotherapie? [What is bibliotherapy?] *Krankendienst*, 44 (3) 1971, 78 – 81.

2018 MUNFORD, W. A. Reading for the visually handicapped, and the National Library for the Blind Austin Books. *In: Print for the visually handicapped reader* ... London, LA, 1971, 26 – 30.

2019 NANNESTAD, Anna (afterwards Anna Nannestad Nicolaysen) *and* STANGE, Ragnhild Holme. The libraries at Ullevål hospital, Oslo; transl. by Eileen E. Cumming. *Book Trolley*, 3 (1) March 1971, 11 – 13. For original in Norwegian *see* no. 1820.
Lisa 1971/864

2020 NATIONAL FUND FOR RESEARCH INTO CRIPPLING DISEASES. *Communication*; *3rd edition*; edited by E. R. Wilshere and others. London, The Fund, 1971. 62 pp. (Equipment for the disabled, 1.)

2021 [NEIL, Alexander, *compiler*.] *Fiction and non-fiction books: for use by the least able pupils in secondary schools*. Glasgow, School Library Association in Scotland, 1971. 69 pp.

2022 NEW YORK STATE. EDUCATION DEPARTMENT. Albany Division for Handicapped Children. *Improving library services for handicapped children: proceedings of the institute (Buffalo, New York, Feb. 1 – 4, 1971)*. New York State Educ. Dept., Albany Div. for Handicapped Children, 1971. 84 pp.

2023 NICHOLAS, Rosslyn M. The day hospital at Pembury and an experiment on the therapeutic use of the talking book. *Book Trolley*, 3 (3) Sept. 1971, 12 – 13.
Lisa 1971/2314

2024 ØRJASÆTER, Tordis. Böckerna och de lässvaga. [Books and dyslexic patients.] *Biblioteksbladet*, 56 (7/8) 1971, 202 – 206.

2025 PEMBERTON, John E. The role of the public library authorities in the development of hospital library services. *Journal of Librarianship*, 3 (2) April 1971, 101 – 119.
Lisa 1971/448

2026 PETKUS, D. *and* PEACOCK, J. Book explosion at Beatty memorial hospital. *Focus on Indiana Libraries*, 25 Sept. 1971, 119 – 121.

2027 PÉTURSDÓTTIR, Kristin H. Library services to the sick and handicapped in Iceland. *Book Trolley*, 3 (3) Sept. 1971, 9 – 12.
Lisa 1971/2284

2028 PLOMAN, Margareta. Biblioteket på Vipeholm. [The library at Vipeholm.] *Biblioteksbladet*, 56 (2 – 3) 1971, 63 – 64.
Lisa 1971/1375

2029 Public library service for the sick and disabled. *Libr. Ass. Rec.*, 73 (1) Jan. 1971, 15.

2030 RITTENHOUSE, David C. Our other customers: prisoners, patients and public libraries. *Wilson Libr. Bull.*, 45 (5) Jan. 1971, 490 – 493.
Lisa 1971/449

2031 ROSANDER, Yngve. Bredda kulturterapin. [Cultural therapy.] *Medicinska Föreningarnas Tidskrift*, (6) 1971, 171 – 173.

2032 RYÖMÄ, Seija. He lukevat sormillaan. [They read with their fingers.] *Kirjastolehti*, 64 (10) 1971, 370 – 371.
Lisa 1972/743

2033 SCHAUDER, D. E. *and* LODDER, N. M. Mechanisation and library co-operation: a new era for SALB. *S. Afr. Libr.*, 39 (1) July 1971, 52 – 55.
Lisa 1971/1374

2034 SELBY, J. R. The library service at the Doncaster Royal Infirmary. *Book Trolley*, 3 (1) March 1971, 3 – 8.
Lisa 1971/863

2035 SEWALL, Lena. *Att arbeta i sjukhusbibliotek: nagrå erfarenheter av arbetet som sjukhusbibliotekarie i Karlstad.* [Hospital library work: some experiences of work as a hospital librarian in Karlstad.] Lund, Bibliotekstjänst, 1971, 158 pp. (SAB – serien 8.)

2036 SEWALL, Lena. Från SSBV. [The special group for library social work.] Bibliography. *Biblioteksbladet*, 56 (10) 1971, 295 – 298.

2037 SHAW, Alison. Reading problems of the visually handicapped. *In: Libraries for health and welfare: papers given to the Hospital Libraries and Handicapped Readers Group conferences in 1968 and 1969.* London, LA, 1971, 42 – 48.

2038 SNELL, Svanhild *and* TANTTU, Orvokki. Lastenkirjastotyötä sairaalassa. [Library service to children in hospital.] *Kirjastolehti*, 64 (10) 1971, 373 – 374.

2039 STIGMARK, Maria. Specialgruppsdagen. [The special group conference.] *Biblioteksbladet*, 56 (7 – 8) 1971, 213 – 214.
Lisa 1972/151

2040 SUTTON, Johanna G. Our other customers – shut ins: consider the confined; methods of reaching in. *Wilson Libr. Bull.*, 45 (5) Jan. 1971, 485 – 489.
Lisa 1971/450

2041 SZÉKELY, S. A betegek könyvtárai. [The hospital libraries.] *Könyvtáros*, 21 (1) 1971, 17 – 19.

2042 TEUTSCH, B. Das fröhliche krankenzimmer: aktion des arbeitskreises für jugendliteratur. [The happy sickroom: action of the working committee for youth literature.] *Buch und Bibliothek*, 23 April 1971, 396 – 397.

2043 TEWS, Ruth M. The role of the librarian on the interdisciplinary team. *In:* Monroe, Margaret E., *editor. Reading guidance and bibliotherapy* . . . Madison, University of Wisconsin, Library School, 1971, 57 – 62.

2044 THORPE, F. A. Books for failing eyesight. *Social Service Quarterly*, XLV July/ Sept. 1971, 16 – 18.

2045 UNITED STATES. JOINT COMMISSION ON ACCREDITATION OF HOSPITALS. Accreditation Council for Facilities for the Mentally Retarded. *Standards for residential facilities for the mentally retarded.* Chicago, Ill., The Commission, 1971, 59 – 63.

2046 URCH, M. E. Hospital libraries – the past and the present. *In: Libraries for health and welfare: papers given to the Hospital Libraries and Handicapped Readers Group conferences in 1968 and 1969.* London, LA, 1971, 12 – 17..

2047 VELLEMAN, Ruth A. The school library in the education of handicapped children. *Rehabilitation Literature*, 32 (5) May 1971, 138 – 140.

2048 VELLEMAN, Ruth A. Serving exceptional children. *School Libraries*, 20 (4) Summer 1971, 27 – 30.
Lisa 1971/1389

2049 VERNON, D. T. A. Information seeking in a natural stress situation: tuberculosis patients' use of books in the patient library. *Journal of Applied Psychology*, 55 Aug. 1971, 359 – 363.

2050 VIG-NIELSEN, Ingeborg. Lydbogsservice på Århus Kommune hospital. [Talking books at the muncipal hospital in Århus.] *Ungdom og Boger*, (1) 1971, 3 – 7.

2051 WEINSTOCK, F. J. Talking books – a free service for the blind and physically handicapped. *Volunteer Leader*, 12 Sept. 1971, 10 – 11.

2052 WOLF, C. *and* MILLER, J. Harwick serves blind. *Am. Libr.*, 2 Dec. 1971, 1193 – 1194.

2053 ZIEGLER, M. Community outreach in Bellingham. *Library News Bulletin (Washington State Library)*, 38 Oct. 1971, 306 – 308.

1972

2054 ALISON, M. J. H. Libraries in hospitals. *Book Trolley*, 3 (6) June 1972, 3 – 10.
Lisa 1972/1683

2055 AMERICAN LIBRARY ASSOCIATION. Round Table on Library Services for the Blind. *Checklist of resources for materials for the blind*. ALA, 1972. 2 pp.

2056 ARBORELIUS, Brita. Artotek – vad är det? [Picture lending what is it?] *Julhälsning: Jultidning för Lasarettet i Lund*, 1972, 19 – 21.

2057 ASSBURY, Edward. Konferencja poświęcona zagadnieniom biblioterapii oraz czytelnictwa chorych. [Conference devoted to questions of bibliotherapy and patients' reading.] *Szpitalnictwo Polskie*, 16 (6) 1972.

2058 BEKKER, Johan. Leesmasjiene en kunsmatige visie – die huidige stand. [Reading machines and artificial vision – the state of the art.] *S. Afr. Libr.*, 39 (5) April 1972, 312 – 321.
Lisa 1972/3160

2059 BJERRE, Aase. Hospitalsbibliotekerne og de somatiske sygehuse i Danmark uden for København. [The hospital libraries and the general hospitals outside Copenhagen.] *Bibliotek 70*, (13) 1972, 277 – 278.

2060 BOKLUND, Vanja *and* PLOMAN, Margareta. *Böcker för lässvaga*. [Books for mentally handicapped and dyslexia patients.] Lund, 1972. 57 pp.

2061 *Book as a therapeutic aid*. [Paper prepared by a Slovak Medical Library for distribution at IFLA 38th session Budapest, 1972.] 1972 (typescript).

2062 BOORER, David. Do mentally handicapped people need books? *Book Trolley*, 3 (5) March, 1972, 11 – 13.
Lisa 1972/1173

2063 BOORER, David. IFLA Libraries in Hospitals Sub-section, hospital library studies 1967 – 71 (7) United Kingdom, 1971: (c) psychiatric hospitals and their need for library services. *Int. Libr. Rev.*, 4 (3) July 1972, 383 – 386.
Lisa 1972/1694

2064 BOORER, David. Serving the mentally ill. *Assistant Librn.*, 65 (7) July 1972, 104 – 106.
Lisa 1972/1693

2065 BOSA, Réal. Les citoyens jugés 'marginaux' en matière de bibliothèque. [Citizens considered 'marginal' in library policy.] *Association Canadienne des Bibliothécaires de Langue Française Bulletin*, 18 (3) Sept. 1972, 198 – 200.
Lisa 1973/113

2066 BROWN, E. G. A library for listeners. *Can. Libr. J.*, 29 (3) May/June 1972, 241 – 244.
Lisa 1972/1750

2067 CAMPFIELD, M. *and* MARSH, J. Carryover of familiar service: the patients' library at the Winnebago state hospital. *Wisconsin Library Bulletin*, 68 May 1972, 167 – 170.

2068 CANADIAN LIBRARY ASSOCIATION. *Public library services for the physically handicapped*. Ottawa, Canadian Library Association, 1972. iii [1] 30 pp. (Adult services section newsletter, spring 1972.)

2069 CHARTERIS, Francis. Library service to the disadvantaged: the aged, the institutionalized, the Aborigines. *Aust. Libr. J.*, 21 (4) May 1972, 156 – 161.
Lisa 1972/1679

2070 CLARK, D. F. Reading in the mental subnormality hospital. *Book Trolley*, 3 (5) March 1972, 3 – 8.
Lisa 1972/1544

2071 COELLN, Alexandra von. Büchereiarbeit für alte menschen. [Library service for the elderly.] *Buch und Bibliothek*, 24 (3) March 1972, 348 – 351.

2072 CONNELLY, J. On being a library intern at a state hospital. *Southeastern Librarian*, 22 Winter 1972, 173 – 175.

2073 CRAMER, C. H. *Open shelves and open minds: a history of the Cleveland public library*. Cleveland, Case Western Reserve Univ. P., 1972, 198 – 204 shut-ins, hospitals and institutions.

2074 CULP, R. W. Mount Sinai hospital library, 1883 – 1970. *Bull. Med. Libr. Ass.*, 60 July 1972, 471 – 480.

2075 CUMMING, Eileen E. Reading for the mentally handicapped: a selective bibliography. *Book Trolley*, 3 (5) March 1972, 14 – 15.
Lisa 1972/1172

2076 CWYNAR, Stanisław. Biblioterapia. [Bibliotherapy.] *Szpitalnictwo Polskie*, 16 (6) 1972, 263 – 265; English summary, 278 – 279.

2077 DALE, Brian *and* DEWDNEY, Patricia. Canadian public libraries and the physically handicapped. *Can. Libr. J.*, 29 (3) May/June 1972, 231 – 236.
Lisa 1972/1691

2078 DEUTSCHER BIBLIOTHEKSVERBAND. Sektion Medizinische Bibliotheken. Untersektion Patientenbibliotheken. *Patientenbibliothek und Bibliotherapie: Bibliotheksarbeit in Krankenhäusern eine Auswahlbibliographie.* [Patients' library and bibliotherapy: library work in hospitals, a select bibliography.] Berlin, D.B.V., 1972 29 pp.

2079 de vos, c. i. Library service for the housebound. *Rehabilitation in South Africa*, 16 (4) Dec. 1972, 115 – 119.

2080 Division for the blind and physically handicapped host to Council for exceptional children session. *Library of Congress Information Bulletin*, 31 March 31 1972, 141 – 142.

2081 DUPLICA, Moya M. The librarian and the exceptional child. *Rehabilitation Literature*, 33 (7) July 1972, 198 – 203.

2082 ELLIOTT, Jon. A housebound reader service. *New Library World*, 73 (861) March 1972, 237 – 238.
Lisa 1972/744

2083 EMERSON, T. L. W. Library service to the disadvantaged child. *Aust. Sch. Librn.*, 9 (4) Dec. 1972, 15 – 25.
Lisa 1973/679

2084 ERICKSON, C. R. *and* LEJEUNE, R. Poetry as a subtle therapy. *Hospital & Community Psychiatry*, 23 Feb. 1972, 56 – 57.

2085 ETTO, Eila. Lasten kirjastotyötä kehitysalueella. Ajankohtaista kirjastoa. 2. Erityistyötä lapsille. [Hospital library service to children in Lapland. Public libraries today. 2. Special service to children.] *Kirjastopalvelu*, 1972, 11 – 20.

2086 FEATHERSTONE, T. M. *and* WINKLEY, S. More for the housebound. *New Library World*, 73 June 1972, 316 – 317.

2087 FISCHER, J. A. A. Ziekenhuizen en de kans om te lezen. [Hospitals and the chance to read – International Institute. London, Aug. 1971.] J. A. A. Fischer, A. Kimmel and F. W. Spijkerboer. *De Openbare Bibliotheek*, 15 (3) March 1972, 86 – 94.
Lisa 1972/1171

2088 Folkebibliotekernes samarbejde med institutioner og persongrupper. Indeholdt i: Biblioteksdirektørens skriftlige årsberetning 1971/72. [Co-operation between the public libraries and institutions *In* the written annual report of the director of the public library 1971/72.] *Bogens Verden*, 54 (12) 1972, 841 – 842.

2089 GILSON, P. A. *and* AL-SALMAN, J. Bibliotherapy in Oklahoma. *Oklahoma Librarian*, 22 July 1972, 12 – 13+

2090 GOLDSMITH, Selwyn. Library planning for the disabled. *Book Trolley*, 3 (8) Dec. 1972, 3 – 7.
Lisa 1973/1361

2091 GOSTYŃSKA, Danuta. Biblioterapia kliniczna i społeczna. [Clinical and social bibliotherapy.] *Szpitalnictwo Polskie*, 16 (6) 1972, 274 – 280; English summary.

2092 GRAY, R. H. *and* KRIS, A. O. Role of a library in an adolescent service: Boston (Mass.) State Hospital. *Hospital & Community Psychiatry*, 23 May 1972, 159 – 161.

2093 Great Lakes health congress: financial support of hospital libraries. *AHIL Quarterly*, 12 Winter 1972, 3 – 6.

2094 HABERER, Isobel J. Reading and the hard of hearing. *Libr. Ass. Rec.*, 74 (9) Sept. 1972, 162 – 164.
Lisa 1972/230

2095 HÅKANSSON, Eva. Litteratur – en väg till kontakt. [Literature – a way to contact.] Stockholm, 1972. 183 pp.

2096 HANNIGAN, Margaret C. New library programs for the elderly. *AHIL Quarterly*, 12 Spring/Summer 1972, 19 – 21.

2097 HINTIKKA, Anna-Maija. Biblioterapiasta. Ajankohtaista kirjastoa. 2. Erityistyötä lapsille. [On bibliotherapy. Public libraries today. 2. Special service to children.] *Kirjastopalvelu*, 1972, 36 – 45.

2098 HÖÖK, Lisbet. Uppsökande biblioteksverksamhet för handikappade ger högre lånefrekvens. [Library work with the handicapped.] *Handikappsamverkan*, 3 (3) 1972, 30 – 35.

2099 HYNES, Jo Catherine. Library work with brain damaged patients: a new mode of bibliotherapy. *Bull. Med. Libr. Ass.*, 60 (2) April 1972, 333 – 339.
Lisa 1972/2362

2100 INTERNATIONAL FEDERATION OF LIBRARY ASSOCIATIONS. Libraries in Hospitals Sub-section. Hospital library studies 1967 – 1971. *Int. Libr. Rev.*, 4 (3) July 1972, 351 – 391. For individual papers *see* nos. 2063, 2115, 2121, 2126, 2129, 2131, 2133, 2138, 2141, 2158.
Hosp. Abstr. 1973/55

2101 JAVELIN, Muriel C. Talking-book service in the libraries of the Nassau Library System. *PLA Bull.*, 27 (2) March 1972, 74 – 78.
Lisa 72/2319

2102 JOHANSEN, Anne. Biblioteksbetjening af læsehæmmede. [Library service to retarded readers: review of Erik Svendsen's Folkebibliotekerne og de læsehæmmede.] *Bibliotek 70*, (17) 1972, 368.

2103 KOEFOED, Ingerlise. De ældre er ikke et fremmed befolkningselement. Hospitalsbibliotekarmødet på Hindsgavl 8 – 9 marts 1972. [Old people are not an unfamiliar element of the population. Meeting for hospital librarians at Hindsgavl 8 – 9 March 1972.] *Bogens Verden*, 54 (6) 1972, 389 – 390.

2104 KOEFOED, Ingerlise. Børn og biblioteker. Samarbejdet med børne-institutionerne: nogle tanker inspireret af en rapport. [Children and libraries. Cooperation with child care centres: some thoughts inspired by a report.] *Bogens Verden*, 54 (8) 1972, 549 – 552.
Lisa 1973/120

2105 KOLODZIEJSKA, Jadwiga. Specjalne zadania bibliotek publicznych. [Special services of public libraries.] *Bibliotekarz*, 39 (11 – 12) 1972, 332 – 337.
Lisa 1973/1196

2106 KOZAKIEWICZ, Wanda. Problemy oganizacji bibliotek szpitalnych. [Problems in the organisation of hospital libraries.] *Szpitalnictwo Polskie*, 16 (6) 1972, 269 – 273; summaries in Russian and English, 278 – 279. Hosp. Abstr. 1973/809

2107 KOZŁOWSKI, Szczepan. Organizacja bibliotek szpitalnych w świetle przepisów prawnych. [Organisation of hospital libraries in the light of legal regulations.] *Szpitalnictwo Polskie*, 16 (6) 1972, 266 – 268.

2108 *Die Krankenhausbücherei. Referate des Fortbildungslehrgangs für Bibliothekare an Krankenhausbüchereien Düsseldorf 1971.* [The hospital library. Papers at a training school for hospital librarians Düsseldorf 1971.] Köln, Greven, 1972. 117 pp. (Veröffentlichung des Bibl. – Lehrinstituts des Landes Nordrhein – Westfalen.)

2109 KRAŚNIEWSKA, Krystyna. Spoleczne ramy biblioterapii. [Social sphere of bibliotherapy.] *Bibliotekarz*, 39 (5) 1972, 149 – 152. Lisa 1972/2854

2110 LAWLER, J. G. Poetry therapy? *Psychiatry*, 35 Aug. 1972, 227 – 237.

2111 LEWIS, M. Joy. Hospital and welfare library services. *In*: Whatley, H. A., editor. *British librarianship and information science, 1966 – 1970.* London, LA, 1972, 560 – 578.

2112 LIBRARY ASSOCIATION. *Hospital libraries: recommended standards for libraries in hospitals – 1972.* London, LA, 1972. 18 pp.

2113 LIBRARY ASSOCIATION *and* NATIONAL ASSOCIATION FOR THE EDUCATION OF THE PARTIALLY SIGHTED. *Clear print: papers and proceedings of a conference sponsored by the Library Association and the National Association for the Education of the Partially Sighted and held on 20 October, 1971* ... London, LA, 1972. 65 pp. (LA research publication, 9.) Lisa 1972/2128

2114 Library services for the disadvantaged and handicapped. *Iowa Library Quarterly*, Jan. 1972 issue.

2115 LUCIOLI, Clara E. *and* BAKER, Elizabeth M. IFLA Libraries in Hospital Sub-section, hospital library studies 1967 – 71 (8) USA, 1967: the role of the public library in hospital library provision. *Int. Libr. Rev.*, 4 (3) July 1972, 387 – 391. Lisa 1972/1690

2116 LUDLOW, [V.] Felicy. A survey of national organisations for the handicapped, based in Toronto. Felicy Ludlow, Joyce Henderson, Laura Murray and Reginald Rawkins. *Can. Libr. J.*, 29 (4) July/Aug. 1972, 310 – 318. Lisa 1972/2318

2117 LUDLOW, V. Felicy. The Toronto public library's service to shut-ins. *Can. Libr. J.*, 29 (3) May/June 1972, 237 – 241. Lisa 1972/1695

2118 MADSEN, Charlotte. Det sociale biblioteksarbejde for løst og dårligt organiseret. [The social extension work is too casual and too badly organised.] *Bibliotek 70*, (17) 1972, 360.

2119 MAIDMENT, William R. Library provision for the visually handicapped. *In*: *Clear print: papers and proceedings of a conference* . . . London, LA, 1972, 41 – 62. (LA research publication, 9.) Lisa 1972/1727

2120 MATTHEWS, David. 1972 and more distant views: chairman's address. *Book Trolley*, 3 (6) June 1972, 17 – 18.

2121 MILLER, A. M. IFLA Libraries in Hospital Sub-section, hospital library studies 1967 – 71 (6) USSR, 1970: the reading matter of patients. *Int. Libr. Rev.*, 4 (3) July 1972, 373 – 377. Lisa 1972/1725

2122 MONEY, Darlene. Volunteers help librarians to serve shut-ins. *Ontario Library Review*, 56 (3) Sept. 1972, 151 – 154. Lisa 1972/2321

2123 MOONEY, Norma S. *Bókasafnspjónusta vid sjúka og vanheila*. [Library services to the sick and the handicapped: survey of present facilities and organisational plan.] Unpublished thesis for BA exam with major in library science, Reykjavik 1972. 81 pp.

2124 MURPHY, D. C. Therapeutic value of children's literature. *Nursing Forum*, 11 (2) 1972, 141 – 164.

2125 NATIONAL BOOK LEAGUE. *Help in reading: books for the teacher of backward children and for pupils backward in reading. An exhibition and booklist selected and annotated by Dr. J. C. Daniels . . . and S. S. Segal . . . ; 5th edition*. London, NBL, 1972. 30 pp.

2126 NIELSEN, Helga. IFLA Libraries in Hospitals Sub-section, hospital library studies 1967 – 71 (1) Denmark, 1968: Danish hospital libraries and the training of hospital librarians. *Int. Libr. Rev.*, 4 (3) July 1972, 351 – 355. Lisa 1972/1688

2127 NYBERG, Mirjam (afterwards Mirjam Grundstroem). Survey of hospital and institutional library activity. *Adult Education* (Helsinki), (1) 1972.

2128 ONUFROCK, B. Appreciative readers by sound, touch and sight: Wisconsin regional library for the blind and physically handicapped. *Wisconsin Library Bulletin*, 68 March 1972, 105 – 106.

2129 PARTINGTON, W. W. IFLA Libraries in Hospitals Sub-section, hospital library studies 1967 – 71 (7) United Kingdom, 1971: (a) the LA Hospital Libraries and Handicapped Readers Group. *Int. Libr. Rev.*, 4 (3) July 1972, 379 – 380. Lisa 1972/1680

2130 PATON, Xenia. Teaching the mentally retarded to read: some personal experiences. *Book Trolley*, 3 (5) March 1972, 9 – 11. Lisa 1972/1545

2131 PAULIN, L. V. IFLA Libraries in Hospitals Sub-section, hospital library studies 1967 – 71 (7) United Kingdom, 1971: (b) current developments in hospital libraries. *Int. Libr. Rev.*, 4 (3) July 1972, 380 – 383. Lisa 1972/1682

2132 PAULIN, L. V. Reorganisation: a prescription for better hospital libraries? *In*: *Proceedings, papers and summaries of discussions at the public libraries conference held at Brighton, 25 Sept. to 28 Sept. 1972*. London, LA, 1972, 25 – 31. Lisa 1972/2827; Hosp. Abstr. 1973/669

2133 PEILLON, Jacqueline. IFLA Libraries in Hospitals Sub-section, hospital library studies 1967 – 71 (2) France, 1971: a voluntary library organization in Lyon and its region. *Int. Libr. Rev.*, 4 (3) July 1972, 357 – 360. Lisa 1972/1687

2134 PETERSEN, Jes. Målrettet opsøgende virksomhed. [Meeting of Danish Special Group for social library work.] *Bogens Verden*, 54 (8) 1972, 542 – 546.

2135 PETROV, I. H. *and* VLAHLIJSKA, L. A. Cultural therapy in the old people's home. *Gerontologist*, 12 Winter 1972, 429 – 434.

2136 PHINNEY, Eleanor. Recognizing the institutional libraries: two decisive decades. *Am. Libr.*, 3 (7) July/Aug. 1972, 735 – 742. Lisa 1972/2314

2137 REIVALA, Raili. Kirjasto ja lukemis – ja kirjoittamishäiriöinen lapsi. [The library and children with difficulties in reading and writing.] Ajankohtaista kirjastoa. 2. Erityistyötä lapsille. [Public libraries today. 2. Special service to children.] *Kirjastopalvelu*, 1972, 21 – 36.

2138 RIMKEIT, Anita. IFLA Libraries in Hospitals Sub-section, hospital library studies 1967 – 71 (3) German Democratic Republic, 1970: the development of patients' libraries. *Int. Libr. Rev.*, 4 (3) July 1972, 361 – 364. Lisa 1972/1685

2139 RIMKEIT, Anita. Patientenbibliotheken in der DDR. [Patients' libraries in the German Democratic Republic.] *Bibliothekar*, 26 (11) Nov. 1972, 728 – 732. Lisa 1973/109

2140 RONGIONE, Louis. Bibliotherapy: its nature and uses. *Cath. Libr. Wld.*, 43 (9) May/June 1972, 495 – 500.

2141 RONNIE, Mary A. IFLA Libraries in Hospitals Sub-section, hospital library studies 1967 – 71 (5) New Zealand, 1971: the professional and the volunteer. *Int. Libr. Rev.*, 4 (3) July 1972, 369 – 372. Lisa 1972/1689

2142 RONNIE, Mary A. IFLA standards: service to hospitals and handicapped readers. *New Zealand Libraries*, 35 (5) Oct. 1972, 295 – 299. Lisa 1973/107

2143 RUSSELL, Jean. Hospital storytelling for children. *Book Trolley*, 3 (8) Dec. 1972, 7 – 9.

2144 SCHMIDT, Hannelore. D.B.V. Arbeitskreis – Krankenhausbüchereien: Aktivitäten, Publikationen, Arbeitsprogramm. [D.B.V. section 'Libraries in hospitals' activities, publications, business – programme.] *Buch und Bibliothek*, 24 (3) March 1972, 341 – 342.

2145 SCHMIDT, Hannelore. Einrichtung und Organisation einer Krankenhausbücherei. [Arrangement and organisation of a hospital library.] *Der Evangelische Buchberater*, 26 (4) Oct./Dec. 1972, 221 – 227.

2146 SCHMIDT, Hannelore. Die Sonderbüchereien der Stadt München: Bericht aus der Praxis. [Special libraries: Libraries in hospitals and in homes for the elderly in Munich. Report on practice.] *Buch und Bibliothek*, 24 (3) March 1972, 344 – 347.

2147 SCHMIDT, L. M., *editor*. Library service to the aging. *AHIL Quarterly*, Spring/ Summer 1972 issue.

2148 SCHULTEIS, Miriam, *sister. Guidebook for bibliotherapy*. Glenview, Ill., Psychotechnics Inc., 1972. 138 pp.

2149 SHAW, Alison. Writing and reading aids for the physically disabled. *Journal of librarianship*, 4 (2) April 1972, 75 – 90, 97.
Lisa 1972/1040

2150 SHIDOKUYO (Council for Securing Reading Rights for the Blind and Visually Handicapped). [Library services for the blind and visually handicapped: a perspective.] *Toshokan – Kai*, 24 (4) Nov. 1972, 162 – 167. (In Japanese.)
Lisa 1973/1198

2151 SIMPSON, Alice. A survey of organizations and institutions serving the physically handicapped in British Columbia. *Can. Libr. J.*, 29 (4) July/Aug. 1972, 319 – 326.
Lisa 1972/2317

2152 SKRZYPEK, Alexander. The Chicago public library services for the blind and physically handicapped. *Illinois libraries*, 54 (4) April 1972, 296 – 300.

2153 STARK, Elisabeth. Bibliotherapie in der Diskussion. [Bibliotherapy in debate.] *Humanitas*, Berlin, 12 (9) 1972, 11.

2154 STEINHOFF, A. Kranke Kinder brauchen Bücher. [Sick children need books.] *Krankenpflege*, 26 (1) 1972, 18.

2155 SVENDSEN, Erik, *editor*. Folkebibliotekerne og de læsehæmmede. [The public libraries and reading for the retarded.] København, 1972.

2156 TANTTU, Orvoki. Lastenkirjastotyötä sairaalassa. [Library work with children in hospital.] Ajankohtaista kirjastoa. 2. Erityistyötä lapsille. [Public libraries today. 2. Special services to children.] *Kirjastopalvelu*, 1972, 1 – 10.

2157 THORPE, F. A. Large print: an assessment of its development and potential. *Libr. Ass. Rec.*, 74 (3) March 1972, 42 – 43.
Lisa 1972/1039

2158 TOMA, Anne. IFLA Libraries in Hospitals Sub-section, hospital library studies 1967 – 71 (4) Hungary, 1970: the organization of hospital libraries. *Int. Libr. Rev.*, 4 (3) July 1972, 365 – 368.
Lisa 1972/1686

2159 UNITED STATES. LIBRARY OF CONGRESS. Division for the Blind and Physically Handicapped. *Aids for handicapped readers*. [Washington] The Division, 1972. 17 pp.

2160 VESTERGAARD, Inger *and* AREVAD, Bodil. Hospitalsvæsenet og det sociale områdes fremtidige struktur. [Hospital service and the future structure of the social field.] *Bibliotek 70*, (9) 1972, 196 – 197.

2161 VETERE, C. La biblioteca in ospedale. [The library in the hospital.] *Ospedali d'Italia*, Como, 9 (9) Sept. 1972, 820 – 824.

2162 WASSNER, Hermann. Haben die Blinden eine öffentliche Bücherei? (Do the blind have a public library?] *Buch und Bibliothek*, 24 (9) Sept. 1972, 854 – 862. Lisa 1972/2830

2163 WOLFF, Hildegard. Aspekte einer Therapie mit dem Buch am Krankenbett. *In: Die Krankenhausbücherei.* [Therapeutic aspects of the book at the hospital bed. *In: The hospital library.*] Köln, Greven Verlag, 1972, 39 – 64.

2164 YAST, Helen. Standards for library service in institutions: B. In the health care setting. *Library Trends*, 21 (2) Oct. 1972, 267 – 285. Lisa 1973/675

A

Aalto, R. 1763, 1850
Ackerknecht, E. 298
Åhlin, G. 453
Ahlnäs, B. 1765
Aitken, W. R. 1939
Alderson, C. I. 488
Aldrich, L. 1214
Aletha, *sister*. 137
Alexander, L. 515, 565, 584, 585
Alexander, R. H. 1601, 1685
Alison, M. J. H. 2054
Allen, E. B. 649
Allsop, K. M. 760, 838
Allum, N. 1166
Al-Salman, J. 2089
Amberg, R. M. 566
American Hospital Association. 299
American Library Association. 38, 44, 1264
American Library Association. Adult services
   division. 1387, 1452
American Library Association. Association of
   hospital and institution libraries. 995, 1033,
   1071, 1120, 1453, 1766, 1851, 1940
American Library Association. Committee on
   hospital libraries. 300, 301, 332, 333, 383,
   384, 454, 455, 489, 516
American Library Association. Hospital librar-
   ies committee. 164
American Library Association. Hospital librar-
   ies division. 614, 650, 651, 675, 676, 715, 716,
   911, 1686
American Library Association. Hospital librar-
   ies round table. 490, 517, 536, 586, 587, 615
American Library Association. Institution
   libraries committee. 178
American Library Association. Library admin-
   istrative division. 1602, 1941
American Library Association. Round table on
   library services for the blind. 2055
American Library Association. War service. 56
Anastasia, M., *sister*. 1167
Andersen, J. B. 179
Andersen, J. M. 588, 717
Andersson, G. 1852
Andreassen, J. 960
Andree, O. 1767
Andresen, L. 1768
Andrewes, J. 1604
Andrews, J. L. 961
Anet, *Mme* P. 456
Aragó, I. 1942
Arbeitskreis 'Krankenhausbüchereien'. 1605,
   1606
Arborelius, B. 877, 1215, 2056
Arevad, B. 1853, 2160
Arnot, J. F. 839, 996
Askwith, *Mrs*. H. 677

Assbury, E. 2057
Avery, C. 1524

B

Baatz, W. H. 761, 800, 1216
Babcock, K. B. 1323
Baber, A. 1854
Bachmann, I. 302
Bacon, A. 205
Baggelaar, A. 997
Bailey, D. H. 878
Baker, E. M. 2115
Baker, M. C. 616, 934
Balme, H. 652
Bangs, J. K. 74
Barber, E. M. 206
Barbour, J. M. 1121
Bare, N. J. 1607
Barker, G. W. 935
Barker, M. H. 75
Barlow, E. 678
Barlow, V. 962
Barry, J. 879
Bartels, H. 1454
Bartine, O. H. 303
Baskin, B. H. 1855
Basset, *Mlle*. 963
Basset, R. S. 1122, 1168
Batie, M. 1943
Baylis, I. M. 148, 149
Beard, R. O. 141
Beasley, J. F. 1944
Beatty, W. K. 1169, 1266, 1388, 1856
Beausejour, M. 180
Becker, M. J. 1857
Beddington, S. 334, 386
Bedwell, C. E. A. 304, 305, 617, 679
Beerens, A.-M. 1170
Bekker, J. 1770, 2058
Belkin, N. 457
Bell, D. 1455
Bellinger, R. C. 1858
Beltman, F. L. Berdenis van Berlekom – *see*
   Berlekom – Beltman, F. L. Berdenis van
Beltman, F. L. Kroese – *see* Kroese – Beltman,
   F. L.
Bereczky, L. 1859
Bergaus, M. V. 207
Berggren, G. 1687
Bergmann, B. 1525
Bergmann, G. 762, 840
Berg-Sonne, V. 1268
Berlekom-Beltman, F. L. Berdenis van. 1052
Berrington, J. 1945
Berry, J. 1171, 1608
Berry, P. 1456
Berset, I. V. 718, 763, 841
Bertelsen, E. 719, 880

Best, D. de 1771
Bialac, V. 1946
Bickel, R. 1123
Biermann, W. 765, 801
Binswanger, O. 336
Birdsall, G. H. 142
Birkholz, U. 1688
Bishop, W. J. 208, 802
Bjerre, A. 1773, 1861, 2059
Blackler, E. W. 337
Blackshear, O. T. 998, 1172
Blake, F. I. 251
Blau, S. A. 1074
Bledsoe, E. P. 109
Blom, M. 1689
Blomquist, H. 965
Blöss, E. 1270
Blume, A. 1690
Boelke, J. 1774
Bogard, H. M. 1458
Boklund, V. 2060
Boldero, H. E. A. 388
Boldt, B. 589
Bolitho, H. 1389
Boorer, D. 1271, 1460, 1609, 1863, 2062, 2063, 2064
Börjeson, O. 1064
Bosa, R. 2065
Böthig, S. 1527
Bourdin, G. 1528, 1610, 1864
Bouton, E. N. 1529
Bow, A. 1327
Bowman, D. 165
Božović, Z. 1124, 1217
Brace, E. A. 766
Bradford, E. C. 151
Bradley, C. E. 538
Brady, D. 1949
Brandt, E. 1461
Branson, W. C. 1125
Bray, R. S. 1272
Brendan, M., *sister*. 1218
Briggs, A. D. 720
Briggs, A. H. 1691
Brink, C. J. van den. 1127
British Library of Tape Recordings for Hospital Patients. 1692
British Red Cross Society. 308, 389, 799
Broadhouse, D. Davies – *see* Davies-Broadhouse, D.
Brock, L. 339
Brodman, E. 458, 539
Broekman, L. 1219
Brom, A. 285
Brooke, G. A. G. 1530
Brooks, E. H. 1273
Brown, E. G. 1950, 2066
Brown, G. 340
Brown, M. 492
Brown, R. 1693
Brown, S. J. M. 252, 804

Bruce, L. R. 653
Bruce-Porter, *Sir* B. 182, 232
Bruun, E. 1128
Bryan, A. I. 459
Bryant, A. 654, 680
Buchanan, *Mrs*. 681
Buggie, S. E. 1601
Bullock, J. Y. 1274
Bullock, M. 493, 494, 540
Bunch, A. J. 1611, 1776, 1865, 1951
Bungenberg de Jong, C. J. 1694
Burgess, D. G. 1531, 1777
Burgoyne, M. H. 39
Burket, R. R. 842, 966, 1034
Burns, L. 1778
Bursinger, B. C. 936
Buswell, C. H. 1952
Butchart, R. 682, 721
Butterworth, M. 1328
Bylund, R. 1866

C

Cable, M. 210
Cahling, U. 1867, 1953
Calame, L. 390
California Library Association. 1612
Camden Public Library. 1695
Campbell, H. C. 1779
Campfield, M. 2067
Canadian Library Association. 2068
Canfield, A. A. 1391
Cantrell, C. H. 1001
Capdeveille, J. 268
Cardinal, J. 805
Cardwell, M. 1075
Carey, M. E. 6, 19, 24, 28, 29, 45, 46, 76, 119, 138
Carlsson, F. 1954
Carner, C. 1533
Cartledge, J. A. 683
Casey, G. M. 1780, 1868, 1955, 1956, 1957
Chadwick, B. 518
Chamberlin, J. A. 1329
Chambers, D. C. 1330
Chance, B. 843
Chandler, G. 1463
Chapman, K. 1869
Chapman, M. T. 460, 541
Charteris, F. 2069
Chastel, G. 1076
Chesshire, K. 542
Chiaromonte, G. 309
Chromse, I. 17
Chudek, K. 1275
Chute, G. 18
Clark, D. F. 2070
Clark, P. O. 30
Clark, R. S. 806
Clarke, E. K. 269, 341
Clarke, J. M. 1534, 1613, 1696, 1958, 1959

Clemmesen, C. 391
Cleveland Public Library. 1697
Cliff, B. 618
Clifton, E. 866
Cloke, J. 882
Clough, H. D. 310
Coachman, D. F. 233
Coates, J. L. 807, 808
Cochran, M. R. 47
Coelln, A. von. 2071
Cohoe, E. 1175
Collins, H. O. 120
Collis, D. 1464
Compton, C. H. 286
Condell, L. 311, 619
Connell, S. M. 684, 767, 768, 769, 770, 809, 810, 844
Connelly, J. 2072
Cooke, A. S. 392
Cooke, M. 845
Cooke, *Mrs.* Paget – *see* Paget-Cooke, *Mrs.*
Copenhaver, M. S. 1035
Corney, R. 1176
Cornwall County Library. 1960
Corson, H. F. 685
Cory, P. B. 1036, 1177
Cosgrove, J. M. 1392
Council of National Library Associations. 1465, 1535, 1614, 1698, 1781
Cowburn, L. M. 1393
Cowern, A. G. 723
Cowles, B. 1276, 1331, 1394
Cowles, R. L. 590
Cowley, A. 57
Cox, E. H. 1699
Cracknell, E. G. 1178
Craigie, A. L. 166
Crain, E. R. 183
Cramer, C. H. 2073
Cramer, G. 234
Creglow, E. R. 152, 211, 235, 496
Cremonesi, G. C. F. 270
Crist, E. 655
Critchley, W. E. G. 1615, 1700, 1961
Croix-Rouge de Belgique. 912, 967, 1002, 1037, 1077, 1129, 1179, 1277, 1278, 1332, 1701
Crooks, S. 1962
Crosby, A. A. 212
Crosley, C. E. 342
Crouch, M. S. 1333
Croucher, L. 567
Culp, R. W. 2074
Cumming, E. E. 1776, 1951, 1963, 2019, 2075
Curtius, F. 591
Cuxart, C. 1964
Cwynar, S. 2076
Czechoslovakia. Ministry of Health. 1466
Czechoslovakia. Ministry of Public Health. 1395

D

Dale, B. 2077

Dale, M. 58
Danebius-Schadee, H. H. 1279
Daniels, J. C. 2125
Danielson, I. 287
Darling, R. L. 1038
Darr, F. 1039, 1180
Darrin, R. 1130
Davie, L. 497
Davies-Broadhouse, D. 544
Davis, E. L. 1536
Day, A. 1467
Delaney, S. Peterson – *see* Peterson-Delaney, S.
Deleon, M. 545
Delisle, M. M., *sister.* 546, 568, 771, 811
Delvalle, J. 1468
Depopolo, M. 1040
Deschamps, M.-C. 1870
De Selliers de Moranville, N. 1220
Deutscher Bibliotheksverband. 2078
Deutscher Büchereiverband. 1616, 1965
Devereux, R. 461
de Vos, C. I. 2079
Dewdney, P. 2077
Dewe, M. 1537
Dick, J. 569
Dijk, C. van. 1326
Distel, H. 343
Dixey, E. 741
Dockhorn, B. 1181, 1182
Dolan, R. 1116, 1678
Dolch, E. T. 1221
Domney, J. M. 1966
Donalies, C. 1538
Donnelly, J. 1116
Dooley, K. 1078
Dopf, K. 393
Doren, E. C. 48
Dorr, M. M. 1644
Doud, M. 59
Douglass, H. 812
Drake, R. B. 87
Dubois, I. 121, 167, 236
Duckitt, D. 394
Dudley, E. 1782
Duffey, K. I. 1396
Duhamel, G. 344
Du Monceau de Bergendal, I. G. 1702, 1783
Dunkel, B. 846
Dunne, M. 1871
Dunningham, A. G. W. 686
Duplica, M. M. 2081
Dux, W. 1376

E

Eason, H. H. 1183
Eastman, L. A. 98, 345
Eaton, E. S. 724, 913, 914
Ebaugh, F. G. 288
Ebert, E. 1222
Edwards, M. 1079

Egas, C. 1872
Eilola, R. 732
Eller, C. S. 620
Elliott, J. 2082
Elliott, J. E. 77
Elliott, P. G. 1131
Ellsworth, R. H. 1617
Ely, V. 968
Emerson, T. L. W. 2083
Engelhardt, D. 969
Eppinger, L. 1470
Epstein, R. 1539
Erickson, C. R. 2084
Eriksson, S. 1703
Esbech, S. 1471
Ethelreda, *sister*. 1223
Etto, E. 2085
Euler, K. F. 1080, 1081, 1101, 1132, 1133, 1184, 1185, 1334, 1335, 1397, 1472, 1473, 1704
Euren, H. R. 1003

F

Fahlbusch, H. Müller – *see* Müller-Fahlbusch, H.
Farrington, A. 570
Farrow, V. L. 1336
Faulds, E. 547
Favazza, A. R. 1540
Featherstone, T. M. 2086
Fédération Internationale des Associations de Bibliothécaires. *See also* International Federation of Library Associations. 213, 237, 271, 272, 312, 313, 395, 396, 397, 687, 688, 725, 773, 847, 915, 916, 917, 970, 1041, 1082, 1134, 1186, 1224, 1280, 1337, 1398, 1541, 1619, 1705, 1785
Fellin, O. A. 656
Fenwick, H. 883
Feydt, A. 1826
Fickel, G. 1281
Fidder, H. 1873
Finckh, G. 765
Fingeret, R. W. 1399
Finzel, S. 1542
Fischer, J. A. A. 2087
Fishbein, M. 273
Fisher, M. 1083
Fitch, W. C. 1543
Fitzgerald, M. E. 1135
Flanagan, J. J., *father*. 1042
Flandorf, V. S. 918, 1004, 1005, 1084, 1085, 1086, 1474, 1475, 1476, 1544, 1620
Fleak, D. H. 1423
Flinn, G. H. 704
Floch, M. 1087, 1088
Foley, M. R. 399, 400
Folz, C. 253
Fonderie-Tierie, E. 1187
Forbes, A. P. 848
Forbes, H. A. 346

Foreman, E. T. 254
Forrest, L. B. 255
Forsdyke, J. 849, 884
Forssell, K. 1225
Forsyth, M. H. 689, 690
Franken, E. Rubbens – *see* Rubbens-Franken, E.
Frary, M. P. 1043
Fraser, A. W. 971
Freeman, M. W. 548
Freiberger, A. 1089
Freiberger, H. 1545
Friendenthal, R. 401
Fröhlich, H. 972
Frommer, E. A. 1621
Frye, D. 1136
Fryer, C. 571
Frykman, [   ]. 1291
Fryksen, B. 1967
Fuller, K. H. 348

G

Gade, E. 726
Gagnon, S. 549, 550
Gale, S. R. 1400, 1477
Gallagher, J. 1090
Gallivan, K. C. 274
Gallozzi, C. 1622
Gardner, F. M. 1188, 1478, 1787, 1788
Gardner, W. P. 402
Garevskii, V. 403
Gariel, E. 1610
Gartland, H. J. 1044, 1091, 1226, 1479, 1789
Gaskell, H. M. 40, 349
Gasking, A. F. J. 1706
Gatliff, J. W. 919
Gaussen, I. 404
Geerdts, H. J. 1227
Geerts, W. 1874
Geiseler, W. 1480
Gelderblom, G. 1092, 1481, 1790
Gerard, E. 405
Germaine, M. 938
Gifford, E. R. 92, 110
Gilkison, E. E. 885
Gilson, P. A. 2089
Gittleman, F. C. 1046
Glazykin, I. 457
Godet, M. 406
Going, M. E. 1045, 1282, 1283, 1338, 1401, 1546, 1707, 1791, 1792, 1875, 1968
Goldsmith, S. 2090
Gostyńska, D. 1547, 1793, 1969, 2091
Gotthardsen, M. O. 1623
Gottschalk, L. A. 727
Göttsche, E. 1182, 1189, 1482
Gould, E. C. 621
Graham, E. C. 1624, 1970
Granger, E. M. 1625
Grannis, F. 1006, 1708, 1794
Grant, G. 475

Graves, J. A. 1190
Gray, J. D. A. 1339
Gray, P. G. 1626
Gray, R. H. 2092
Great Britain. Department of Health and Social Security. 1876, 1877
Great Britain. Department of Health for Scotland. 850
Great Britain. Ministry of Health. 813, 939, 1228, 1548
Great Britain. Scottish Education Department. 1795
Greco, C. M. 1878
Green, E. 60, 61, 70, 110
Greenaway, E. 1229, 1549
Greenslade, L. K. 315
Grieson, V. E. 592
Grills, M. A. 774
Grogan, J. 1709
Gronseth, O. A. 1093
Gross, R. 1046
Grove, H. H. 1284
Grove, L. 1191
Grundstroem, M. – *see* Nyberg, M. (afterwards M. Grundstroem)
Gubalke, W. 1340, 1402
Guex, S. 407
Guild of Hospital Librarians. 657, 775, 814, 851, 886
Günnel, P. 1403
Gunness, V. 852
Günther, J. 1710
Gut, W. 408
Guthrie, D. 1285, 1483
Guzik, K. 1230
Gyde-Pedersen, M. 289, 316, 350, 409, 658, 728, 729, 853

H

Haas, D. B. 1550
Haberer, I. J. 2094
Haffenden, J. W. 463
Haggerty, C. E. 973
Hagle, A. D. 1627
Hahn, H. 1711
Håkansson, E. 2095
Hallqvist, M. 1484
Hamilton, A. 1712
Hamlin, D. R. 88
Handel, R. S. 887
Hankar, [ ]. 776
Hannah, R. G. 974
Hannigan, M. C. 940, 975, 1007, 1286, 1287, 1341, 1404, 1713, 1797, 1798, 1972, 1973, 2096
Hansen, M. B. 1974
Hansen, O. R. B. 1231
Happ, F. W. 1799
Harding, G. 1714
Harney, H. Müller – see Müller-Harney, H.

Harris, J. D. 1047
Harris, N. G. 1975
Harrison, K. C. 1232, 1342, 1800
Hart, J. A. 1976
Hartzenberg, M. 1945
Harvey, B. C. 1233
Harvey, M. L. 572
Hasler, D. 1094
Havens, S. 1551
Haycraft, H. 1288, 1405, 1715
Hays, D. O. 706
Heathfield, S. 1628
Hedemann, A.-G. 1879
Heintze, I. 1095
Heinze, H. 1192
Heinze, L. 593, 622
Henderson, J. 2116
Henderson, J. M. 730
Henderson, W. T. 1341
Henriot, G. 256, 275, 317
Henry, R. P. 1289
Hensel, H. 318
Hering, L. C. 319
Hervey, G. S. 594
Hewitt, M. 1629
Hill, A. M. 1343
Hill, W. 815
Hilliard, J. 1977
Hillson, N. 816, 817
Himwich, W. A. 1096
Hintikka, A.-M. 2097
Hirn, S. 1801
Hirsch, L. 818, 920, 1008
Hjelmqvist, B. 1485
Hodge, H. A. 351
Hodock, I. 1978
Hoffman, K. F. 1290
Hofrén, M. 352
Høgh, H. 1902, 1979
Hök-Lundin, E. 731
Holland, C. 31
Hollway, M. 732
Holm, A. D. 551, 623, 733
Holmsten, U. 734
Holmström, B. 1048, 1802
Höök, L. 1716, 1717, 2098
Hoover, A. F. 117
Hopkins, T. W. 659
Horcasitas, C. 777
Houël, H. 412, 466
Hounsome, J. 820
Howard, A. L. 596, 854
Howard, V. 633
Huettenbuegel, J. 1718
Huguenor, H. H. 1682
Hulmann, M. 413
Hunt, E. 1234
Hunter, J. 1194
Huri, *Mme.* 963
Huri, N. 1049
Husby, J. 1486

Hussey, E. R. J. 521
Hutchinson, L. C. 597
Huxley, F. A. 78
Hvardal, M. 1502
Hyatt, R. 502
Hynes, J. C. 2099

I

Ignatius, E. 735
Il'inskaia, O. 736
Illinois Department of Mental Health. 1554
Illinois State Library. 1554
Interassociation Hospital Libraries Committee. 1407
International Federation of Library Associations. *See also* Fédération Internationale des Associations de Bibliothécaires. 1195, 1235, 1803, 1880, 1981, 1982, 2100
International Guild of Hospital Librarians. 320, 414, 415, 416, 417
International Guild of Hospital Librarians. British section. 356, 418, 467, 503, 554, 598, 626, 660
Ireland, G. O. 168, 188
Irish Republic. Hospital Library Council. 419, 504, 1408, 1631
Irving, J. A. 821, 822
Isom, M. F. 66

J

Jack, A. 1632
Jackson, J. A. 123
Jackson, W. S. 1881
Jakob, H. 1805
James, M., *sister.* 1196
Jameson, M. 276
Jamieson, J. 823
Janes, L. A. 124
Janicki, A. 1882
Jankowska, E. 1806
Jannasch, C. 1487
Jansen, M. 1555
Janssen, C. E. 976, 1009, 1236
Javelin, M. C. 2101
Jeanneret, R. 420
Jeffreys, G. L. O. 505
Jekić, U. 1345
Jensen, F. 888
Jensen, K. M. 824, 1010
Johansen, A. 1884, 2102
Johns, H. 941
Johnson, B. C. 1197
Johnson, C. W. 1011
Johnston, N. 1488
Johrden, J. A. 1409
Jones, A. F. 573
Jones, C. 79
Jones, E. B. 153
Jones, E. K. 12, 13, 14, 15, 19, 20, 23, 25, 26, 32, 33, 34, 41, 42, 49, 99, 100, 111, 125, 189, 468

Jones, J. W. 1556
Jones, L. E. 889, 1237
Jones, P. 101, 112, 113, 126, 127, 128, 169, 190, 215, 238, 258, 321, 358, 599, 600, 661, 737
Jong, C. J. Bungenberg de – *see* Bungenberg de Jong, C. J.
Jordan, D. 942
Judge, A. 627
Jung, H. D. 1557
Junge, R. 1489
Junier, A. J. 1138, 1292

K

Kabell, M. 1346
Kamman, G. R. 277, 421, 469
Kanninen, M. 601, 738
Kappes, M. L. 628
Karjalainen, V. 1807
Karsakoff, H. 247
Karsakoff, P. 247
Kauppi, H. 943, 1139, 1558, 1633
Kayser, F. 359
Kearns, M. M. 1050, 1238
Kellaway, H. 422
Kellner, B. 1491, 1719, 1885
Kemme, A. P. F. M. 1433
Kenchington, S. 1983
Kennedy, M. E. 423
Kent, M. L. 692, 693
Kent County Council. Education committee. 1198, 1411
Kenyon, X. 936
Kerslake, J. F. 781
Kersten, H.-H. 1347
Kerwin, P. F. 855, 1099
Kewley, P. D. 1632
Keyes, A. W. 977
Kildal, A. 890
Kimmel, A. 2087
Kindelsperger, B. E. S. 322, 323
King, E. A. 555
King, F. A. 360
King, J. E. 978
King, M. E. 1348
King Edward's Hospital Fund for London. 1140
Kingsland, G. S. 694
Kinney, M. M. 662, 693, 1141, 1293, 1559
Kinos, H. 602
Kircher, C. J. 695
Kirstein, K. 1886
Kjerrström, U. 1720, 1721, 1887
Klages, W. 1412
Klumb, *Mrs.* D. 1984
Knibbe, W. 944
Knight, N. H. 1722
Knox, D. 239
Knox, J. B. 945
Koch, T. W. 43, 50, 67
Koefoed, I. 1985, 2103, 2104

Koelher, E. 80
Kolmodin, T. 629
Kolodziejska, J. 2105
Koolhaas, A. A. 1326
Koumans, F. P. 757
Kovács, P. 1888
Kozakiewicz, W. 1724, 1889, 1890, 2106
Kozłowski, S. 2107
Kraśniewska, K. 2109
Kraus, E. 1294
Kris, A. O. 2092
Křivinková, J. 1051, 1199, 1200, 1201, 1349, 1350, 1634, 1986
Kroese-Beltman, F. L. 1414
Kruzan, R. 1100
Kuehn, M. 1987
Kuhlmann, F. 1560
Kulczycki, M. 1988
Kuntz, E. 1081, 1101
Künzel, D. 1561
Kurtz, M. E. 191

L

La Bauve, L. F. 1810
Lafay, F. 1240
Lamb, S. D. 154
Landau, R. A. 1891
Lange, [ ]. 856
Lange, K. 1142, 1295
Langfeldt, J. 1202
Laquer, B. 7
Larsen, J. 1241
Larsson, E. 1415
Latini, L. A. 782
Lattanzi, A. D. 1012, 1013, 1636, 1892
Laur, G. Liebrich – *see* Liebrich-Laur, G.
Laurie, G. 1416
Lavinder, C. H. 102
Lawler, J. G. 2110
League of Library Commissions. 10
Ledgard, D. 1726
Leeuwenburgh, P. B. 1417, 1811, 1893, 1894, 1895, 1990
Leich, H. G. R. 1492, 1637, 1638
Leith, M. 1639
Lejeune, R. 2084
Lemaître, H. 271, 278, 312, 324, 397, 427, 428, 472, 506
Lemke, [ ]. 429
Lentz, R. T. 1493
Lepalczyk, I. 1102
Leszczyński, J. 1014
Leuschner, L. K. 1562
Lewis, C. 430
Lewis, M. J. 1053, 1297, 1298, 1351, 1352, 1418, 1419, 1494, 1495, 1537, 1563, 1564, 1565, 1727, 1728, 1788, 1812, 1813, 1814, 1815, 1991, 1992, 2111
Leys, D. 1353, 1420
Library Association. 192, 216, 217, 240, 259,

260, 362, 431, 783, 784, 785, 1496, 1993, 2112, 2113
Library Association. County libraries group, Wales. 1994
Library Association. Hospital libraries and handicapped readers group. 1422, 1497, 1640, 1641, 1729, 1995
Library Association. Hospital libraries committee. 218, 219
Library Association. West Midland branch. 1896
Liebig, M. 1997
Liebrich-Laur, G. 432
Lilly, E. 290
Limper, H. K. 1245, 1568
Lind, J. E. 143
Lindblad, I. 1354
Linde, I. 170, 193
Lindem, S. 205, 220
Lindem, S. M. 522
Linder, G. 363
Linderberg, K. 1355, 1998
Linnovaara, L. 1569
Lipchak, A. C. 1054
Little, L. T. 171
Lockett, W. J. 891
Lodder, N. M. 2033
Logan, M. 1999
Lohmann, V. L. 1816
London, W. A. 1897
Long, D. E. 825
Loo, K. J. M. van de. 1433
Loomis, M. L. W. 4
Lord, E. 857
Lozano, C. D. R. 1055
Lucioli, C. E. 664, 1246, 1299, 1423, 1570, 1571, 1643, 1644, 1730, 1898, 2000, 2001, 2115
Ludlow, V. F. 1779, 1817, 2116, 2117
Lund, E. 632
Lundeen, A. 633, 1103, 1104, 1247
Lundin, E. Hök – *see* Hök-Lundin, E.
Lundström, B. 2002
Lyell, L. 364
Lyman, H. H. 1524, 2003
Lyngen, G. 740
Lyon, E. 2004
Lyons, G. J. 1356, 1645

M

Maas, G. 473, 523, 524, 556
McAlister, C. 826
McArthur, T. 1357
Macaskill, H. 696
McCardle, S. E. 129
McClaskey, H. C. 1818
McColvin, L. R. 1248
McCorkle, R. 827
McCrossan, J. A. 1731, 1899
McCuaig, M. E. 979
McCullough, F. 1900

McDaniel, W. B. 1015
McDowell, D. J. 2005
McFarland, J. H. 858, 892
McFarlane, D. M. 433
McInnes, E. M. 1358
McKenna, C. E. 922
Mackenzie, C. 634
Mackenzie, N. 697
MacKown, M. 741
Maclean, F. 2006
Maclean, M. 35
McNamara, M. E. 1056
McNutt, R. J. 828
McPeake, J. G. 1016
Macrum, A. M. 194, 195, 221, 241, 261, 262
Madsen, C. 1901, 1902, 2118
Mahlow, J. 1359
Mahon, M. W. 1360
Mahon, S. H. 859
Mahoney, A. 860
Mahoney, S. M. 1572
Mahout, *Mme.* 1017
Maidment, W. R. 2119
Manucharova, E. V. 861
Marchi, L. 1361
Markus, F. 893, 1300
Marsh, J. 2067
Marshall, M. R. 2007
Martin, W. A. 923
Mary Christine, *sister.* 1498
Mary Concordia, *sister.* 1362
Mary Germaine, *sister.* 1203
Mason, M. F. 525, 557, 635, 665
Masters, A. 1249
Mathews, K. R. 742
Matthews, A. 1363
Matthews, D. A. 1646, 1647, 1903, 2120
Matthews, G. M. 2008
May, M. 2009
Mayden, P. M. 894
Menninger, K. 1250
Menninger, W. C. 365
Meri, S.-L. 895, 946, 1018, 1144, 1301, 1302, 1364
Methven, M. L. 526, 666, 1019
Meyer, J. R. 2010
Meyers, A. S. 2011
Meyling, A. 1425
Michaels, J. J. 667
Michell, R. A. 1648
Milam, C. H. 68, 81, 89
Miles, N. M. 1204
Milkovich, M. 743
Miller, A. M. 2121
Miller, J. 2052
Miller, M. M. 155
Miller, M. P. D. 114
Miller, N. 291
Millward, R. H. 1303, 1365
Minić, V. 2012
Minkiewicz, M. 1565

Minnesota Association of Hospital, Medical and Institution Librarians. 558
Minto, J. 242
Miralda, M. 279
Mitchell, D. 1426
Mitchell, J. 1116
Mohrhardt, F. E. 862, 924, 947
Moisio, A. H. 434
Molenaar, Th. K. 1904
Molin, B. 1905
Molin, L. 1905
Money, D. 2122
Monroe, M. E. 1819, 2013, 2014, 2015, 2016
Montelin, T. 1304
Montojo, C. 280
Moody, E. P. 863, 896
Moody, M. 1145
Moody, M. T. 1305, 1428, 1429, 1732, 1733
Mooney, N. S. 2123
Moore, A. C. 11
Moore, S. 925
Moore, T. V. 574
Moran, A. 1906
Morris, E. F. 172
Morris, E. L. 1366
Morrissey, M. R. 156, 173, 474
Morrow, W. A. 1306
Moses, H. A. 1762
Mounce, M. W. 1782
Mounts, A. 1251
Mullen, F. A. 1501
Mullen, M. M. 1734
Müller, C. 1205
Muller, R. J. 1735
Müller-Fahlbusch, H. 2017
Müller-Harney, H. 1907
Munck af Rosenschöld, K. 744, 864
Munford, W. A. 1020, 1106, 1107, 1367, 1430, 1573, 2018
Munro, J. 1206
Murison, W. J. 980
Murphy, D. C. 2124
Murphy, E. F. 1545
Murray, L. 2116
Mushake, K. 698

N

Nagórska, I. 1252
Nand, M. 575
Nannestad, A. (afterwards A. N. Nicolaysen). 1502, 1820, 2019
Närhi, M. K. 897
National Association for the Education of the Partially Sighted. 1993, 2113
National Association of Group Secretaries. 1574
National Book League. 1736, 2125
National Fund for Research into Crippling Diseases. 2020
National Institutes of Health. 1207

Neelameghan, A. 898, 926
Nefedčenko, M. 1908
Neil, A. 2021
Nenadovič, L. 1253, 1307
Nepustil, B. 1109
Ness, C. H. 1146
Neuman, S. 899
Nevermann, C. 948
New York State. Education department. 2022
New York State. Interdepartmental health and
  hospital council. 1503
Nicholas, R. M. 2023
Nicolaysen, A. N – *see* Nannestad, A. (after-
  wards A. N. Nicolaysen)
Nielsen, H. 787, 865, 1368, 1504, 1821, 2126
Nielsen, H. G. 1575
Nielsen, I. Vig – *see* Vig-Nielsen, I.
Nielsen, N. T. 1909
Nielsen, O. 1254
Nieman, D. E. 1147, 1910
Niemeijer, J. 1738
Nieminen, R. 1911
Nieuwenborgh, P. van 900
Nikolussi, R. 1148
Nilsson, A. 1954
Nistri, M. 901
Noakes, E. H. 1576
Noe, B. 745
Nohrström, K. 601
Norrie, J. 699, 746
Northern Ireland. Ministry of Education. 1577
Nowell, C. 366
Nuiver, J. 1739
Nunn, M. L. 1021
Nyberg, M. (afterwards M. Grundstroem).
  1369, 1578, 1650, 1651, 1740, 1822, 1823,
  1824, 2127
Nyborg, K. 1308
Nye, P. W. 1432, 1741
Nyquist, R. H. 866
Nyren, J. S. 1891

O

Oathout, M. C. 949, 950
O'Connell, J. A. 636
O'Connor, R. A. 90, 91, 103, 174, 222
Odescalchi, E. K. 1652, 1742
Oliver, B. 637, 1579
Olsen, D. 1505
Olsson, K. 1743
Onufrock, B. 2128
Opdahl, S. 1825
Order of St. John. 308, 389, 799
Ørjasæter, T. 1826, 2024
Ormerod, J. 263
Orr, J. M. 1580
Ørvig, A. 1150
Ostenfeld, E. 157, 196, 197, 223, 325, 391, 435,
  729, 747
Östling, G. 224

O'Toole, M. 1505
Oxener, R. A. 1370

P

P., E. M. 225
Paget, S. J. 1434
Paget-Cooke, *Mrs.* 700
Paine, M. M. 475
Paine, P. M. 475
Palivec, V. 476, 701
Panse, F. 1435, 1653
Parland, O. 1581
Partington, W. W. 1582, 1583, 1912, 2129
Paton, W. B. 1744
Paton, X. 2130
Patten, K. 69
Patterson, D. 867
Paulin, L. V. 1506, 2131, 2132
Payne, J. 1913
Payne, K. 527
Peacock, J. 2026
Peart, D. R. 1256
Pedersen, M. Gyde – *see* Gyde-Pedersen, M.
Peifer, D. B. 1745
Peillon, J. 2133
Peltier, M. 1257
Pemberton, J. E. 2025
Pepino, J. 748
Perheentupa, L. 1827, 1828
Périer, G. D. 437
Pers, M. 1746
Persson, E. 1829, 1914
Persson, L.-C. 1537
Peters, I. 868
Peters, M. 1507
Petersen, J. 2134
Petersen, M. C. 438
Peterson, M. 1501
Peterson, M. V. 788
Peterson-Delaney, S. 198, 439, 507
Petkus, D. 2026
Petrov, I. H. 2135
Pétursdóttir, K. H. 1747, 2027
Philbrook, L. F. 478
Phillips, E. 749
Philomene, *sister*. 1309
Phinney, E. 1057, 1151, 1310, 2136
Pieters, E. 604
Piper, A. C. 219
Pleasants, M. G. 638
Pleijel, S. 1728
Plenge, J. 367
Pleskii, G. 440
Ploman, M. 2028, 2060
Plumb, R. W. 130
Podgóreczny, J. 1436
Poindron, P. 725, 829, 916
Pomeranz, E. B. 508
Pomeroy, E. 116, 144, 226, 243, 264, 368, 479,
  576

Poort, E. M. van der. 1922
Porter, *Sir* B. Bruce – *see* Bruce-Porter, *Sir* B.
Powell, J. W. 830
Powell, M. J. 244
Powers, R. K. 369
Pöysälä, P. 1655, 1656, 1830
Preble, M. C. 668
Presar, M. A. 927
Preston, N. K. 51
Price, P. P. 1584
Priller, R. 1152
Pritchard, F. C. 281
Protočková, V. 1153
Przybylski, F., *father*. 831
Puyn, U. 1681

Q

Quint, M. D. 605

R

Radford, D. 1658
Rainey, M. 158, 159, 227
Ranganathan, S. R. 480
Rankin, E. J. 82
Rantasalo, V. 1154
Raussendorf, C. 1373
Rawkins, R. 2116
Raymond, E. 1508
Raymond, H. 326
Raymond, V. 370, 441, 669
Reb, C. L. 606
Rees, L. M. 1659
Reichsstelle für das Büchereiwesen. 510
Reivala, R. 2137
Reixach, K. 1831
Research Institute for Consumer Affairs. 1832, 1916
Retief, H. J. M. 1917
Reumer, D. 1433
Richards, J. S. 951
Richardson, J. A. 1976
Richter, K. H. 1059
Ricker, E. L. 1060
Riddell, M. A. 512
Rieff, D. 1510
Riemsdijk, G. A. van 982, 1061, 1062, 1311
Rigden, M. S. 1587
Rimkeit, A. 2138, 2139
Rittenhouse, D. C. 2030
Roberts, M. E. 201, 228, 229, 230, 245, 246, 247, 371, 372, 373, 374, 375, 414, 415, 442, 513, 514, 528, 670, 702, 750, 751, 752
Roberts, O. W. 703
Robinson, C. E. 704
Robinson, G. C. 871
Robinson, G. S. 36
Robinson, J. A. 16, 19, 27
Roche, M. M. 983
Rochester General Hospital. 160
Rockall, F. W. 1706

Rodot, P. Vallery – *see* Vallery-Rodot, P.
Rogan, O. F. 607
Rogers, J. A. 1661
Romani, D. 1918
Rongione, L. 2140
Ronnie, M. A. 1588, 2141, 2142
Roome, W. H. 705
Roos, S. de 1313
Rosander, Y. 2031
Rose Mary, *sister*. 483
Ross, J. 789
Rossell, M. 327
Rossem, J. van. 1833
Rossini, G. 1662
Rourke, H. L. 529
Rozenblum, S. E. 952
Rubbens-Franken E. 1023, 1111
Rucks, P. 1155
Ruhberg, G. A. 202
Russell, J. 2143
Russell, W. L. 118
Russell, W. R. 1438
Rutherford, *Mrs.* H. W. 1374
Ryan, M. J. 1063
Rydberg, B. 1024
Rynell, A. 1663, 1749
Ryömä, S. 1919, 2032

S

Saarnio, L. 1025
Sainte-Leonie, *sister*. 1439
St. John, F. R. 706, 790
Salmon, W. H. 5
Salum, I. 1064
Sanders, B. M. 1440, 1589
Šapošnikov, A. E. 1511
Sauer, J. L. 328
Schadee, H. H. Danebius – *see* Danebius-Schadee, H. H.
Schädelin, I. Schmid – *see* Schmid-Schädelin, I.
Scharioth, J. 1834
Schauder, D. E. 1835, 1920, 2033
Schauffler, R. H. 131
Schenk zu Schweinsberg, C. 1112
Schenström, B. 484
Schick, F. L. 1921
Schiller, M. B. 640
Schmid-Schädelin, I. 915, 917, 929, 984, 985, 1157, 1186, 1224, 1258, 1337, 1375
Schmidt, B. 577
Schmidt, H. 1209, 1210, 1512, 1590, 1665, 2144, 2145, 2146
Schmidt, L. M. 2147
Schmitz, T. 1513
Schneck, J. M. 641, 642, 643
Schöne, H. 1666
Schonebaum, A. 1922
Schroers, H. 1441, 1442
Schueller, H. 1026
Schulteis, M., *sister*. 2148

Schüller, M. 376
Schultze, E. 9
Schulz, K. 293
Schulz, M. 175
Schulze, [ ]. 578
Schumacher, M. 530, 579
Schuster, E. 1438
Schwab, S. I. 70, 92
Schyra, B. 1591
Scott, B. L. 161
Scott, C. E. 37
Scottish Hospital Centre. 1667, 1923
Scougall, J. 1924
Scrivens, B. 1443
Scullin, V. 953
Seaman, F. H. 248
Secchi, M. 1925
Seegers, W. Th. 1926
Segal, S. S. 2125
Selby, B. 1150
Selby, J. R. 2034
Severin, E. 954
Severin, V. 869
Sevriugina, E. 903
Sewall, L. 2035, 2036
Sexton, K. 1259
Sexton, L. A. 176
Shapleigh, D. R. 707, 708
Shaw, A. 1668, 1669, 1836, 1837, 2037, 2149
Shaw, L. J. 986
Shellenberger, G. 71
Shidokukyo, 2150
Shiels, *Sir* D. 644
Shore, H. 1670
Shorey, K. 378
Showell, G. F. G. 1027
Siemen, U. 1376
Silcock, G. M. 560
Simon, B. V. 753
Simpson, A. 2151
Simpson, V. 1377
Sindik, N. 1378
Singley, L. 115
Sioux City, Iowa. Public Library. 132
Sirovs, J. 987, 1065
Sjögren, H. 955
Skinner, M. E. 671
Skrefsrud, G. 1066
Skrzypek, A. 2152
Smith, A. M. 1260
Smith, B. A. 561
Smith, D. 1838
Smith, E. P. 956
Smith, F. W. 1592
Smith, J. W. 608
Smith, M. S. 672
Smith, M. Watt – *see* Watt-Smith, M.
Smith, X. P. 580
Smokoski, F. J. 1751
Snell, S. 2038

Söderbergh, M. L. 363
Söderblom, H. 1927
Soderström, S. 1954
Sohon, J. A. 294, 444
Sonne, V. Berg – *see* Berg-Sonne, V.
Southerden, M. G. H. 645, 792, 904
Spångberg, M. 988, 1158, 1211
Sperry, R. S. 162
Spijkerboer, F. W. 2087
Spohn, A. J. 832
Spokes, A. 1314
Spore, V. 609
Standlee, M. W. 610, 709
Stange, R. H. 1820, 2019
Staniszewski, I. 710
Stark, E. 1373, 2153
Steele, U. M. 1928
Steffens, M. 930
Stegmann, [ ] von. 1514
Stein, B. 1514
Stein, E. A. 833
Steinhoff, A. 2154
Stenersen, G. 363
Stephens, M. 1315
Stern, W. B. 961
Stewart, H. G. 231
Stewart, N. 445
Stigmark, M. 2039
Stockett, J. C. 104, 105, 133, 134, 135, 145, 283
Stockhausen, J. Wirth – *see* Wirth-Stockhausen, J.
Stokes, L. Z. 1572
Stokes, R. 711
Stone, J. E. 905
Stovall, M. W. 1379
Strager, H. 562
Strauss, H. 93
Stresno, [ ]. 1593
Strong, T. 582
Stubkjaer, M. 1028
Stuckey, E. 1328
Stuckey, E. C. 834
Sturt, R. 1212, 1380, 1444, 1445, 1594, 1752, 1839, 1929
Stürup, G. K. 563
Sullivan, M. R. 794
Sumner, C. W. 72, 84, 85, 94, 136, 146, 249
Sumner, J. J. 835
Sutinen, K. 1840
Sutton, J. G. 2040
Svendsen, E. 2155
Svensson, M. 1515
Sweet, L. 95, 106, 147, 177
Swenson, R. P. 1671
Swift, H. P. 1262
Swinnerton, F. A. 646
Sydenham, J. H. 1672, 1673
Sytz, F. 265
Székely, S. 2041
Szymánska, G. 1252

T

Taffel, R. 1841
Tait, L. 1516, 1753
Talbot, G. 1067
Talboys, R. St. C. 446
Tanttu, O. 2038, 2156
Tappert, K. 52
Tartre, P. E. 139
Taylor, N. B. 871
Tebbel, J. 1754
Teirich, H. R. 1316, 1446
Teutsch, B. 2042
Tews, R. M. 611, 990, 1114, 1159, 1317, 1318, 1674, 1931, 2043
Thayer, *Mrs.* N. 96
Thiekötter, H. 1029, 1115, 1160, 1517
Thomas, B. 1675
Thompson, A. M. C. 932, 957
Thompson, G. 1518
Thompson, V. A. 906
Thornton, J. L. 796, 872, 1381
Thorpe, F. A. 1842, 2044, 2157
Thorsteinsdóttir, K. 1747
Thulin, K. 1755, 1843, 1932
Ticknor, W. E. 1030, 1161
Tierie, E. Fonderie – *see* Fonderie-Tierie, E.
Tilanus, A. D. W. 1324
Tighe, J. 907
Todd, J. E. 1626
Tofan, A. 1676
Toma, A. 2158
Toma, I. 1844, 1845, 1846
Tomlinson, J. A. 564
Tone, M. 958
Tooker, G. C. 1966
Toulson, S. 1519
Trammell, G. R. 754
Treutwein, I. 933
Trog, *Mlle.* 1041
Tuck, L. C. 22
Tucker, W. B. 1031
Tüllmann, A. 329, 583
Turk, H. M. 532
Turner, G. 713
Turner, P. B. 447, 485
Tyler, A. S. 330
Tylor, D. 3
Tynell, K. O. L. 486
Tyrihjell, M. 755, 756

U

Underwood, M. B. 991
United Hospital Fund of New York. 1068, 1595, 1596, 1757
United States. Joint Commission on Accreditation of Hospitals. 2045
United States. Library of Congress. 1758, 2159
United States. Veterans Administration. 908, 909, 992, 1116, 1319, 1447, 1677, 1678
United States. Veterans Bureau. 140, 203

United States. War Department. 648
Unkila, E. 1162
Upton, M. E. 1163, 1759
Urch, M. E. 1320, 1382, 2046

V

Vallery-Rodot, P. 873
Vanderburg, M. A. 1117
Van der Riet, F. G. 1934
Varga, A. M. 1847
Vedsted, I. 1448, 1935
Veggeland, U. 1449
Velleman, R. A. 1597, 2047, 2048
Vernon, D. T. A. 2049
Vestergaard, I. 2160
Vetere, C. 2161
Vig-Nielsen, I. 1679, 2050
Vlahlijska, L. A. 2135
Vogulys, B. R. de. 1164
Volin, L. K. 1321
Vollans, R. F. 714, 1936
Von Oesen, E. 1639
Voorthuysen, R. L. van 757
Vrhovac, N. 1598

W

Wahrow, L. A. 993
Wallace, M. L. 534, 874
Wallis, J. 1599, 1680
Walmer, J. D. 1520
Walsh, M. A. 1848
Walter, F. K. 448
Walz, H. 994
Washington State Library. 1937
Wassner, H. 2162
Watson, H. E. 449
Watt-Smith, M. 266
Waugh, F. 19
Webb, G. B. 295, 296
Webster, C. 53, 86, 97, 107, 108
Webster, H. E. 758
Wechselberg, K. 1681
Wegener, S. 1760
Weimerskirch, P. J. 1521
Weinstock, F. J. 2051
Welch, H. F. 674
Wendt, H. 1938
Wetlesen, J. M. 267, 331, 450
White, R. W. 1383
Wight, B. L. 1522
Wiles, J. Z. 1263
Williams, M. J. 875, 1165
Williams, N. 54
Wilshere, E. R. 2020
Wilson, B. 1761
Wilson, B. K. 759
Wilson, K. 1322, 1450
Wingborg, O. 1118, 1213
Winkley, S. 2086
Winnberg, A. M. 1384

Winnick, P. 1682
Winowich, N. 1385
Wirth-Stockhausen, J. 297
Wirz, H. G. 417, 451
Wisconsin University. 1683
With, T. K. 876
Wolf, C. 2052
Wolff, H. 1600, 1684, 1849, 2163
Wood, J. E. 910
Woodman, E. 381
Woodman, R. 250
Wright, C. H. 204
Wright, R. W. 73
Wright, Z. 382
Wrobel, A. M. 1119

Wyatt, A. S. 1451
Wyrsch, J. 452

Y

Yast, H. T. 797, 1032, 1070, 1257, 2164
Yelland, M. 1523
Yockey, R. M. 798

Z

Zaccaria, J. S. 1762
Zangerle, J. 1386
Zemis, S. 959
Ziegler, M. 2053

GEOGRAPHICAL INDEX/
INDEX PAR RÉGION GÉOGRAPHIQUE/
GEOGRAPHISCHES REGISTER

Australia
673, 839, 907, 987, 996, 1065, 1194, 2083

Austria
1386

Belgium
437, 456, 624, 764, 776, 805, 900, 912, 967, 976,
1002, 1009, 1037, 1077, 1102, 1105, 1129, 1170,
1179, 1220, 1236, 1277, 1278, 1332, 1701, 1702,
1783

Canada
148, 364, 433, 465, 515, 565, 585, 742, 821, 822,
845, 978, 979, 1196, 1315, 1390, 1426, 1439,
1509, 1779, 1817, 1950, 2065, 2066, 2068, 2077,
2116, 2117, 2122, 2151

Czechoslovakia
701, 1051, 1109, 1153, 1199, 1200, 1201, 1349,
1350, 1395, 1466, 1634, 1986, 2061

Denmark
157, 196, 197, 216, 223, 267, 284, 289, 302, 314,
316, 325, 350, 361, 367, 391, 409, 435, 436, 531,
551, 562, 563, 588, 623, 632, 658, 702, 717, 719,
726, 729, 733, 747, 853, 865, 876, 880, 888, 890,
930, 960, 1010, 1045, 1150, 1231, 1254, 1322,
1368, 1415, 1448, 1450, 1486, 1500, 1504, 1555,
1575, 1617, 1623, 1679, 1711, 1773, 1802, 1821,
1853, 1884, 1886, 1901, 1902, 1909, 1935, 1947,
1974, 1979, 1985, 2050, 2059, 2088, 2102, 2103,
2104, 2118, 2126, 2134, 2155, 2160

Finland
601, 602, 734, 735, 738, 895, 897, 943, 946, 1018,
1025, 1128, 1137, 1139, 1144, 1154, 1162, 1301,
1302, 1364, 1369, 1415, 1558, 1569, 1578, 1581,
1633, 1651, 1655, 1656, 1740, 1763, 1765, 1801,
1802, 1807, 1822, 1824, 1827, 1828, 1830, 1840,
1850, 1911, 1919, 2032, 2038, 2085, 2097, 2127,
2137, 2156

France
256, 275, 306, 317, 324, 335, 344, 404, 412, 413,
466, 472, 524, 779, 829, 873, 963, 1017, 1049,
1122, 1168, 1240, 1528, 1610, 1864, 1870, 2133

Germany (to 1945)
7, 9, 17, 93, 170, 193, 293, 297, 298, 329, 343,
359, 376, 393, 429, 473, 482, 509, 510, 511, 523,
524, 556, 578, 583, 591

Germany (Democratic Republic)
748, 944, 948, 972, 1059, 1205, 1227, 1281, 1373,
1376, 1441, 1442, 1457, 1470, 1480, 1489, 1525,
1527, 1538, 1542, 1557, 1561, 1760, 1767, 1786,
1796, 1805, 1938, 2078, 2138, 2139, 2153

Germany (Federal Republic)
762, 765, 801, 840, 856, 868, 933, 969, 994, 1026,

1029, 1039, 1080, 1081, 1092, 1101, 1112, 1115,
1132, 1133, 1148, 1160, 1180, 1181, 1182, 1184,
1185, 1189, 1192, 1202, 1208, 1209, 1210, 1239,
1265, 1270, 1290, 1312, 1316, 1334, 1335, 1340,
1347, 1359, 1397, 1402, 1413, 1435, 1437, 1454,
1462, 1472, 1473, 1481, 1482, 1487, 1490, 1492,
1507, 1512, 1513, 1514, 1517, 1560, 1590, 1600,
1605, 1606, 1616, 1618, 1625, 1637, 1638, 1653,
1664, 1665, 1666, 1681, 1684, 1688, 1690, 1704,
1718, 1748, 1775, 1790, 1804, 1808, 1834, 1849,
1907, 1965, 2042, 2071, 2108, 2144, 2145, 2146,
2154, 2162, 2163

Hungary
1719, 1844, 1845, 1846, 1847, 1859, 1885, 1888,
2041, 2158

Iceland
1747, 2027, 2123

India
307, 480, 575, 898, 926

Irish Republic
252, 353, 355, 357, 398, 419, 504, 804, 879, 1408,
1631

Italy
270, 309, 901, 1012, 1013, 1636, 1662, 1892,
2161

Japan
2150

Jordan
1649

Netherlands
285, 757, 997, 1023, 1052, 1061, 1062, 1073,
1111, 1127, 1173, 1187, 1219, 1242, 1267, 1269,
1296, 1311, 1313, 1324, 1325, 1326, 1370, 1371,
1414, 1417, 1421, 1424, 1425, 1433, 1585, 1694,
1738, 1739, 1771, 1833, 1860, 1872, 1873, 1874,
1894, 1897, 1904, 1922, 1926

New Zealand
492, 505, 564, 631, 686, 696, 699, 746, 883, 1206,
1588, 2141, 2142

Norway
179, 331, 663, 718, 740, 755, 756, 763, 841, 870,
890, 1045, 1066, 1069, 1142, 1255, 1415, 1449,
1502, 1768, 1820, 1825, 1826, 1879, 2019

Poland
959, 1014, 1230, 1252, 1275, 1547, 1724, 1793,
1806, 1882, 1889, 1890, 1969, 2057, 2076, 2091,
2105, 2106, 2107, 2109

Romania
1676

Russia (to 1922) *see also* USSR
5

Scandinavia *see also* individual countries
931, 1024, 1045, 1268, 1295, 1304, 1308, 1415,
1800, 1802

South Africa, Republic of
501, 910, 1539, 1593, 1770, 1835, 1917, 1920,
1934, 1945, 2033, 2058, 2079

Spain
268, 279, 327, 1942, 1964

Sweden
224, 267, 282, 287, 292, 352, 363, 379, 380, 425,
426, 443, 453, 484, 486, 577, 589, 629, 731, 744,
750, 824, 836, 837, 864, 877, 954, 955, 988, 989,
1045, 1048, 1064, 1095, 1113, 1118, 1158, 1211,
1213, 1215, 1232, 1279, 1291, 1354, 1355, 1410,
1415, 1484, 1485, 1491, 1515, 1663, 1687, 1689,
1703, 1714, 1716, 1717, 1719, 1720, 1723, 1743,
1746, 1749, 1750, 1755, 1772, 1809, 1829, 1843,
1852, 1866, 1867, 1887, 1905, 1914, 1927, 1932,
1943, 1948, 1953, 1954, 1967, 1998, 2002, 2024,
2028, 2031, 2035, 2036, 2039, 2056, 2060, 2095,
2098

Switzerland
336, 390, 401, 407, 408, 420, 432, 451, 452, 791,
929, 984, 1157, 1375

Union of Soviet Socialist Republics *see also*
Russia
403, 440, 457, 736, 861, 869, 903, 952, 1017,
1511, 1908, 2121

United Kingdom
1, 2, 3, 8, 31, 40, 43, 67, 181, 182, 184, 185, 187,
192, 199, 200, 201, 204, 209, 214, 216, 217, 218,
219, 225, 228, 232, 240, 242, 247, 257, 259, 260,
266, 276, 281, 304, 305, 308, 326, 334, 337, 339,
347, 349, 351, 356, 362, 366, 370, 377, 386, 388,
389, 392, 394, 405, 418, 422, 427, 428, 430, 431,
441, 442, 449, 461, 462, 463, 464, 467, 470, 471,
477, 481, 491, 493, 494, 495, 498, 500, 503, 513,
519, 520, 521, 528, 533, 535, 537, 538, 540, 542,
543, 544, 547, 554, 555, 559, 560, 567, 572, 581,
598, 612, 613, 625, 626, 630, 634, 637, 639, 644,
645, 647, 652, 657, 659, 660, 670, 677, 679, 680,
681, 682, 683, 689, 691, 697, 700, 702, 703, 711,
712, 713, 714, 720, 721, 722, 730, 760, 766, 772,
775, 778, 783, 784, 785, 789, 792, 793, 796, 799,
802, 803, 806, 807, 808, 812, 813, 814, 816, 820,
834, 835, 838, 849, 850, 851, 859, 872, 878, 882,
884, 890, 891, 904, 921, 925, 928, 932, 935, 939,
942, 956, 957, 962, 971, 980, 986, 1000, 1016,
1017, 1020, 1027, 1053, 1075, 1106, 1107, 1108,
1140, 1143, 1166, 1174, 1178, 1188, 1193, 1198,
1212, 1214, 1228, 1248, 1249, 1271, 1282, 1283,
1285, 1297, 1303, 1314, 1320, 1328, 1329, 1333,
1338, 1339, 1342, 1343, 1344, 1346, 1348, 1352,
1358, 1365, 1367, 1372, 1380, 1381, 1382, 1401,
1418, 1419, 1422, 1427, 1430, 1434, 1440, 1443,

1444, 1445, 1451, 1455, 1456, 1459, 1460, 1463,
1464, 1467, 1483, 1494, 1495, 1496, 1506, 1508,
1509, 1516, 1518, 1519, 1530, 1531, 1534, 1546,
1548, 1552, 1553, 1565, 1566, 1567, 1573, 1574,
1577, 1579, 1580, 1582, 1583, 1587, 1589, 1592,
1594, 1599, 1604, 1609, 1611, 1613, 1615, 1621,
1626, 1628, 1629, 1632, 1635, 1640, 1641, 1642,
1647, 1648, 1650, 1658, 1659, 1661, 1667, 1669,
1672, 1673, 1675, 1680, 1692, 1693, 1695, 1696,
1700, 1707, 1719, 1727, 1728, 1729, 1744, 1752,
1753, 1776, 1777, 1784, 1787, 1791, 1792, 1795,
1813, 1815, 1832, 1836, 1839, 1863, 1876, 1877,
1893, 1896, 1903, 1906, 1912, 1913, 1923, 1925,
1929, 1930, 1939, 1951, 1958, 1960, 1961, 1963,
1976, 1983, 1994, 1995, 2006, 2007, 2009, 2023,
2025, 2034, 2046, 2054, 2062, 2063, 2064, 2070,
2090, 2111, 2112, 2119, 2120, 2129, 2130, 2131,
2132, 2143

United States of America
6, 10, 11, 12, 13, 14, 15, 16, 18, 20, 21, 22, 23, 24,
25, 26, 27, 28, 29, 32, 33, 35, 36, 37, 38, 39, 41,
42, 44, 45, 46, 47, 48, 49, 50, 51, 52, 53, 54, 55,
56, 57, 58, 61, 62, 63, 64, 65, 67, 68, 69, 71, 72,
73, 75, 76, 78, 79, 81, 82, 83, 84, 85, 86, 87, 88,
90, 92, 94, 95, 96, 97, 98, 99, 100, 101, 102, 103,
104, 105, 106, 108, 109, 111, 112, 113, 114, 115,
116, 117, 118, 119, 120, 121, 122, 123, 124, 125,
126, 127, 128, 129, 130, 132, 133, 134, 135, 136,
137, 138, 141, 142, 143, 144, 145, 146, 147, 152,
153, 155, 156, 158, 159, 160, 161, 162, 164, 166,
167, 168, 169, 173, 174, 175, 176, 177, 178, 180,
183, 191, 198, 202, 203, 205, 206, 207, 210, 211,
212, 216, 220, 222, 226, 227, 231, 233, 234, 235,
236, 239, 241, 243, 248, 249, 250, 251, 254, 261,
263, 264, 273, 274, 277, 283, 286, 288, 290, 294,
295, 296, 299, 300, 301, 303, 311, 315, 318, 319,
321, 322, 323, 328, 330, 332, 333, 338, 340, 341,
342, 345, 346, 354, 364, 365, 368, 369, 378, 381,
382, 383, 384, 385, 399, 400, 402, 411, 421, 423,
427, 434, 438, 439, 444, 445, 446, 448, 450, 454,
455, 458, 459, 460, 468, 469, 474, 475, 478, 483,
487, 488, 489, 490, 496, 497, 499, 502, 507, 508,
512, 516, 517, 518, 522, 525, 526, 527, 529, 530,
532, 534, 536, 539, 541, 545, 546, 548, 549, 550,
552, 557, 558, 561, 568, 569, 574, 576, 580, 582,
586, 587, 590, 592, 595, 597, 604, 605, 606, 607,
608, 609, 610, 611, 614, 615, 616, 618, 619, 620,
621, 627, 628, 633, 635, 636, 638, 640, 648, 650,
651, 656, 664, 665, 666, 672, 674, 675, 676, 684,
685, 690, 693, 694, 695, 698, 704, 705, 706, 707,
708, 709, 710, 715, 716, 723, 724, 727, 741, 743,
745, 749, 753, 754, 758, 759, 761, 771, 777,
782, 786, 787, 788, 790, 794, 797, 798, 800, 810,
818, 823, 825, 826, 831, 832, 833, 842, 846, 848,
852, 857, 858, 860, 862, 867, 874, 885, 887, 889,
890, 892, 893, 896, 899, 902, 906, 908, 911, 913,
914, 918, 919, 920, 922, 923, 924, 927, 934, 936,
938, 941, 945, 947, 949, 951, 953, 958, 961, 965,
966, 968, 973, 974, 975, 977, 983, 991, 993, 995,
998, 999, 1003, 1005, 1006, 1007, 1008, 1011,

United States of America—*contd.*

1015, 1017, 1019, 1021, 1028, 1030, 1031, 1032, 1033, 1035, 1036, 1038, 1040, 1042, 1044, 1047, 1050, 1054, 1055, 1056, 1057, 1060, 1063, 1067, 1068, 1070, 1071, 1074, 1079, 1083, 1084, 1085, 1087, 1088, 1089, 1090, 1091, 1093, 1096, 1100, 1103, 1104, 1110, 1114, 1117, 1119, 1120, 1121, 1123, 1125, 1126, 1130, 1131, 1135, 1136, 1138, 1141, 1146, 1149, 1151, 1155, 1159, 1161, 1163, 1165, 1167, 1169, 1172, 1176, 1177, 1183, 1190, 1191, 1197, 1203, 1204, 1207, 1216, 1222, 1223, 1225, 1226, 1233, 1234, 1237, 1238, 1243, 1244, 1245, 1247, 1251, 1257, 1259, 1262, 1264, 1272, 1273, 1274, 1276, 1284, 1286, 1287, 1288, 1289, 1292, 1293, 1294, 1298, 1299, 1300, 1306, 1309, 1310, 1317, 1318, 1323, 1327, 1330, 1331, 1336, 1341, 1356, 1357, 1360, 1361, 1362, 1363, 1366, 1374, 1377, 1379, 1383, 1384, 1385, 1387, 1388, 1391, 1392, 1394, 1396, 1399, 1400, 1407, 1423, 1428, 1429, 1431, 1447, 1452, 1453, 1458, 1461, 1465, 1468, 1474, 1475, 1476, 1477, 1488, 1493, 1498, 1499, 1501, 1503, 1520, 1521, 1522, 1524, 1526, 1529, 1532, 1535, 1536, 1543, 1544, 1549, 1550, 1551, 1554, 1556, 1559, 1562, 1568, 1570, 1571, 1572, 1576, 1584, 1586, 1595, 1596, 1597, 1601, 1602, 1603, 1607, 1608, 1612, 1614, 1622, 1624, 1639, 1643, 1644, 1645, 1652, 1654, 1660, 1670, 1671, 1674, 1677, 1682, 1683, 1685, 1686, 1697, 1698, 1699, 1709, 1713, 1722, 1730, 1731, 1732, 1733, 1734, 1737, 1742, 1745, 1751, 1757, 1758, 1759, 1761, 1762, 1764, 1766, 1769, 1778, 1780, 1781, 1782, 1789, 1794, 1797, 1798, 1799, 1810, 1816, 1818, 1819, 1831, 1838, 1841, 1848, 1851, 1854, 1855, 1856, 1857, 1858, 1865, 1868, 1869, 1878, 1881, 1883, 1898, 1899, 1918, 1924, 1928, 1933, 1937, 1940, 1941, 1944, 1946, 1949, 1952, 1955, 1956, 1957, 1962, 1966, 1970, 1971, 1972, 1973, 1975, 1977, 1978, 1984, 1987, 1996, 1997, 1999, 2000, 2001, 2003, 2004, 2008, 2013, 2014, 2015, 2016, 2022, 2026, 2030, 2040, 2043, 2045, 2047, 2048, 2051, 2052, 2053, 2055, 2067, 2072, 2073, 2074, 2080, 2081, 2084, 2089, 2092, 2093, 2096, 2101, 2114, 2115, 2124, 2128, 2135, 2136, 2147, 2148, 2152, 2159, 2164

Yugoslavia

1022, 1124, 1156, 1217, 1253, 1307, 1345, 1378, 1598, 2012

SUBJECT INDEX HEADINGS

Bibliographies and Reading Lists
Bibliotherapy
Blind and Partially Sighted
Book Selection
Children
Deaf
Dumb
Education and Training
Hospital Libraries, Services to Patients in General
Hospital Libraries, Services to Patients in Chest Hospitals, including TB Sanatoria
Hospital Libraries, Services to Patients in Psychiatric Hospitals
Hospital Libraries, War Service
Housebound Readers
Infection
International Federation of Library Associations
Large Print
Mentally Handicapped
Old People
Physically Handicapped
Picture Lending
Planning (Library Accommodation)
Publicity
Reading Aids
Reading Interests
Staff
Standards
Talking Books and Newspapers
Trolleys
Voluntary Helpers
Voluntary Organisations

TABLE DES MATIERES

Appareils d'aide à la lecture — *voir* Reading Aids
Aveugles et amblyopes — Blind and Partially Sighted
Bibliographies et listes de livres à lire — Bibliographies and Reading Lists
Bibliothèques d'hôpitaux, Services aux malades en général — Hospital Libraries, Services to Patients in General
Bibliothèques d'hôpitaux, Services aux malades dans les hôpitaux spécialisés en maladies respiratoires y compris sanatoria pour tuberculeux — Hospital Libraries, Services to Patients in Chest Hospitals, including TB Sanatoria
Bibliothèques d'hôpitaux, Services aux malades en instituts psychiatriques — Hospital Libraries, Services to Patients in Psychiatric Hospitals
Bibliothèques d'hôpitaux, Service en temps de guerre — Hospital Libraries, War Service
Bibliothérapie — Bibliotherapy
Chariots — Trolleys
Contagion — Infection
Education et formation — Education and Training
Enfants — Children
Fédération Internationale des Associations de Bibliothécaires — International Federation of Library Associations
Handicapés mentaux — Mentally Handicapped
Handicapés Physiques — Physically Handicapped
Intérêts littéraires — Reading Interests
Livres en grands caractères — Large Print
Livres et journaux parlés — Talking Books and Newspapers
Malades à domicile — Housebound Readers
Muets — Dumb
Normes — Standards
Organisations bénévoles — Voluntary Organisations
Personnel — Staff
Personnel bénévole — Voluntary Helpers
Personnes âgées — Old People
Planification (installation matérielle) — Planning (Library Accommodation)
Prêt de reproductions de tableaux — Picture Lending
Publicité — Publicity
Sélection des livres — Book Selection
Sourds — Deaf

Alte Menschen	*siehe*	Old People
Ausbildung und Fortbildung		Education and Training
Ausleihe von Bildern		Picture Lending
Bibliographien und Bücherverzeichnisse		Bibliographies and reading lists
Bibliotherapie		Bibliotherapy
Blinde und Sehbehinderte		Blind and Partially Sighted
Buchauswahl		Book Selection
Bücher und Zeitungen auf Tonbändern		Talking Books and Newspapers
Bücherwagen		Trolleys
Freiwillige Helfer		Voluntary Helpers
Freiwillige Organisationen		Voluntary Organisations
Geistig Behinderte		Mentally Handicapped
Grossdruck		Large Print
Hausbebundene Lesser		Housebound Readers
Infektion		Infection
Internationaler Verband Der Bibliothekar-Vereien		International Federation of Library Associations
Kinder		Children
Körperbehinderte		Physically Handicapped
Krankenhausbibliotheken, Dienste für Patienten in Allgemeinen Krankenhäusern		Hospital Libraries, Services to Patients in General
Krankenhausbibliotheken, Dienste für Patienten in Krankenhäusern für Lungen-krankheiten, einschliesslich TB-Sanatorien		Hospital Libraries, Services to Patients in Chest Hospitals, including TB Sanatoria
Krankenhausbibliotheken, Dienste für Patienten in Militärkrankenhäusern		Hospital Libraries, War Service
Krankenhausbibliotheken, Dienste für Patienten in Psychiatrischen Krankenhäusern		Hospital Libraries, Services to Patients in Psychiatric Hospitals
Lesehilfen		Reading Aids
Leseinteressen		Reading Interests
Öffentlichkeitsarbeit		Publicity
Personal		Staff
Planung (Unterbringung der Bibliothek)		Planning (Library Accommodation)
Richtlinien		Standards
Stumme		Dumb
Taube		Deaf

Bibliographies and Reading Lists
208, 262, 447, 485, 641, 642, 771, 833, 909, 992, 1072, 1116, 1169, 1171, 1191, 1204, 1257, 1266, 1294, 1319, 1336, 1407, 1409, 1465, 1535, 1537, 1595, 1614, 1678, 1698, 1710, 1721, 1774, 1781, 1856, 2010, 2075, 2078

Bibliotherapy
7, 33, 70, 92, 101, 109, 114, 123, 144, 165, 168, 177, 183, 188, 202, 211, 215, 236, 358, 365, 368, 382, 408, 437, 438, 439, 452, 459, 469, 479, 483, 487, 505, 508, 539, 568, 574, 640, 641, 642, 643, 644, 649, 662, 673, 684, 695, 710, 727, 730, 749, 758, 788, 818, 826, 831, 833, 848, 857, 892, 901, 907, 909, 920, 940, 943, 949, 952, 953, 955, 960, 975, 992, 995, 996, 1007, 1008, 1015, 1018, 1021, 1033, 1038, 1050, 1063, 1064, 1065, 1071, 1087, 1088, 1101, 1103, 1116, 1123, 1138, 1139, 1161, 1167, 1171, 1216, 1223, 1227, 1238, 1250, 1266, 1273, 1286, 1287, 1291, 1292, 1293, 1294, 1305, 1306, 1316, 1317, 1318, 1319, 1330, 1336, 1353, 1386, 1388, 1409, 1412, 1420, 1428, 1431, 1446, 1457, 1458, 1470, 1472, 1480, 1489, 1509, 1520, 1521, 1525, 1527, 1533, 1538, 1540, 1542, 1557, 1561, 1562, 1601, 1604, 1608, 1633, 1637, 1674, 1678, 1685, 1690, 1710, 1714, 1719, 1732, 1733, 1760, 1762, 1767, 1793, 1819, 1840, 1875, 1882, 1931, 1940, 1969, 1974, 2005, 2013, 2017, 2031, 2057, 2076, 2084, 2089, 2091, 2097, 2099, 2109, 2110, 2121, 2124, 2140, 2153, 2163

Blind and Partially Sighted
276, 285, 302, 309, 314, 327, 367, 428, 457, 472, 488, 512, 729, 731, 735, 740, 803, 806, 843, 867, 869, 887, 900, 903, 910, 914, 941, 951, 959, 961, 962, 972, 982, 1006, 1017, 1019, 1020, 1023, 1029, 1047, 1061, 1075, 1076, 1106, 1107, 1108, 1115, 1127, 1128, 1135, 1146, 1148, 1160, 1229, 1240, 1255, 1259, 1272, 1275, 1288, 1296, 1348, 1361, 1366, 1367, 1377, 1383, 1393, 1405, 1426, 1430, 1432, 1455, 1464, 1511, 1517, 1524, 1532, 1545, 1550, 1551, 1556, 1572, 1573, 1602, 1626, 1639, 1646, 1647, 1649, 1655, 1657, 1658, 1668, 1669, 1691, 1707, 1708, 1709, 1713, 1715, 1731, 1735, 1737, 1741, 1754, 1758, 1768, 1774, 1784, 1786, 1794, 1805, 1810, 1814, 1825, 1828, 1833, 1835, 1836, 1837, 1842, 1852, 1858, 1867, 1873, 1915, 1920, 1928, 1934, 1939, 1950, 1993, 2012, 2032, 2033, 2037, 2051, 2052, 2055, 2058, 2066, 2083, 2088, 2105, 2111, 2113, 2119, 2128, 2150, 2152, 2162

Book Selection
19, 34, 46, 59, 91, 110, 140, 150, 154, 167, 171, 172, 178, 196, 203, 212, 221, 234, 236, 253, 254, 255, 265, 269, 273, 291, 296, 341, 346, 348, 354, 360, 466, 478, 483, 484, 502, 509, 510, 515, 527, 545, 546, 557, 600, 655, 665, 678, 684, 714, 722, 749, 811, 848, 897, 926, 950, 975, 1004, 1028, 1034, 1081, 1085, 1086, 1121, 1125, 1152, 1171,

1173, 1185, 1198, 1208, 1247, 1252, 1264, 1284, 1288, 1291, 1312, 1326, 1362, 1405, 1411, 1437, 1452, 1462, 1499, 1505, 1523, 1555, 1558, 1575, 1580, 1588, 1596, 1620, 1664, 1695, 1702, 1708, 1712, 1715, 1736, 1740, 1748, 1749, 1763, 1788, 1794, 1796, 1808, 1826, 1850, 1891, 1976, 2007, 2021, 2024, 2060, 2125

Children
11, 18, 28, 35, 75, 139, 151, 158, 159, 227, 267, 274, 276, 382, 399, 400, 446, 557, 678, 710, 766, 772, 774, 778, 786, 834, 845, 852, 875, 906, 918, 958, 1004, 1005, 1035, 1036, 1038, 1043, 1046, 1047, 1054, 1067, 1084, 1085, 1086, 1094, 1112, 1131, 1136, 1165, 1175, 1177, 1207, 1213, 1221, 1245, 1260, 1327, 1333, 1336, 1356, 1361, 1366, 1383, 1392, 1409, 1474, 1475, 1476, 1484, 1495, 1501, 1529, 1537, 1544, 1549, 1556, 1563, 1568, 1597, 1620, 1621, 1629, 1644, 1648, 1656, 1661, 1681, 1695, 1712, 1730, 1736, 1737, 1757, 1808, 1841, 1884, 1886, 1914, 1927, 1932, 1963, 1967, 1979, 1985, 1994, 2022, 2032, 2038, 2042, 2047, 2048, 2080, 2083, 2085, 2097, 2104, 2124, 2137, 2143, 2154, 2156

Deaf
11, 22, 51, 726, 1036, 1177, 1568, 1829, 1911, 1978, 1985, 2083, 2094

Dumb
11, 726

Education and Training
49, 142, 210, 448, 450, 474, 499, 526, 587, 597, 612, 615, 661, 712, 753, 787, 824, 842, 937, 1024, 1226, 1268, 1293, 1295, 1301, 1304, 1308, 1450, 1542, 1663, 1711, 1783, 1789, 1813, 1818, 1830, 1903, 1909, 1924, 1933, 2108, 2126

Hospital Libraries, Services to Patients in General
2, 3, 4, 9, 17, 25, 29, 37, 38, 42, 44, 54, 55, 60, 61, 62, 63, 65, 68, 72, 77, 78, 79, 82, 84, 85, 86, 89, 90, 93, 94, 96, 97, 99, 102, 103, 104, 105, 107, 108, 111, 112, 117, 118, 120, 122, 126, 129, 132, 136, 141, 146, 148, 149, 157, 162, 164, 170, 174, 176, 179, 180, 182, 186, 187, 189, 190, 192, 193, 194, 197, 201, 205, 207, 216, 217, 218, 219, 220, 222, 223, 224, 225, 226, 229, 231, 232, 237, 239, 241, 242, 244, 245, 246, 247, 249, 251, 252, 256, 257, 260, 261, 263, 264, 266, 267, 268, 275, 278, 279, 280, 281, 282, 283, 284, 287, 289, 292, 294, 297, 298, 299, 300, 301, 304, 305, 306, 310, 315, 316, 317, 318, 320, 321, 324, 325, 328, 330, 331, 332, 333, 334, 335, 336, 337, 344, 350, 356, 359, 362, 363, 366, 370, 371, 372, 373, 374, 375, 376, 378, 380, 383, 384, 390, 392, 393, 403, 404, 405, 407, 409, 411, 412, 513, 414, 415, 416, 417, 418, 421, 424, 425, 426, 430, 431, 432, 434, 435, 436, 440, 442, 443, 451, 453, 454, 455, 458, 460, 461, 464, 465, 467, 468, 470, 471, 473, 475, 476,

480, 481, 484, 486, 489, 490, 492, 496, 501, 503, 514, 516, 517, 522, 523, 524, 530, 531, 536, 551, 554, 557, 562, 565, 566, 571, 576, 577, 578, 583, 584, 586, 589, 593, 598, 599, 601, 603, 604, 609, 613, 614, 618, 620, 621, 623, 628, 630, 632, 635, 650, 651, 652, 654, 657, 658, 660, 666, 672, 674, 675, 676, 679, 682, 696, 699, 700, 701, 703, 708, 711, 713, 715, 716, 718, 720, 721, 723, 724, 728, 733, 737, 738, 742, 744, 745, 746, 748, 750, 754, 757, 761, 765, 775, 781, 783, 784, 789, 791, 792, 793, 796, 797, 801, 802, 813, 814, 819, 825, 837, 839, 840, 841, 851, 853, 856, 859, 860, 864, 865, 868, 870, 872, 874, 878, 879, 882, 883, 885, 889, 890, 895, 898, 899, 908, 919, 921, 922, 923, 924, 925, 927, 929, 931, 932, 933, 938, 939, 944, 945, 946, 948, 956, 957, 964, 969, 979, 980, 984, 985, 986, 988, 989, 990, 994, 1003, 1011, 1012, 1013, 1016, 1026, 1032, 1040, 1042, 1044, 1045, 1053, 1060, 1066, 1069, 1070, 1080, 1091, 1092, 1097, 1104, 1109, 1113, 1114, 1122, 1137, 1140, 1142, 1143, 1144, 1149, 1150, 1153, 1154, 1157, 1158, 1159, 1163, 1164, 1168, 1180, 1181, 1182, 1185, 1188, 1189, 1193, 1194, 1196, 1197, 1200, 1202, 1205, 1206, 1210, 1211, 1212, 1223, 1225, 1228, 1231, 1239, 1244, 1246, 1256, 1262, 1263, 1265, 1270, 1274, 1279, 1281, 1282, 1283, 1291, 1298, 1302, 1309, 1320, 1322, 1331, 1334, 1335, 1338, 1339, 1340, 1342, 1347, 1354, 1357, 1359, 1364, 1368, 1373, 1374, 1375, 1376, 1380, 1381, 1382, 1384, 1385, 1391, 1394, 1395, 1400, 1401, 1402, 1403, 1406, 1408, 1415, 1418, 1419, 1422, 1427, 1436, 1439, 1440, 1442, 1443, 1444, 1445, 1449, 1451, 1463, 1466, 1478, 1479, 1481, 1482, 1490, 1491, 1492, 1494, 1497, 1500, 1502, 1504, 1512, 1516, 1519, 1522, 1528, 1531, 1534, 1536, 1539, 1546, 1548, 1552, 1553, 1565, 1566, 1567, 1570, 1571, 1574, 1577, 1578, 1582, 1583, 1584, 1588, 1589, 1590, 1594, 1596, 1598, 1600, 1605, 1610, 1611, 1612, 1613, 1618, 1625, 1628, 1634, 1638, 1640, 1641, 1642, 1643, 1651, 1654, 1656, 1659, 1662, 1665, 1666, 1667, 1676, 1679, 1684, 1688, 1696, 1703, 1707, 1716, 1718, 1720, 1723, 1725, 1728, 1729, 1743, 1746, 1747, 1750, 1753, 1761, 1766, 1773, 1776, 1777, 1779, 1780, 1787, 1790, 1791, 1792, 1795, 1802, 1804, 1809, 1814, 1815, 1817, 1820, 1821, 1822, 1838, 1839, 1844, 1845, 1846, 1847, 1848, 1849, 1859, 1864, 1865, 1877, 1885, 1888, 1889, 1890, 1893, 1894, 1896, 1900, 1908, 1912, 1923, 1925, 1935, 1939, 1942, 1951, 1957, 1958, 1983, 1986, 1995, 1996, 2019, 2025, 2027, 2034, 2035, 2039, 2041, 2046, 2054, 2059, 2061, 2073, 2087, 2088, 2106, 2107, 2111, 2115, 2118, 2127, 2129, 2131, 2132, 2136, 2138, 2139, 2141, 2142, 2144, 2145, 2146, 2148, 2160.

Hospital Libraries, Services to Patients in Chest Hospitals, including TB Sanatoria
80, 95, 106, 115, 152, 153, 163, 175, 191, 195, 221, 235, 267, 286, 295, 296, 322, 323, 336, 401, 420, 449, 508, 518, 529, 588, 627, 631, 633, 638, 647, 707, 717, 747, 756, 763, 817, 877, 893, 1030, 1031, 1049, 1051, 1101, 1161, 1168, 1329, 1569, 1623, 1699, 1821, 2049, 2126

Hospital Libraries, Services to Patients in Psychiatric Hospitals
6, 12, 13, 14, 21, 23, 36, 87, 98, 100, 119, 133, 135, 138, 143, 156, 168, 173, 178, 206, 212, 215, 250, 277, 288, 311, 339, 351, 358, 365, 377, 381, 385, 391, 402, 427, 452, 478, 497, 507, 532, 534, 549, 550, 596, 605, 619, 642, 643, 649, 667, 685, 698, 719, 730, 734, 741, 751, 755, 759, 760, 780, 800, 807, 808, 812, 820, 821, 822, 830, 838, 846, 863, 877, 880, 886, 888, 894, 896, 904, 930, 936, 940, 942, 943, 949, 950, 953, 968, 971, 974, 975, 983, 991, 993, 1008, 1010, 1025, 1027, 1063, 1064, 1090, 1119, 1130, 1132, 1155, 1162, 1170, 1171, 1182, 1192, 1214, 1216, 1237, 1249, 1251, 1271, 1292, 1297, 1328, 1341, 1343, 1379, 1404, 1429, 1435, 1441, 1456, 1460, 1467, 1503, 1508, 1510, 1520, 1554, 1559, 1588, 1601, 1609, 1617, 1645, 1651, 1685, 1726, 1763, 1778, 1797, 1821, 1850, 1854, 1863, 1881, 1882, 1902, 1964, 1977, 1999, 2006, 2063, 2064, 2072, 2092, 2095, 2126

Hospital Libraries, War Service
5, 31, 43, 45, 48, 50, 52, 53, 56, 57, 58, 64, 66, 67, 69, 71, 73, 116, 349, 462, 491, 493, 494, 495, 498, 500, 513, 519, 520, 528, 533, 535, 538, 540, 542, 543, 548, 552, 572, 580, 594, 606, 607, 608, 610, 616, 648, 656, 823

Housebound Readers
338, 340, 342, 345, 369, 664, 736, 794, 798, 978, 1048, 1095, 1176, 1303, 1355, 1423, 1434, 1451, 1592, 1599, 1615, 1624, 1628, 1632, 1641, 1652, 1680, 1693, 1700, 1727, 1742, 1755, 1782, 1795, 1815, 1843, 1869, 1879, 1899, 1913, 1922, 1943, 1960, 1961, 2011, 2040, 2053, 2065, 2069, 2073, 2077, 2079, 2082, 2086, 2117, 2122, 2142

Infection
387, 631, 815, 881, 1059, 1098, 1261, 1469

International Federation of Library Associations
213, 230, 237, 271, 272, 278, 312, 313, 395, 396, 397, 414, 415, 506, 687, 688, 725, 773, 847, 915, 916, 917, 970, 1041, 1082, 1134, 1186, 1195, 1224, 1235, 1258, 1280, 1337, 1398, 1471, 1541, 1564, 1619, 1630, 1705, 1785, 1803, 1861, 1880, 1895, 1921, 1959, 1981, 1982, 1990, 1992, 2100

Large Print
1459, 1523, 1627, 1635, 1691, 1697, 1735, 1754, 1770, 1796, 1891, 1936, 1989, 1991, 1998, 2044, 2157

Mentally Handicapped
27, 1079, 1118, 1136, 1198, 1327, 1411, 1452, 1505, 1555, 1575, 1712, 1717, 1736, 1751, 1799, 1853, 1855, 1857, 1886, 1914, 1937, 1946, 1947, 1962, 1973, 1975, 1976, 1984, 1985, 1997, 2002, 2004, 2007, 2008, 2010, 2021, 2028, 2045, 2060, 2062, 2070, 2075, 2081, 2088, 2102, 2125, 2130, 2155

Old People
445, 973, 978, 997, 998, 1023, 1052, 1057, 1073,
1074, 1095, 1111, 1126, 1145, 1151, 1172, 1173,
1183, 1187, 1242, 1243, 1267, 1269, 1276, 1299,
1303, 1310, 1311, 1313, 1314, 1324, 1325, 1326,
1342, 1346, 1360, 1365, 1369, 1370, 1387, 1414,
1417, 1421, 1423, 1425, 1433, 1448, 1468, 1488,
1507, 1543, 1585, 1586, 1592, 1593, 1599, 1607,
1628, 1651, 1655, 1656, 1680, 1727, 1738, 1739,
1765, 1814, 1824, 1834, 1860, 1872, 1873, 1879,
1883, 1894, 1897, 1917, 1918, 1922, 1926, 1952,
1956, 1987, 2011, 2065, 2069, 2071, 2096, 2103,
2135, 2146, 2147

Physically Handicapped
1035, 1043, 1067, 1229, 1254, 1321, 1327, 1423,
1501, 1515, 1597, 1622, 1639, 1709, 1713, 1715,
1731, 1737, 1745, 1752, 1774, 1779, 1798, 1814,
1858, 1870, 1878, 1892, 1896, 1914, 1919, 1927,
1928, 1932, 1944, 1954, 1970, 2002, 2048, 2077,
2083, 2090, 2098, 2116, 2151, 2152

Picture Lending
905, 1906, 2056

Planning (Library Accommodation)
343, 410, 477, 617, 739, 1068, 1201, 1321, 1349,
1372, 1447, 1530, 1576, 1603, 1675, 1677, 1752,
1772, 1776, 1807, 1887, 1954, 2090

Publicity
444, 768, 1300, 2035

Reading Aids
692, 732, 816, 828, 835, 849, 866, 875, 876, 884,
891, 954, 981, 1058, 1105, 1120, 1147, 1285,
1291, 1352, 1389, 1399, 1416, 1432, 1438, 1483,
1545, 1689, 1706, 1734, 1741, 1812, 1832, 1862,
1871, 1904, 1910, 1916, 2020, 2058, 2149, 2159

Reading Interests
46, 147, 166, 233, 348, 368, 512, 515, 547, 558,
611, 809, 810, 893, 913, 1014, 1135, 1547, 1724,
1725, 1905, 1968, 2024, 2057

Staff
243, 248, 303, 386, 645, 653, 671, 770, 1110,
1309, 1493, 1503, 1868

Standards
482, 511, 587, 615, 752, 902, 911, 947, 1117,
1141, 1195, 1258, 1323, 1496, 1503, 1506, 1518,
1587, 1602, 1606, 1616, 1636, 1686, 1701, 1776,
1803, 1811, 1823, 1851, 1861, 1868, 1965, 1973,
2045, 2112, 2164

Talking Books and Newspapers
982, 1029, 1061, 1062, 1146, 1160, 1178, 1241,
1275, 1289, 1410, 1486, 1526, 1692, 1768, 1827,
1831, 1929, 1930, 1953, 2023, 2050, 2051, 2088,
2101

Trolleys
196, 379, 1351, 1722, 1756, 1812

Voluntary Helpers
160, 377, 460, 525, 541, 557, 570, 579, 622, 625,
635, 637, 639, 645, 668, 677, 681, 683, 770, 854,
855, 934, 977, 1099, 1453, 1461, 1477, 1596,
1941, 1971, 2009, 2141

Voluntary Organisations
40, 184, 186, 187, 204, 228, 247, 270, 308, 326,
329, 347, 349, 356, 364, 375, 388, 389, 418, 441,
467, 491, 498, 503, 520, 521, 530, 533, 554, 559,
598, 625, 626, 637, 639, 657, 660, 670, 677, 680,
764, 775, 799, 805, 814, 851, 859, 912, 928, 935,
967, 976, 987, 1002, 1009, 1016, 1022, 1037,
1077, 1124, 1129, 1156, 1166, 1179, 1217, 1220,
1236, 1277, 1278, 1307, 1332, 1344, 1345, 1380,
1579, 1672, 1673, 1694, 1701, 1707, 1876, 1906,
2133, 2141